In collaboration with:

Konstantin Gugleta

Daniela Hauenstein-Stümpfig

Maneli Mozaffarieh

Peter Schneider

Glaucoma

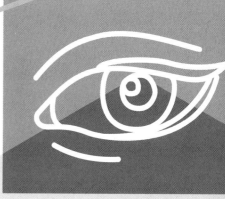

The 1st English edition

was translated by:

Kathleen Bucher

Arthur Funkhouser

Ronald Gerste

HOGREFE

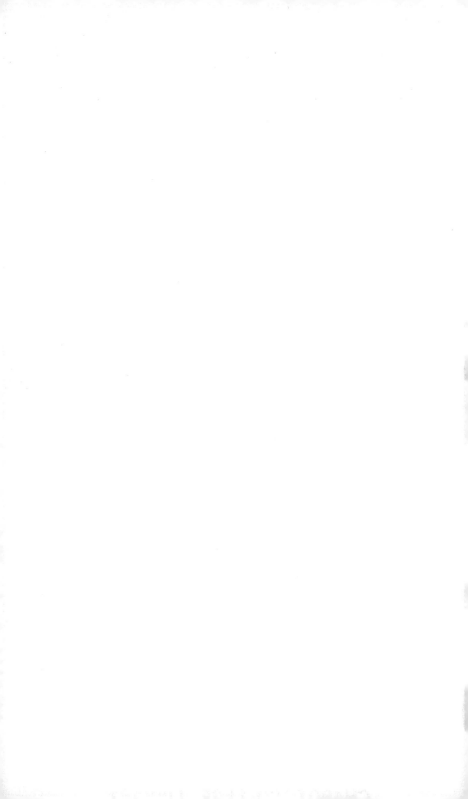

Josef Flammer, M. D.

GLAUCOMA

A Guide for Patients
An Introduction for Care-Providers
A Quick Reference

3rd revised edition

Hogrefe

Correspondence address:
Josef Flammer, M.D.
Prof. and Head
Department of Ophthalmology
University of Basel, Eye Institute
Mittlere Strasse 91
CH-4031 Basel (Switzerland)
e-mail: info@glaucoma-meeting.ch

In collaboration with:
Konstantin Gugleta, M.D., Ophthalmology Senior Physician
Daniela Hauenstein-Stümpfig, Research Technician
Maneli Mozaffarieh, M.D., Ophthalmology Resident
Peter Schneider, Professional Medical Illustrator

Translated from the 2nd German into the 1st English edition by:
Kathleen Bucher, B.A., Medical Translator and Editor at BioConsult GmbH
Arthur Funkhouser, Ph.D., Psychotherapist and Physicist
Ronald Gerste, M.D., Ph.D., Medical Writer and Ophthalmologist

Library of Congress Cataloging-in-Publication Data
is available via the Library of Congress Marc Database under the
LC Control Number 2006928639

Library and Archives Canada Cataloguing in Publication

Flammer, J. (Josef)
    Glaucoma : a guide for patients : an introduction for care-providers :
a quick reference / Josef Flammer. — 3rd rev. ed.

Originally published in German under title: Glaukom.
Includes bibliographical references and index.
ISBN 0-88937-342-6

    1. Glaucoma—Popular works. I. Title.

RE871.F5313 2006   617.7'41   C2006-903362-5

ISBN 0-88937-342-6

Hogrefe & Huber Publishers, Seattle Toronto Bern Göttingen
© 2006 by Hogrefe & Huber Publishers

USA: P.O. Box 2487, Kirkland, WA 98083-2487, Phone (425) 820-1500, Fax (425) 823-8324,
e-mail hh@hhpub.com
CANADA: 12 Bruce Park Avenue, Toronto, Ontario M4P 2S3, Phone (416) 482-6339,
e-mail hh@hhpub.com
SWITZERLAND: Länggass-Strasse 76, CH-3000 Bern 9, Phone 031 300-4500, Fax 031 300-4590
GERMANY: Rohnsweg 25, D-37085 Göttingen, Phone (0551) 496090, Fax (0551) 4960988,
e-mail hhpub@hogrefe.de

Printed in Germany

Foreword to the 3rd English edition

The Glaucoma book was first published in German language back in the year 2000. This first German edition was sold out so quickly, that we published a second revised German edition in the same year. The second German edition was then translated into French, Italian and English. The English edition served as the basis for translation to many other languages. This book was written as a guide for patients and an introduction for healthcare-providers. Meanwhile it is also very popular among physicians as a first introduction into the field of glaucoma.

We have received feedbacks from patients from all over the world. They often express satisfaction that their complaints and symptoms are reflected in this book. They are more confident to cope with glaucoma on their own and have more hope for the future. They can ask their physicans more specific questions and the discussions among patients is facilitated. We are also very pleased, that the International Glaucoma Association decided to use this glaucoma book as the reference.

Since the second English edition in 2003 there is some progression in the field of glaucoma. Therefore chapters on pathophysiology of glaucomatous damage and vascular dysregulation were rewritten for this new edition.

Even after many editions and translations it is still possible that the reader may find some errors. We are very thankful for all kinds of feedback. We hope that this 3rd edition will further support physicans, health-providers and in particular all patients.

Basel 2006   Josef Flammer

UNI
BASEL

Foreword to the 1st edition

Glaucoma is a disease that poses a serious threat to vision. When a patient is confronted with this diagnosis, his first reaction is usually one of disbelief. After a while, he begins to realize that there are many others confronted with the same fate, and that it is possible to live, even comfortably, with this disease. Gradually, with acceptance, comes the desire for more information about this condition. The patient seeks to know how the disease originates, whether he did something "wrong" to cause it, whether a change in his lifestyle can improve it and which treatment options are available. These questions are quite understandable because this disease will accompany the patient for the rest of his life.

The most important partner for discussing this disease is the patient's ophthalmologist. The patient should develop a close, long-term and trusting relationship with this healthcare professional.

Unfortunately, there is often too little time during the patient's consultation to discuss in sufficient detail the various complexities of the disease, and to relate to the patient those aspects that are important at that moment. This is thus the primary objective of this book. Naturally a book cannot replace the dialogue between patient and physician, but it should enhance and complement it. In the Table of Contents, there are boxes placed next to the various topics. Here the physician can simply check those areas that are pertinent to, and should be read by, the individual patient. The patient can then take his time reading the information presented in the book; perhaps certain aspects will even be understood that were originally not fully grasped when first presented. At the next consultation, the patient can then ask about those aspects still unclear.

The amount of information wanted and needed varies from patient to patient. Some are quite satisfied with just a modest explanation, such as that found in standard pamphlets, while others will even delve into medical textbooks. This book seeks to create a bridge between the professional and the interested lay reader. Information that is usually only found in professional literature is reduced to the essentials and presented in a form that is simple and easy to understand.

Today, medical science develops at an incredibly rapid pace. This will mean that certain parts of this book will inevitably be dated and obsolete; nevertheless, the basic knowledge that is available about the disease process will not soon be replaced. The treating physician will certainly provide the patient with information about new developments not mentioned in this book if he feels they could prove helpful or useful.

It is the hope of the authors that this book will provide patients, relatives and friends, as well as care-providers and even those simply interested in this topic, with a better understanding of the clinical picture of glaucoma. The authors are convinced that this will serve the patient by helping him to better accept his diagnosis, understand his treatment and live with his disease.

January 2001   Josef Flammer

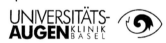

UNIVERSITÄTS-
AUGENKLINIK
BASEL

Table of Contents

1 Introduction

1.1 Purpose of the Book

This book was written to provide the reader with an overview of glaucoma, the different forms of this complex group of diseases and the various treatment options. Although it is based on current scientific knowledge, the authors realize that there are conflicting views on certain aspects of this disease. In order to make the book clearer and more readable, some areas have been simplified. Numerous illustrations and diagrams have been included to help in understanding the often complex issues.

Main Section and Supplementary Chapters. The book is structured to resemble an assembly kit: There is a main section that deals specifically with glaucoma, and a section with supplementary chapters ("S") providing additional information and explanations on certain topics. Reading the additional chapters is not essential to understanding the main section, but may be of particular value to those readers whose interest in glaucoma and ophthalmology has been sparked and who wish to delve deeper into a certain topic.

Which Chapters are Important for Me? The structure of this book makes it easy to read just some of the chapters. Because there are many forms of glaucoma and corresponding treatments, boxes have been placed by the Table of Contents so your physician can mark those that are of special importance to you. This enables you to quickly find information about your particular type of glaucoma and its therapy without having to read the entire book – but all the better if your curiosity is piqued while reading and you want to read more! At the end of the longer chapters in the main section, there is a summary that stresses the most important points covered therein.

Additional Reading. At the end of the book (A 3), there is a list of reference books and articles for additional reading. Most of these publications were written for health care professionals and may prove somewhat difficult for the lay reader. Here, too, the rule applies: You may read everything, but you certainly don't have to. For health care professionals: This bibliography does not claim to be comprehensive, but is just a small selection of the current literature on glaucoma.

Your Ophthalmologist. Should you have questions that are not satisfactorily answered by this book, do not hesitate to contact your ophthalmologist who is familiar with your personal situation. Your doctor should certainly be your primary source for explanations and advice. There are also various organizations that focus on glaucoma (see A 4).

Problems with Medical Terminology. When lay readers study health-related literature, they often become confused by the medical terms. To solve this problem, a) these terms are explained in the text as far as is practical; b) a glossary has been added (A 1) that lists and defines the most important terms in alphabetical order; and c) the etymological basis of the term is provided in square brackets within the text. (Etymology is the study of the historical origins of words.) First the foreign language that gave rise to the word is listed, be it Greek (Gr.), Latin (Lat.) or French (Fr.), then the root word in italics, and finally the English definition. As an example: [Gr. *ophthalmos:* the eye].

Gender. Just as there are male and female patients, so are there male and female ophthalmologists. To make the book more readable, only the masculine form is mentioned, for example, "The patient sees his doctor and receives his treatment"; but naturally, all patients and all practitioners are included, regardless of gender.

1.2　What is Glaucoma?

The term "glaucoma" covers a wide range of diseases. Unfortunately, the word is not always universally used in the same sense, and this can be quite confusing for those confronted with this disease for the first time. Some books, usually from continental Europe, define glaucoma as a group of conditions having one thing in common: an elevated intraocular pressure (IOP). Other articles, mainly from the English-speaking world, define glaucoma as only those cases where there is damage to the optic nerve and a loss of visual function.

In the routine practice of ophthalmology, it has proven useful to apply the term glaucoma to all patients having an increased intraocular pressure (with or without glaucomatous damage), as well as to all patients suffering from glaucomatous damage (with or without a high IOP). In this book, glaucoma is used in the broadest sense of the word.

The term, glaucoma, originates from the ancient Greek word, *glaukos,* meaning "gray-blue." Unfortunately, medical history does not tell us why (or when) the term glaucoma was introduced.

In order to understand this disease, it is important to distinguish between the risk factors that can lead to damage and its progression, and the damage itself (cf. Fig. 1.1).

As a simple example from another field of medicine, heart attacks (myocardial infarctions) can be used. This common cardiac disease is caused by an inadequate blood flow through the coronary

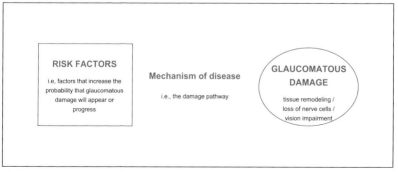

Fig. 1.1: Glaucomatous damage develops when a patient has risk factors.

arteries, thus leading to cell death. Certain risk factors are known to increase the likelihood of a heart attack, e.g. smoking, high lipid levels in the blood, increased blood pressure, etc. Just as with heart attacks, in glaucoma, one has to distinguish between the damage itself – specifically, the loss of neural cells – and the contributing risk factors. Among these risk factors for glaucomatous damage are an increased (elevated) intraocular pressure but also, for instance, a low systemic blood pressure. The following chapters explain exactly what glaucomatous damage is and how it occurs. In Chapter 4, the risk factors that lead to glaucomatous damage are discussed in detail.

1.3   What is Glaucomatous Damage?

The act of seeing (vision) transpires in several steps: light enters the eye; the retina then "transforms" this light into electrical nerve impulses that the brain can process. The light is absorbed by the retinal photoreceptors – the rods and cones – and the information transmitted to retinal ganglion cells (axons). All this visual information is then sent as nerve impulses through the optic nerve to the part of the brain called the visual cortex (cf. S 1). All retinal ganglion cell axons converge at the optic disc (also called the papilla or the optic nerve head), from where the optic nerve (*nervus opticus*) emerges. The optic nerve connects the eye with the brain (Figs. 1.2 and 1.3). The optic disc contains only axons but no photoreceptors. This small section of the retina is thus not able to "see" anything and makes up the *physiological* "blind spot." This small area of missing information is hardly noticed because, to a certain degree, the brain compensates for the absent parts of the overall picture. Nevertheless, blind spots can be identified during the visual field examination (cf. Chapter 6.5).

In glaucoma, the nerve cells and nerve fibers progressively die. As a consequence, the connection between the eye and brain, so crucial for vision, is gradually severed. The eye still "sees" the light because the rods and cones are still working, but the transmission of visual information to the brain is interrupted. This is the core of the problem and is termed "glaucomatous damage." The process that

Fig. 1.2: Nerve fibers (*) in the retina.

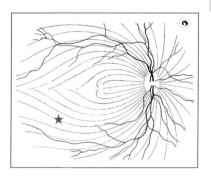

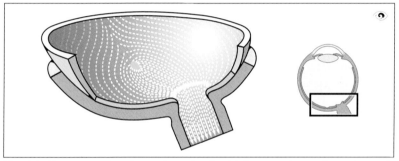

Fig. 1.3: The nerve fibers leave the retina by joining together to form the optic nerve, which exits at the optic disc.

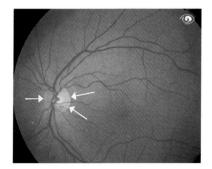

Fig. 1.4: The posterior segment of an eye (fundus) showing a normal optic disc (→).

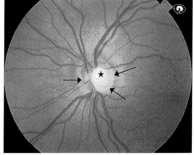

Fig. 1.5: The posterior segment of an eye (fundus) showing an excavated (*) optic disc (→).

leads to the death of the nerve cells will be comprehensively explained in Chapter 2.2.

The loss of nerve fibers is particularly apparent at the optic disc. The ophthalmologist can look directly at this situation with his instruments, thus enabling an assessment of the damage (discussed in more detail in Chapter 6).

Figure 1.4 shows the optic disc of a healthy eye while Figure 1.5 is a disc with marked glaucomatous damage. There is a clearly visible cupping in the center of the optic disc; nerve fibers are missing here. Doctors call this an excavation [Lat. *cavum:* cave]. In addition to the loss of nerve fibers, there are other changes in the optic nerve that will be discussed later (cf. Chapter 2.1).

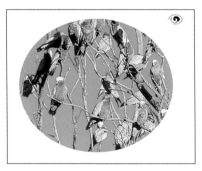

Fig. 1.6: The image as seen by a healthy person.

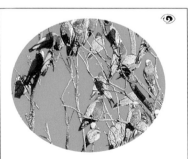

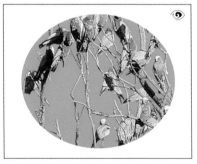

Fig. 1.7: The image as seen by someone with incipient glaucomatous damage.

Fig. 1.8: The image as seen by someone with moderate glaucomatous damage. Some birds are missing, but the patient is unaware that they are not observed.

1.4 What are the Consequences of Glaucomatous Damage?

In the early stages of the disease, when the first nerve cells and their "extensions" are dying, visual function often remains surprisingly intact. As the condition progresses, increasingly severe defects arise in the patient's vision. Though the patient is often still unaware of these defects, they can be detected by an ophthalmologist. This is what makes glaucoma dangerous: When the patient becomes aware of the visual field loss, the disease is already in an advanced stage. While the patient might be happy that visual acuity remains unaffected, this can provide a false sense of security – visual field loss can be severe, even with 20/20 vision (cf. Chapter 2.1.3).

To illustrate this point, Figure 1.6 shows how a normal person sees his environment; Figures 1.7 and 1.8 provide a rough idea of how a glaucoma patient with moderate damage perceives this same image. However, this is just an approximate illustration of what the glaucoma patient sees in the early disease stage. Just as a healthy person doesn't notice his physiological blind spot (cf. Chapter 1.3), the glaucoma patient is unaware of the increasing number and size of pathological "blind spots" (also called scotomata) that are caused by progressive nerve cell loss. The reason for this is the brain's ability to somehow compensate for the missing elements in the picture. Subjectively, vision is normal; objectively, vision is impaired. Diagnosing glaucoma therefore cannot wait until the patient complains of visual loss. Early detection is crucial! If eye examinations take place soon enough and the required treatment is started early, visual impairment or blindness can usually be prevented.

1.5 How Common is Glaucoma?

It is difficult to give an accurate answer to this question. The numbers of those afflicted actually depend on the definition of glaucoma, on the ethnic group being studied and on the population's mean age. Figures indicate that, on average, 3% of the general population is afflicted with glaucoma. When only older populations are considered, the numbers are significantly higher (cf. Chapter 4).

It is estimated that about 70 million people worldwide have relevant glaucomatous damage, but only half are aware of the diagnosis, and an even smaller percentage receive adequate treatment. At least seven million glaucoma patients are blind in both eyes and this number is increasing.

Summary

Glaucoma is a group of diseases that is often – though by no means always – associated with an elevated intraocular pressure. Glaucomatous damage is defined as the loss of retinal nerve cells and their fibers (which make up the optic nerve). As a result, defects in the visual fields develop which, in the beginning, go unnoticed by the patient. Early detection of glaucoma is crucial as treatment is available.

2   Glaucomatous Damage

As mentioned in the Introduction, there is a distinction made between glaucomatous damage and the risk factors that lead to glaucomatous damage.

2.1   Phenomenology of Glaucomatous Damage

Phenomenology (the description and classification of phenomena) only describes what a certain damage looks like without considering its cause [Gr. *phainomenon*: appearance]. With glaucomatous damage, there are two phenomenological aspects: one is morphological and the other functional. The morphological aspect describes the visible changes at the optic nerve head, and specifically for glaucoma, this is cupping (cf. S 1) or excavation [Gr. *morphae*: form; Gr. *logos*: science of or knowledge about something]. Functional changes provide information about visual loss, manifested in glaucoma as visual field defects. It is therefore of paramount importance that the ophthalmologist examine the optic discs and, if necessary, test the visual fields.

2.1.1 Nerve Fiber Loss in Glaucoma

As mentioned earlier, in glaucoma, the retinal nerve cells and their fibers slowly die, eventually severing the connection between the eye and brain. Figure 1.2 is a drawing showing the course of nerve fibers; Figure 2.1 also shows nerve fibers, but as seen in an ordinary photograph. Because nerve fibers are transparent, they can barely be seen. For Figures 2.2 and 2.3, a small trick was used: the pictures were taken in light where all red had been filtered out. The fibers now become almost discernible. Figure 2.2 shows the nerve fibers of a healthy individual, and Figure 2.3, the nerve fiber layer of a patient with glaucoma.

Each eye is connected to the brain by approximately one million nerve fibers. These fibers fan out through the innermost layer of the retina, come together at the optic disc and leave the back part of

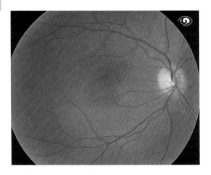

Fig. 2.1: Picture of a fundus. The nerve fibers are barely visible.

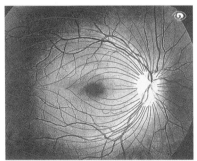

Fig. 2.2: Picture of a fundus. The nerve fibers are sketched in red.

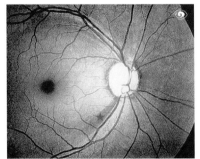

Fig. 2.3: This picture, taken in red-free light, reveals the loss of a nerve fiber bundle (*).

the eye in bundles, the optic nerve. Throughout the course of a lifetime, even a healthy person will lose some nerve fibers as part of the natural aging process. In glaucoma patients, the nerve fiber loss occurs at a faster rate, somewhat analogous to time-lapse photography.

2.1.2 Glaucomatous Tissue Loss

"Atrophy" is another name for tissue loss, and the original definition means "not nourished" [Gr. *trophein*: to nourish]. Atrophy of the papilla (also called the optic disc or the optic nerve head) is a partial or complete demise of those nerve fibers that form the optic nerve.

Other causes besides glaucoma can lead to papillary atrophy, and these are then termed "bland papillary atrophy" which underscores their non-glaucomatous origin. Causes of bland papillary atrophy include accidents in which the optic nerve has been cut, certain hereditary diseases, and even some vitamin deficiencies.

How can bland papillary atrophy be distinguished from glaucomatous papillary atrophy? Figure 2.4 shows a normal papilla, Figure 2.5 a bland atrophy and Figure 2.6 a glaucomatous atrophy. The picture on the left shows a papilla taken from someone living, and that in the middle is from the eye of a cadaver. Why would a cadaver eye be any different? As there is no blood flowing in someone deceased, the retina is no longer transparent. The yellow area of the posterior segment, the fovea, thus becomes clearly visible since the

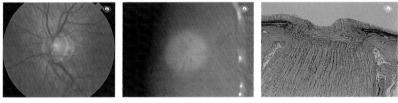

Fig. 2.4: Normal optic disc: in a healthy person (left), in the eye of a cadaver (middle), and a histological section (right).

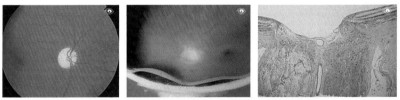

Fig. 2.5: Bland atrophy of the optic disc: the eye of a patient (left), of a cadaver (middle), and a histological section (right).

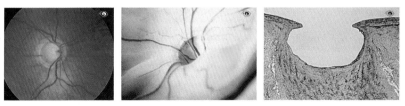

Fig. 2.6: Glaucomatous atrophy of the optic disc: the eye of a patient (left), of a cadaver (middle), and a histological section (right).

reddish tone that arises from circulating blood in the living eye is no longer present. On the right, there is a histological cross-section of the papilla [Gr. *histion*: tissue]. Histology is the field of medicine that examines different types of tissues under a microscope after the specimen has been specially prepared and cut into extremely thin slices. The tissue can additionally be stained with various dyes that permit certain structures to be more easily visible. For example, nerve tissues absorb dyes differently than muscle cells; inside a particular tissue, glucose deposits look different than lipids, etc.

Bland papillary atrophy is characterized by a loss of nerve fibers without a simultaneous loss of other tissues that make up the papilla.

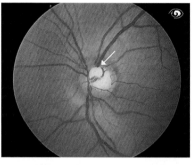

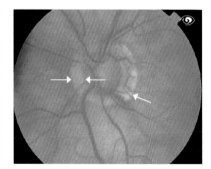

Fig. 2.7: The blood vessels appear to be "bayoneted" at the rim of the excavation (→).

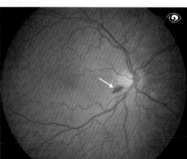

Fig. 2.8: Small hemorrhage at the rim of the optic disc (→).

Fig. 2.9: Peripapillary choroidal atrophy (→).

Glaucomatous papillary atrophy is characterized by the following:

- The optic disc begins to develop a typical cupping, also called excavation. Besides nerve fibers dying, there is also a marked loss of the supporting glial cells and of blood vessels; underlying structures, such as the lamina cribrosa, are remodeled in an outward fashion. This is a very slow process that can take years or even decades.

- In the area of the excavation, the blood vessels may bend sharply backwards ("bayoneting") as they cross the excavation margin (Fig. 2.7). Local constriction of the blood vessels (vasoconstriction) may occur as well as small hemorrhages at the rim of the optic disc (Fig. 2.8), or there may be peripapillary atrophy (Gr. *peri:* around, in the vicinity of) of the choroid (Fig. 2.9). This is a sign of tissue loss around the disc. Photoreceptors and pigment epithelial cells (cf. S 1) in the part of the retina that borders on the papilla are also threatened.

2.1.3 Functional Loss in Glaucoma

As would be expected when nerve fibers die, the patient experiences a decrease in visual function. But what is surprising is that such a large number of axons have to disappear before the ensuing visual defect is noticed. Vision is an extremely complex process involving many different aspects, such as stereoscopic vision, color vision, motion perception, etc. All these functions may be affected in the glaucoma patient. At a relatively early stage, there are disturbances in color vision, contrast sensitivity and adaptation to darkness. To reiterate, as this disease develops very slowly, the patient will hardly notice these changes. At a later stage in the disease, some patients are quite bothered by glare from light.

Defects in the visual field are the most common functional loss. The visual field of an eye comprises all the areas that it can see at any given moment while staring at a fixed point. Defects in the field are called scotomata (singular: scotoma) (Fig. 2.10). These are, so to speak, "holes" in one's visual field. One differentiates between abso-

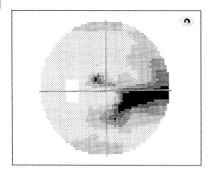

Fig. 2.10: Visual field of a glaucoma patient. The black areas represent scotomata.

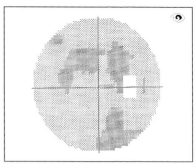

Fig. 2.11: Visual field of a glaucoma patient with early relative scotomata.

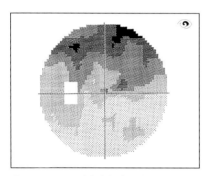

Fig. 2.12: Visual field of a glaucoma patient with moderately severe damage.

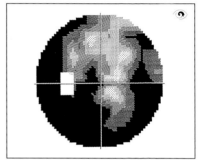

Fig. 2.13: Visual field of a glaucoma patient with very severe damage.

lute scotomata and relative scotomata. An absolute scotoma is a complete loss of function in a given part of the visual field; a relative scotoma is defined as a reduced ability to see in that part of the visual field (Fig. 2.11). Most scotomata go unnoticed by the patient. Just as someone with normal vision is not aware of his blind spot, a glaucoma patient discovers his scotomata either late in the disease course or not at all. Once again, it must be stressed that visual acuity usually remains normal even in cases with advanced visual field losses. A visual acuity of 20/20 in an eye examination does not mean that the patient's vision is perfect. Under certain circumstances, a glaucoma patient with severe visual field defects might be able to read even the smallest print without difficulties or read a clock far away.

Figure 2.12 shows a moderate, and Figure 2.13, a severe visual field defect. Chapter S 10 provides more information on the measurement of the visual fields and how they are evaluated. Visual field defects will be covered in more detail in Chapter 6.5.

2.2   How does Glaucomatous Damage Arise?

Glaucomatous damage is defined as the loss of retinal ganglion (nerve) cells and their axons that lead from the optic nerve to the brain. Additionally, there is also involvement of the glial cells (supporting cells) in the disease process.

Glaucoma patients lose nerve and glial cells [Gr. *glia:* glue] as their disease progresses. Glial cells provide support and nourishment to the nerve cells so they can function properly. When a cell dies without an accompanying inflammatory reaction, basically a "simple" cell death, it is known as cell apoptosis [Gr. *apoptein*: to fall down]. Dying cells were compared to leaves falling from a tree in autumn, and thus the expression was introduced into medical terminology.

However, it is now known that each cell has the ability to initiate its own demise. A healthy cell requires information from its environment that tells the cell that it is still needed. If this positive feed-back ceases or is even substituted by negative information telling the cell that it is a nuisance, the cell might start its own destruction: the cell turns on its "apoptosis program." Under normal conditions, this only happens when the cell is past its prime or has become superfluous.

Two "system errors" are feasible in this model: the potential for apoptosis could be either too strong or too weak. Both are signs of disease. Tumor cells, for instance, characteristically often lack the ability for apoptosis: The tumor spreads unchecked and disconnected from natural control mechanisms, thus displacing healthy, functional tissue.

Equally unwelcome is a pathological cell loss caused by excessive apoptosis. This happens in several neurodegenerative diseases of the brain, such as Alzheimer's disease.

In glaucoma, the loss is primarily found in retinal ganglion cells. Not all the details of this process are known, for example, how it is triggered or what the exact mechanism is. The current concept is summarized in Chapter 5.

However, there are a number of factors that are known to increase the likelihood of occurrence or progression of glaucomatous damage; these are called risk factors. There are risk factors that can be influenced, such as an elevated intraocular pressure, low systemic blood pressure, and the dysregulation of blood vessels (called vasospasms, cf. S 11). But there are other risk factors that are beyond control, such as age, gender, refractive errors, etc. The importance of the various factors is still a matter of controversy among ophthalmologists. While some experts still regard glaucoma as solely a problem of increased IOP, other research groups emphasize the importance of circulatory problems in the development of glaucoma. This is a contradiction only at first glance. For most diseases there are different causes that work together and, depending on his particular experience and point of view, the doctor attributes more importance to certain factors. Below is an allegory of this from everyday life.

2.2.1 The Problem of Causality

There are often discussions about why something has happened, what has caused [Lat. *kausa*: reason] a particular event. Quite different points of view might appear to oppose each other:

Every morning, Mr. Smith drives to his workplace located on the other side of the river. He has been doing this for years. He must cross a bridge that is quite exposed to weather conditions and is often icy. On one particular winter morning, the frozen surface is covered in places by snow. As usual, Mr. Smith is running a bit late and doesn't slow down while crossing the bridge. His car starts to skid and he veers off the road; his car becomes entangled in the railing and is badly damaged.

And now, the question arises: What actually caused the accident and the damage to the vehicle? Various opinions can be voiced. Perhaps Group A would maintain that the unequivocal cause of the accident was that the speed was not adjusted to the actual road conditions. Had Mr. Smith been driving slowly, perhaps even very slowly, there would most probably not have been an accident. No one can strongly dispute Group A's opinion. Speed certainly played a role. But perhaps Group B is made up of car industry professionals and they take a different view. They insist that the accident would not have happened had Mr. Smith been driving a better car. Group B is also correct because, indeed, on the very same day, many other cars traveling at a similar speed crossed the bridge without having an accident – however, these cars were equipped with anti-locking brake systems and winter tires. And then Group C voices yet another opinion: They place the blame on the community. They claim that had snowplows removed ice and snow from the bridge in time, there would not have been an accident. For them, the cause of the accident was the icy bridge and the fact that the road had not been properly cleared. Indeed, there are many other factors that could have also been critical, such as the driver's reaction time, etc.

This example underscores the fact that events are usually caused by a variety of contributing factors working together. Depending on the observer's point of view, one or the other factor will be emphasized or perhaps the problem is even reduced to just one single cause.

If this example were applied to understanding glaucomatous damage, the IOP could be substituted for the car's speed. As noted, if the driver had maintained a speed that compensated for the hazardous road conditions (meaning had driven very slowly), probably no accident would have occurred. The same applies to intraocular pressure. If each eye's IOP were specifically adapted to its individual needs (in some cases, even an extremely low IOP), then glaucomatous damage would hardly ever occur. But just as driving slowly does not totally remove the risk of an accident, it is still possible to develop glaucoma even at very low IOP levels, but fortunately, this is a very rare event. For practical purposes, a certain speed has to be maintained and other factors have to be taken into account as well: Both reliable snow removal from the roads and high-quality cars significantly reduce accident risks without completely slowing down traffic. Along the same lines, improving reduced blood circulation can protect some patients' eyes so that even "normal" intraocular pressure is no longer damaging.

This example also demonstrates that one cause alone can lead to damage if that factor is extreme. Even the best car – driving in good conditions – can get into an accident if the speed is dangerously high. Likewise, an elevated IOP can lead to damage even in a healthy eye. But just as an icy road can be so slippery that even a very cautious driver might skid off the road, there are glaucoma patients who develop optic nerve damage even when the IOP is low, sometimes very low. The need for evaluating the other risk factors thus becomes clear. The aim of this allegory is to emphasize that most diseases, just as with glaucoma, are caused by several factors working together, and that one factor by itself, however, if extreme, can also cause damage. To focus on one single risk factor is not right or wrong, but merely a simplification. To properly evaluate the situation, all factors should be taken into consideration and their effects measured against each other (cf. Chapter 5).

An elevated intraocular pressure is an extremely important risk factor for glaucoma. Since this factor can be both easily monitored and treated, it has been the focus of attention for several decades. The various mechanisms of an increase in IOP are described in Chapter 3, Chapter 4 deals with additional risk factors and Chapter 5 demonstrates how the different factors work together to induce glaucomatous damage.

2.2.2 The Significance of Intraocular Pressure

From a physical point of view, the pressure that exists inside the eye's globe is nothing but the difference between the absolute IOP and the atmospheric pressure at any given moment. Therefore, what is actually meant by intraocular pressure is, in fact, this difference in pressures, the relative IOP. But what components make up the IOP?

To facilitate understanding, the eye is divided into several parts, including an anterior chamber and a posterior chamber. Inside these chambers, there is a circulating, water-like fluid called the aqueous humor. It is produced by the eye's ciliary body and initially excreted into the posterior chamber (cf. S 1), and then flows through the pupil into the anterior chamber (Fig. 2.14).

Part of the aqueous humor is directed via the trabecular meshwork into the canal of Schlemm. This circular canal, located at the transition from cornea to sclera, is connected to veins that course through the scleral surface. This venous plexus serves as the aqueous humor's exit out of the eye and into the bloodstream.

Another portion of the aqueous humor flows through interstitial spaces of the iris and the ciliary body under the sclera. The aqueous humor diffuses through the sclera, which is permeable to fluid, into the connective tissue of the orbit, and then drains via blood vessels into the general circulation. And yet some of the aqueous humor is directly absorbed by the blood vessels of the choroid, the layer behind the retina. These exit routes are termed the uveoscleral outflow path [Lat. *uvea:* grape]. The choroid, consisting mainly of blood vessels, resembles a grape.

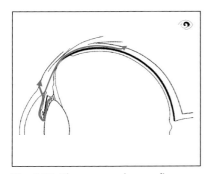

Fig. 2.14: The aqueous humor flows from the posterior chamber into the anterior chamber; it leaves the eye through the trabecular meshwork or through the uvea and sclera.

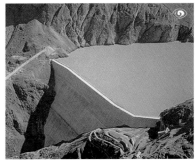

Fig. 2.15: As in a dam, the desired pressure can only be maintained if there is equilibrium between inflow and outflow.

Aqueous humor is actively produced (i.e. secreted) by the eye while the outflow has to overcome a certain amount of resistance (cf. S 1). This is the source of the intraocular pressure. Since the globe can only minimally expand in any direction, the IOP results from the balance between the production and outflow of the aqueous humor. Decreased production and/or an easier outflow results in a decrease in the IOP. On the other hand, the intraocular pressure rises when the ciliary body produces more aqueous humor and/or the resistance to outflow increases (cf. Figure 2.15).

What is the Purpose of the IOP?

1. The intraocular pressure maintains the eye in a stable form. When changing the direction in which the eye's gaze is directed, the muscles of the eye exert a strong force on the globe. The eyelids also put pressure on the eye. A certain amount of IOP is a reliable protection against deformation of the globe whenever there is eye movement or a blink. Such deformations would affect the quality of the retinal image (cf. S 4). Intraocular pressure thus literally keeps the eye in shape.

2. Intraocular pressure is also necessary to prevent certain eye tissues from swelling. In fact, the IOP actually replaces oncotic pressure [Gr. *ogkos:* swelling]. Oncotic pressure is the suction exerted on the fluids in neighboring tissues by protein molecules that circulate in the bloodstream. With this "force of attraction" the protein molecules can actively dehydrate the tissues surrounding the blood vessels and remove "cell garbage." There are, however, small pores in the vessel walls of the choroid. The smaller protein molecules can leave the blood vessels through these pores, thus removing the oncotic suction. But given these facts, and considering that the eye does not have lymphatic vessels for drainage, how can the eye be freed from the end products of its metabolism, its "garbage," and tissue swelling be avoided? This is where intraocular pressure comes back into the picture: The IOP forces the fluid containing the end products back into the blood circulation.

3. The circulating aqueous humor constantly bathes the different tissues of the eye, including the lens and the internal layer of the cornea (cf. S 1). Both the lens and the cornea are "avascular" [Lat. *vas*: vessel], meaning neither has its own blood vessels. If they were supplied by blood vessels, they would lose their transparency and this would impair visual function. To survive without blood vessels, they have to be constantly irrigated and nourished by the aqueous humor.

In short: Intraocular pressure is a necessity. If the IOP is too low for a prolonged period, disturbances arise, such as swelling of the choroid. The ophthalmologist calls this a choroidal effusion. In such cases, the visual function is impaired. Under normal circumstances, however, vision is quickly restored if the IOP again rises to normal. Figure 2.16 shows a diagram of what happens to a normal eye when the intraocular pressure is too high or too low.

How High is Normal Eye Pressure? The answer depends on what one considers normal. From a statistical point of view, "normal" is an IOP range that is most frequently measured in healthy eyes. Even among the non-glaucomatous population, many differences in eye pressure are recorded. Most people have an average IOP between 9–21 mmHg, with a mean IOP of approximately 15 mmHg. There are also healthy individuals with an IOP lower than 9

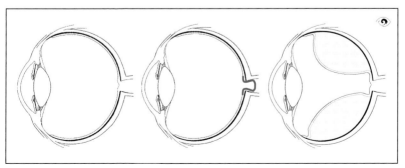

Fig. 2.16: If the intraocular pressure is too high, glaucomatous damage will develop (middle); if it is too low, the choroid swells (right).

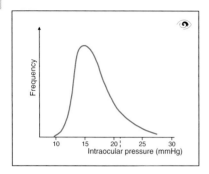

Fig. 2.17: Frequency distribution of IOP values among the healthy population.

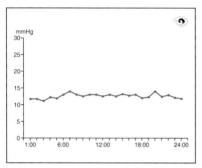

Fig. 2.18: During a 24-hour period, there are slight fluctuations in the IOP of a healthy person.

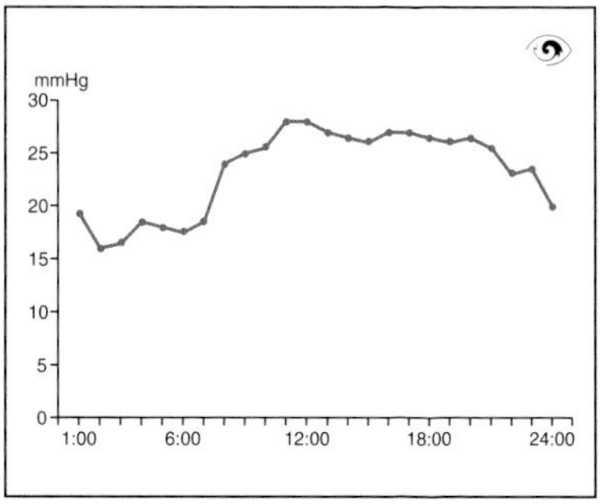

Fig. 2.19: A glaucoma patient, by contrast, experiences more pronounced fluctuations of IOP.

mmHg or higher than 21 mmHg, although these cases are rare (Fig. 2.17).

The fact that most healthy people have an IOP less than 22 mmHg does not automatically mean that this is a threshold beyond which glaucomatous damage inevitably begins. As will be seen later, optic nerve damage can occur at IOP levels below 21 mmHg. On the other hand, there are people who do not have glaucomatous damage who live perfectly well with an IOP above 21 mmHg. The IOP level that is still tolerated or the threshold beyond which damage occurs varies according to the individual and depends upon other risk factors (cf. Chapters 4 and 5).

Just as is seen with blood pressure, the intraocular pressure goes up and down. These fluctuations vary from person to person (Fig. 2.18). In glaucoma patients, not only is the intraocular pressure increased, but it also fluctuates more than in healthy eyes (Fig. 2.19). To monitor these fluctuations and the IOP peaks in particular, one single IOP measurement is not sufficient. Several measurements at various times of the day are needed.

Note: Intraocular pressure is measured in "mmHg." Hg is the chemical abbreviation for mercury. The pressure is thus determined by recording the change in height in mm of a mercury column.

2.2.3 The Significance of Ocular Perfusion

Like the brain, the eye is supplied with blood by the carotid artery (*arteria carotis*) (cf. Figure 2.20). The ophthalmic artery, a branch of the carotid, continues into the orbit and supplies the eye and its surroundings with blood (Fig. 2.21). Many words (such as ophthalmology, for instance) have the root term, "ophtha," which comes from the ancient Greek, *ophthalmos,* meaning "eye." Therefore, ophthalmology is the study of the eye.

The anterior segment of the eye is supplied by the blood vessels of the eye's muscles. For the posterior segment, there are two different systems of blood circulation. The central retinal artery (*arteria centralis retinae*) enters the globe together with the optic nerve and supplies the retina [Lat. *rete:* net], and this is known as the retinal circulation (cf. Figure 2.22). The choroid (cf. S 1) is supplied by branches of the short posterior ciliary arteries. These ciliary vessels

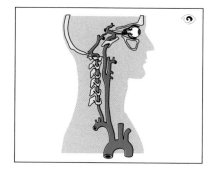

Fig. 2.20: The carotid artery supplies the eye and the anterior parts of the brain with blood; the vertebral arteries supply the posterior segments of the brain.

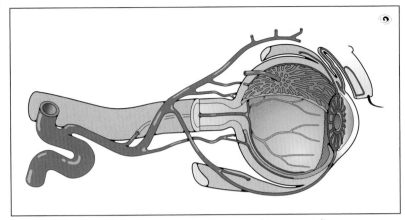

Fig. 2.21: The ophthalmic artery supplies the eye and its surroundings.

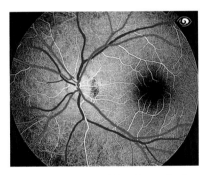

Fig. 2.22: The retinal blood vessels: To help distinguish between the vessels, the arteries are shown in red, the veins in blue.

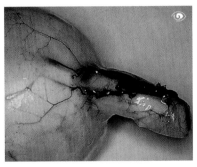

Fig. 2.23: In this picture, the posterior ciliary arteries have been stained with a dark dye.

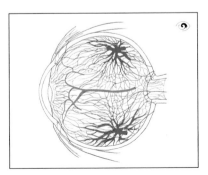

Fig. 2.24: The blood flows from the choroid into the vortex veins.

enter the eye's posterior pole through the sclera (Fig. 2.23). This is called the choroidal circulation.

Venous blood leaves the retina via the central retinal vein (*vena centralis retinae*). Just as the central retinal artery, this vein enters the center of the papilla and follows the course of the optic nerve for a short distance. Venous outflow from the choroid uses the vortex venous systems. "Vortex" means "a whirled arrangement" which aptly describes the shape of these veins (cf. Figure 2.24).

With regard to its circulation, the papilla (optic disc) is in a unique position: The papilla's surface is arterially supplied by the retinal circulation, the underlying parts by the same vessels as the choroid. The venous outflow completely merges into the retinal circulation, i.e. the central retinal vein. The optic disc's circulation thus shares characteristics with both the retinal as well as the choroidal vasculature (Fig. S 1.52). Vasoactive substances, meaning drugs that can influence the diameter of the vessels, can reach the papilla via the choroid. This explains why the papilla is so susceptible to circulatory problems. These will be covered in detail in Chapter 5.

Glaucoma patients often suffer from a decreased ocular perfusion. This is a very important risk factor and will be discussed extensively in Chapter 4.2.7. As Chapter 5 will demonstrate, a reduced blood flow increases the eye's sensitivity to intraocular pressure.

Summary

The loss of retinal ganglion cells and their axons is called glaucomatous damage. When it comes to glaucomatous papillary atrophy, glial cells and blood vessels are irreversibly damaged along with nerve fibers in the optic disc, a development that leads to disc excavation. As a consequence, visual field defects occur, but the patient hardly notices these in the early stages of the disease. Several factors contribute to glaucomatous damage, most notably an elevated intraocular pressure and a reduced ocular blood flow.

3 Classification of the Various Types of Glaucoma

Traditionally, the cause of IOP elevation has been used as the basis for classifying the various types of glaucoma. By far the most common reason for an increase in intraocular pressure is a reduced outflow capacity of the aqueous humor, usually located at the anterior chamber angle and the trabecular meshwork (cf. S 1). Disturbances of the trabecular outflow pathway may, in turn, have a variety of causes, as discussed later in this chapter.

Although the chance of developing an elevated IOP significantly rises as one ages, an increase in the intraocular pressure can occur at any age. Indeed, congenital glaucoma affects babies who are born with high IOP or develop an increase shortly after birth. An elevated IOP during childhood is defined as infantile glaucoma; and when this condition occurs during adolescence, the proper term is juvenile glaucoma.

3.1 Congenital Glaucoma

Affected infants may be born with a high intraocular pressure or may develop an increased IOP within the first weeks of life.

The Cause. Congenital glaucoma is a rare form of glaucoma. Both eyes are usually involved, but to varying degrees; boys are affected slightly more frequently than girls. A hereditary factor is occasionally present. The genes responsible for the development of the eye and the mutations inducing glaucoma and other genetic defects are currently being researched, and there has already been some progress made in their identification (cf. S 3). However, there are also sporadic cases, meaning found among children who do not have a hereditary tendency for developing congenital glaucoma.

The IOP elevation is caused by the failure of the anterior chamber angle and the trabecular meshwork to develop appropriately during intrauterine development (cf. S 2). In these infants, the aqueous humor does not properly drain, but since the production of aqueous humor is nevertheless normal, the intraocular pressure is high.

Figure 3.1 shows a regularly developed chamber angle, whereas in Figure 3.2, the trabecular meshwork has not yet fully developed and is still partially covered by a membrane.

Consequences of an Increased IOP during Infancy. Depending on the IOP level, glaucomatous damage is inevitable after weeks, months or even years. This basically occurs via the same mechanisms as in the adult. In addition to optic nerve damage, the globe (eyeball) enlarges because the sclera in the eye of a baby is distensible.

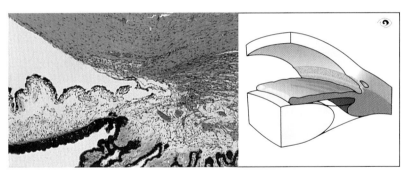

Fig. 3.1: The normal chamber angle: on the left is a histological cross-section; on the right is a drawing of the same.

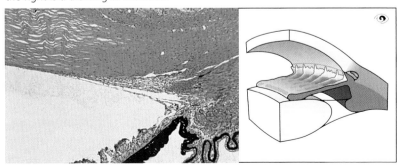

Fig. 3.2: An underdeveloped chamber angle.

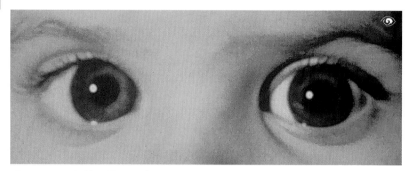

Fig. 3.3: A child suffering from congenital glaucoma with characteristically enlarged eyeballs.

All segments of the outer eye, but especially the cornea and sclera, expand. The eyes of these afflicted children are thus large (Fig. 3.3).

However, certain layers of the cornea are not very elastic, and stretching may result in small tears that cause a certain degree of corneal opacification (Fig. 3.4).

If the IOP is lowered, this opacity is partially reversible. As a result of the optic nerve damage and/or corneal opacity, children with congenital glaucoma may be permanently visually impaired.

As mentioned earlier, the eyes, optic nerves and certain segments of the brain participate in the visual process. At the time of birth, this visual system is not yet fully developed. During the first years of life, this system can complete its development only if there is normal binocular vision. If one eye does not see properly during childhood (for example, because of a unilateral lens opacification),

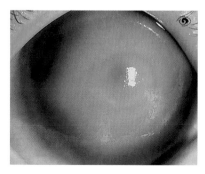

Fig. 3.4: Opacified cornea in an eye afflicted with congenital glaucoma.

maturation of the visual apparatus on this side is threatened. Without appropriate therapy, it is likely that vision will be permanently impaired because full development has never been achieved (i.e. amblyopia) [Gr. *amblys:* blunt; Gr. *opsein:* to see]. Amblyopia can only be treated during childhood, correction as an adult is not possible. It is therefore of utmost importance that young glaucoma patients be able to use both eyes and that they have normal binocular vision as soon as possible.

Diagnosis of Congenital Glaucoma. Fortunately, congenital glaucoma is not a common disease: only about one in ten thousand newborns is affected. Early detection of this ailment is essential; these children can be helped if diagnosed in time.

What are the specific signs and symptoms that lead one to suspect congenital glaucoma?
First of all, enlarged eyes; tear flow is often increased and photophobia (avoidance of light) causes these babies to squeeze their eyes shut. Often, they also rub their eyes.

How is Congenital Glaucoma Diagnosed?
Examining newborns and infants is a bit more difficult than checking an adult's eye. If glaucoma is suspected, a thorough examination under general anesthesia is necessary. This is the only way to measure the IOP without putting too much stress on the baby and to avoid blepharospasm (spasmodic closure of the eyes). Blepharospasm can, in turn, lead to a transient rise in the IOP. Besides measuring the IOP, anesthesia allows a thorough investigation of all segments of the eye and, in particular, the optic disc.

Treatment of Congenital Glaucoma. Treatment depends on the severity of the disease. In moderate cases, one might start with IOP-lowering eye drops. But usually, especially in advanced disease stages, surgery is required to reduce the intraocular pressure. The ophthalmic surgeon will decide when and which type of procedure is necessary.

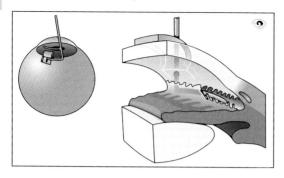

Fig. 3.5: Trabeculotomy in congenital glaucoma.

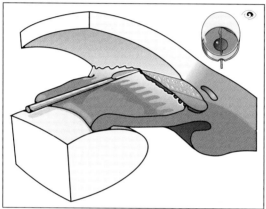

Fig. 3.6: Goniotomy in congenital glaucoma.

Several surgical procedures are possible. Figure 3.5 shows a trabeculotomy, and Figure 3.6, a goniotomy. Another option is a trabeculectomy, described under procedures for adult glaucoma patients (cf. Chapter 7.4). The purpose of all these techniques is to improve the aqueous humor outflow and thus lower the IOP to normal levels.

Because the intraocular pressure can again increase at any time, even after a successful operation, frequent follow-up examinations by the ophthalmologist are necessary. Should the IOP again increase, medication must be started or the operation repeated. It is not only possible to do surgery again and again, it is sometimes inevitable. Congenital glaucoma can be associated with additional birth defects of the eye or other parts of the body. When certain signs occur together, they often make up a "syndrome" (for example, Axenfeld-Rieger Syndrome, Peters' anomaly, aniridia, neurofibromatosis, etc.). In particular, this means that every child born with congenital glaucoma has to be examined for other diseases or birth defects. Likewise, a child having any of these birth defects must have his IOP examined as early as possible so glaucoma can be identified or excluded.

3.2   Infantile Glaucoma

In the broadest sense of the term, infantile glaucoma is also congenital glaucoma. However, the term infantile is used because the intraocular pressure starts to rise at some time during the first years of life. The cause for this IOP increase is basically the same as in congenital glaucoma, but it occurs later since the anterior chamber angle is more mature than when glaucoma is present at birth. Due to the more advanced developmental stage of the outflow system, the IOP may be normal during the first years of childhood and then gradually increase.

Diagnosis of Infantile Glaucoma. The classical features of congenital glaucoma are not present in infantile glaucoma. The eyes are not enlarged and symptoms, such as epiphora (excessive tear flow), photophobia (aversion to light) and opaque cornea, are lacking. This type of glaucoma is occasionally diagnosed during routine screening or when the child is examined because of a family history of glaucoma.

For other children, glaucoma is accompanied by impaired vision and strabismus (crossed eyes). When this is the case, advanced glaucomatous damage is already present. This again underscores the necessity of having a thorough ophthalmologic evaluation for all visual problems in childhood, including squinting. The types of glaucoma that appear during childhood are often inherited.

The Consequences of an Increased IOP in Childhood. The consequences are basically the same as those in adult glaucoma patients, i.e. optic disc cupping and visual field defects. Since these children are usually healthy otherwise and they have normal blood circulation, their prognosis is relatively good after the IOP returns to normal. Once again, detection and the earliest possible treatment of glaucoma are crucial.

Treating Infantile Glaucoma. Treatment does not basically differ from that for other types of glaucoma. If medical therapy does not adequately reduce the IOP, then laser treatment is considered. Because the anterior chamber angle has not yet completely matured, this angle can sometimes be opened by a procedure known as laser membranotomy. The result is similar to that achieved with a goniotomy used in congenital glaucoma. If the outcome with laser treatment is not satisfactory, meaning that the IOP is still elevated and/or there is already tissue damage, then surgery should be performed as soon as possible. The surgeon will decide which procedure is best. Even after successful surgery, it is possible that the intraocular pressure again increases, and thus regular eye examinations are necessary.

3.3 Juvenile Glaucoma

Juvenile [Lat. *juvenilis:* youthful] glaucoma is an IOP increase that occurs in an older child or young adult and is often inherited. During a thorough examination, the ophthalmologist may find discreet evidence of an incomplete maturation of the chamber angle, and as treatment, a laser goniotomy (cf. S 13) can be performed. The clinical features as well as treatment of juvenile glaucoma are quite similar to adult chronic open-angle glaucoma (cf. Chapter 3.4), and will therefore not be discussed in detail here.

As a closing remark, it should be noted that children can also be afflicted with other forms of glaucoma, for example, secondary glaucoma as a result of accidents or inflammations. These forms of glaucoma are similar to those seen in adults and will be discussed later.

3.4   Primary Chronic Open-Angle Glaucoma (POAG)

Increased IOP is usually caused by inadequate drainage. Most of the aqueous humor leaves the eye via the trabecular meshwork that leads to Schlemm's canal, from where it enters the bloodstream (cf. S 1). If the anterior chamber angle is not completely developed, the aqueous humor's access to the trabecular meshwork is partially blocked, and the consequence is congenital glaucoma (cf. Chapter 3.1). When the IOP rise occurs at a later age, it is termed infantile glaucoma (cf. Chapter 3.2). When the outflow channels in the chamber angle are blocked by the iris, angle-closure glaucoma develops (cf. Chapter 3.5). Secondary glaucoma results from the drainage being impaired as a result of a different eye disease (cf. Chapter 3.6).

When the chamber angle is normally developed and not blocked by the iris and, furthermore, there is no other apparent cause for an increased IOP, then one speaks of primary chronic open-angle glaucoma. It is termed "open-angle" glaucoma because the chamber angle is open; "chronic" because it takes years to develop; and "primary" because it is not the result of any other eye disease. Because this is by far the most common form of glaucoma, it will be discussed in detail. The common abbreviation is POAG and the Latin name is *glaucoma chronicum simplex.*

POAG has been traditionally divided into: a) eyes having glaucomatous damage and high IOP (i.e. high-tension glaucoma); b) eyes having glaucomatous damage but normal IOP (i.e. normal-ten-

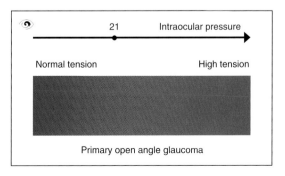

Fig. 3.7: Primary open-angle glaucoma: There is a gradual transition from normal-tension glaucoma to high-tension glaucoma; there are no precisely defined pressure levels that separate the two.

sion glaucoma, also known as normal-pressure glaucoma); and c) eyes having an elevated intraocular pressure but with no visible optic nerve damage. This classification is somewhat arbitrary (Fig. 3.7) as these three types are just various manifestations of one single disease. Because this classification is still used in most textbooks, it will also be followed here. However, it must be emphasized that there is no clear dividing line that separates these forms.

The higher the IOP, the greater the risk for glaucomatous damage; however, there is no clear, definitive threshold beyond which the IOP causes damage. There is, nevertheless, a shift in the emphasis of the various risk factors. The lower the intraocular pressure when tissue damage occurs, the more likely that other risk factors, such as low systemic blood pressure or vascular dysregulation, are involved and have contributed to the damage.

Besides the level of the intraocular pressure, normal-tension glaucoma and high-tension glaucoma differ slightly in their morphological appearance. On average, glaucoma patients with a normal IOP develop optic disc hemorrhages more frequently, and have a more pronounced peripapillary atrophy (tissue loss around the optic disc), somewhat shallower cupping and less displacement of the disc vessels (Figs. 3.8 and 3.9). Alterations of conjunctival blood vessels and the appearance of shiny retinal spots (called "gliosis-like alterations" in ophthalmic literature) are also more common with normal-tension glaucoma.

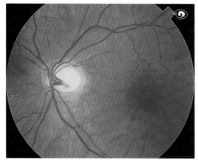

Fig. 3.8: Optic disc clearly showing glaucomatous damage in a patient with increased IOP.

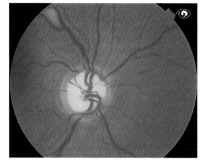

Fig. 3.9: Optic disc clearly showing glaucomatous damage in a patient with normal IOP.

As mentioned, the artificial divide between normal and high-tension glaucoma is usually set at 21 mmHg. Due to the often pronounced circadian IOP fluctuations, the chance of surpassing this limit increases with the number of measurements taken. If a patient undergoes frequent eye examinations, chances are higher that an occasional IOP above 21 mmHg will be registered. This applies to a healthy person as well, although less frequently. Again, this underscores just how relative this classification actually is.

3.4.1 POAG with Increased Intraocular Pressure

This is chronic open-angle glaucoma (*glaucoma chronicum simplex*) in the narrowest sense of the term. Also called high-tension or high-pressure glaucoma, it is characterized by a slow loss of retinal ganglion cells with optic disc cupping and ensuing visual field defects (cf. Chapter 2.1). The main risk factor is increased intraocular pressure, but additional risk factors may also be present (cf. Chapter 4). The IOP is usually slightly increased, ranging between 20 and 30 mmHg, but may occasionally reach levels between 30 and 40 mmHg. Because an IOP even this high does not cause pain and visual defects are not noticed at first, the patient is not aware that he has glaucoma. Diagnosis is often made during a routine eye exam. The ophthalmologist not only measures the IOP but also carefully examines the optic disc. If the appearance of the papilla is not quite

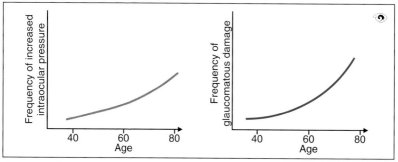

Fig. 3.10: The intraocular pressure increases with age. Glaucomatous damage can occur at any time. Since it is irreversible, the number of patients having glaucomatous damage increases among the older population.

normal or if there are already signs of glaucomatous damage, then additional examinations will be made (cf. Chapter 6).

Although primary chronic open-angle glaucoma may be present in the young, it becomes more frequent with advancing age (Fig 3.10), and is by far the most common form of glaucoma.

Up to 10 percent of the elderly population suffer from chronic open-angle glaucoma, and among those of African heritage, percentages are even higher. In contrast to normal-tension glaucoma, both men and women are equally affected (cf. Chapter 3.4.2).

The Causes of Increased IOP. Open-angle glaucoma means that when the ophthalmologist examines the anterior chamber angle, he sees nothing that could block the aqueous humor outflow, but nevertheless, the IOP is elevated.

The actual cause is the increase in the outflow resistance at the trabecular meshwork itself. The aqueous humor has to flow through this meshwork to reach Schlemm's canal (cf. Figure 3.11). In glaucoma patients, the meshwork becomes increasingly laden with substances (Fig 3.12) that impair aqueous humor drainage.

It is not known why these deposits accumulate. When cells are subjected to a certain amount of stress (such as being exposed to increasingly higher levels of free radicals), they produce these substances. Future research projects will investigate whether, and if so, then how, this happens in glaucoma patients.

Another observation that is quite typical for open-angle glaucoma: Not only is there an increase in the average IOP, but the IOP level also undergoes more marked fluctuations. Unfortunately, these ups and downs are particularly damaging, even more damaging than an increased, but stable, IOP level. The question then arises, "What treatment options are available?"

Treatment. As soon as glaucomatous damage is identified, the intraocular pressure should be significantly lowered with any of three basic methods: medical therapy, laser therapy or surgery. In most cases, if the glaucomatous damage is not too advanced, the initial approach attempted is usually with medication (cf. Chapter 7.2).

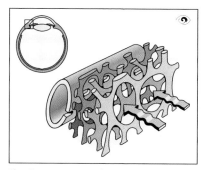

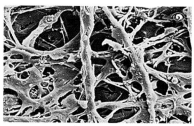

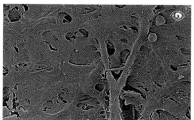

Fig. 3.11: Aqueous humor (green) drains through the trabecular meshwork into Schlemm's canal.

Fig. 3.12: Trabecular meshwork (magnified) of a healthy individual (above) and a glaucoma patient (below).

However, if the IOP remains high or the damage progresses despite a normalized IOP, then surgery is almost always the next option. The operation has both advantages and disadvantages (as discussed in Chapter 7.4), but the prognosis for the visual field is especially good when the IOP is surgically lowered. This is probably due to the fact that an operation not only reduces the IOP but also keeps it relatively stable. Laser treatment (cf. Chapter 7.3) does not play a significant treatment role in this type of glaucoma. Occasionally laser trabeculoplasty is used to lower the intraocular pressure but the pressure fluctuations still continue (though at a lower level), and the IOP almost inevitably rises again after a few years. Therefore, to avoid subjecting the patient to two procedures, surgery is usually performed with IOP not controlled by medication or when advanced optic nerve damage is present.

Other risk factors are frequently involved in the damage. If tissue loss has occurred with only moderately increased IOP or if it gets worse despite pressure normalization, then these other risk factors have to be seriously evaluated.

3.4.2 POAG with Normal Intraocular Pressure

If there is glaucomatous damage (optic disc excavation and/ or visual field loss) even though the IOP has been normal on repeated measurements, then the patient has normal-tension glaucoma. Again, it must be emphasized that there is no fundamental difference between normal-tension glaucoma and high-tension glaucoma. The difference is simply in the level of the IOP, but keep in mind that there is no rigid limit. Since there is no clear division between the two, it is sometimes difficult to definitively assign the patients to either group. But, in reality, this is not critical because both high-tension and normal-tension POAG basically have the same diagnostic evaluation and treatment.

As mentioned, there are certain risk factors that contribute to developing glaucomatous damage (cf. Chapter 4). If there is tissue loss while the IOP is normal or just slightly increased, there will certainly be other risk factors besides IOP that are present (cf. Chapter 5). Glaucomatous damage in patients with high IOP is almost identical to that observed in individuals having normal pressure. There are only minor differences that have already been discussed. Just to repeat, patients with normal-tension glaucoma more often have the following changes: optic disc hemorrhages, peripapillary atrophy, a shallow excavation and occasionally a pale neuroretinal rim (Figs. 3.8, 3.9), gliosis-like alterations of the retina, as well as changes in the conjunctival vessels (Chapter 6.6). All these symptoms can be observed by the ophthalmologist and are clues that other factors, in addition to just an increased IOP, are involved in the mechanism of damage.

Therapy. The goal of treatment and the treatment itself are basically the same for normal and elevated-pressure POAG, that is, to achieve a lower and, even more importantly, a stable IOP. In normal-pressure POAG, the level considered "safe" for the patient – also called the "target pressure" – is lower than in high-pressure glaucoma. A reduction to less than 15 mmHg is often the treatment goal. If vascular problems are involved, therapy strives to achieve normal ocular perfusion, as discussed in Chapter 7.5.

Prognosis. Basically, the prognosis for normal-tension glaucoma is quite similar to that for high-tension glaucoma. High-tension glaucoma without adequate tension-lowering therapy can lead to blindness. However even though there is frequently severe visual impairment in patients having normal-tension glaucoma, total blindness is rare. This is probably due to the fact that vascular risk factors relevant to glaucoma (low blood pressure and vascular dysregulation) tend to decrease with age. Nevertheless, normal-tension glaucoma must be taken very seriously to prevent visual impairment or blindness.

3.4.3 POAG without Discernible Glaucomatous Damage

When intraocular pressure exceeds the – purely statistically defined – threshold value of 21 mmHg without visible damage, it is then called ocular hypertension (cf. Chapter 1.2). Although there is no glaucomatous tissue loss present, we define it as glaucoma. Indeed, there is no actual damage present that can be monitored, but there is a higher risk that it will develop later. This does not mean damage will occur at levels above 21 mmHg, and no damage will occur at lower values. Both are possible. There is no clear pressure level beyond which glaucomatous damage occurs. It can happen at any IOP level, however, the likelihood that it will occur increases with elevated tension.

Therapy. At precisely which point an elevated IOP deserves treatment is hotly debated by experts. Depending on the clinical features, the IOP level and the presence of additional risk factors, the ophthalmologist must make the decision as to when treatment is reasonable. When there are frequent follow-up examinations of the visual fields and optic discs, treatment can usually be postponed. Regular eye examinations in short intervals provide the physician with the opportunity to detect even the slightest of changes. However, should regular follow-ups not be possible or if one wants to err on the side of safety, then it might be prudent to lower an elevated intraocular pressure earlier in some patients than in others. With pressures of 25 mmHg or more, IOP-reducing therapy is usually started.

3.5   Primary Angle-Closure Glaucoma

Primary angle-closure glaucomas are usually associated with a pronounced increase in the intraocular pressure. These diseases share a complete or partial physical barrier to aqueous humor outflow that is created by the iris. One must differentiate between the predisposition for angle-closure glaucoma and the disorder itself [Lat. *praedispositio:* state of mind or body favorable to, sensitivity to]. Someone having a particular predisposition has a certain risk of developing acute angle-closure glaucoma at some time. The predisposing and triggering factors will be discussed below.

3.5.1 Acute Angle-Closure Glaucoma

There are two mechanisms that can lead to primary angle-closure glaucoma and these are: a) pupillary block mechanism (cf. Chapter 3.5.1.1) and b) plateau iris mechanism (cf. Chapter 3.5.1.2).

3.5.1.1 Pupillary Block Mechanism

Primary pupillary block occurs only in eyes that have a narrow anterior chamber angle, the angle formed by the cornea and the iris (cf. S 1). A narrow angle is found in hyperopic (far-sighted) individuals because their eyes are shorter and the anterior chamber is therefore comparatively shallow. The depth and volume of the anterior chamber and angle decrease steadily throughout life due to the continuous thickening of the lens with age. The presence of just one risk factor seldom leads to acute angle-closure glaucoma. Therefore, younger, far-sighted – or older, normal-sighted – people rarely suffer from pupillary block. But when a hyperopic patient gets older, the likelihood significantly increases. The classical case of pupillary block glaucoma is that of an older, hyperopic individual. In general, the risk is greater among women because their anterior chambers are usually shallower than those of men.

Predisposition to Pupillary Block. Figure 3.13 is a cross-section of a healthy anterior segment; Figure 3.14 (top) shows the same segment belonging to an elderly emmetropic (no refractive error) person. The thickening of the lens has reduced the anterior chamber depth and pushed the iris forward.

Figure 3.14 (bottom) shows a cross-section of the anterior segment of a hyperopic eye. As this far-sighted eye ages, the lens

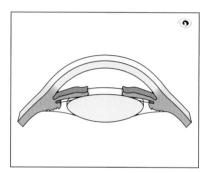

Fig. 3.13: Open chamber angle of a young adult.

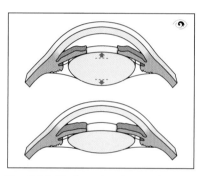

Fig. 3.14: Shallow chamber angle: an elderly person with a thick lens (top), a young hyperope (bottom).

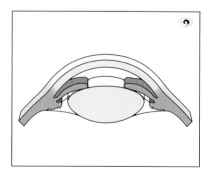

Fig. 3.15: Extremely shallow chamber angle of an elderly, hyperopic patient.

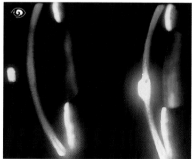

Fig. 3.16: Picture taken at the slit-lamp: a normal chamber angle (left), an angle with a shallow anterior chamber (right).

becomes thicker and the anterior chamber will become even more shallow (Fig. 3.15). This reduction in volume and depth is visible in a slit-lamp examination (Fig. 3.16). In this situation, depicted here, the outflow can still be quite normal. Although the iris is located in close proximity to the trabecular meshwork, drainage is still possible.

Acute Attack of Angle-Closure Glaucoma. In patients having the above-mentioned predisposition, the backside of the iris exerts pressure on the lens. With strong forces induced by the simultaneous contraction of the iris sphincter muscle (that reduces pupil size) and the iris dilator muscle (that increases pupil size), the net result is that the pupil is maintained in an intermediate position. However, the iris and the pupil are then forcefully pushed towards the lens surface (Fig. 3.17). When the iris is pushed against the lens, the aqueous humor can barely pass from the posterior chamber

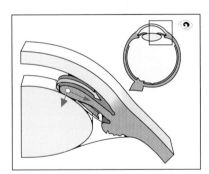

Fig. 3.17: The pressure exerted by the iris on the lens impedes aqueous humor outflow.

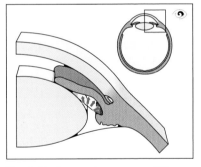

Fig. 3.18: Due to the pressure difference, the iris is pushed forward.

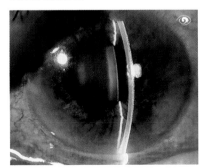

Fig. 3.19: Slit-lamp picture: shallow chamber angle and an iris that has been pushed into an anterior position.

through the pupil to the anterior chamber: a pressure gradient starts to build up. As a consequence, the intraocular pressure in the posterior chamber will be higher than the IOP in the anterior chamber. This pressure difference then pushes the iris forward at its weakest part, the peripheral segment (Figs. 3.18 and 3.19). The trabecular meshwork thereby becomes blocked by the iris. This leads to a sudden and extreme rise in IOP called "acute angle-closure glaucoma" or simply "glaucoma attack."

Precipitating Events. Constriction of the pupil is performed by the sphincter muscle in the iris that is controlled (i.e. innervated) by the so-called parasympathetic part of the autonomic nervous system. Dilation of the pupil is performed by the dilator muscle of the iris that is innervated by the sympathetic part of the autonomic nervous system. There are situations when both iris muscles are active at the same time, that is, work in opposite directions, and thereby exert pressure on the lens. This occurs, for example, when there is emotional stress or shock, and also potentially when one is dreaming. One short example: While replacing a light bulb in a store, an electrician falls off a ladder. Naturally, this gives him quite a scare. He is rushed to the emergency room, examined and, finding no serious injuries, released. Back at home about an hour later, he develops an increasingly severe headache that is accompanied by nausea, vomiting and redness of the eyes. He returns to the hospital where he is diagnosed with acute bilateral angle-closure glaucoma. By the way, the patient, who is approaching retirement, has been severely far-sighted (hyperopic) since childhood.

Symptoms. In acute glaucoma, the intraocular pressure rapidly rises from normal to extremely high levels, thereby causing severe headaches and eye pain. Extraocular symptoms, such as stomach cramps, nausea and vomiting, are sometimes – though not always – part of the picture. The eye suffering the attack is extremely red (Fig. 3.20) and the patient's vision is blurred. During an acute attack, sources of light appear unfocussed and surrounded by colored halos (Fig. 3.21).

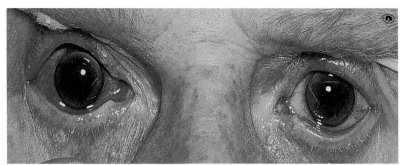

Fig. 3.20: Acute angle-closure glaucoma seen on the left. The eye is markedly red.

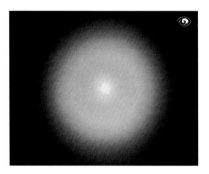

Fig. 3.21: A patient with corneal edema sees colored halos around light sources.

These visual problems are due to edema of the anterior corneal layers caused by the increased IOP. Since the deeper layer, the corneal stroma, cannot expand backward during an increase in the IOP, all the fluid is pushed into the cornea's superficial layer, the epithelium (Fig. 3.22). These fine intraepithelial droplets of water act like little lenses and change the light's direction. This not only impairs the patient's vision (causing blurriness) but also makes the cornea appear less shiny than normal and rather dull during an episode of acute glaucoma.

Treatment. Because the IOP is so high and the patient suffers from severe symptoms, emergency treatment is necessary (cf. Chapter 7). The main goal is to remove the iris from the trabecular meshwork and thus facilitate aqueous humor outflow. The first step is to equalize the pressure in the anterior and posterior chambers. To

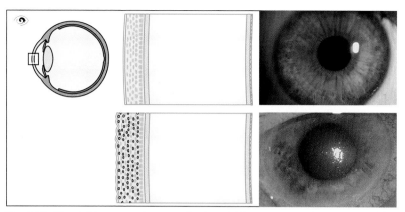

Fig. 3.22: Top right: a normal cornea, in the middle, a cross-section. Bottom right: corneal edema that makes the cornea appear slightly opaque.

achieve this, a new, artificial hole is cut into the base of the iris. The aqueous humor now has a new pathway and no longer has to go through the pupil to reach the anterior chamber. This small opening can be easily created with a laser (cf. S 13) or in a surgical procedure. The first procedure is called a laser iridotomy, the latter, a surgical iridectomy [Gr. *temnein:* to cut; Gr. *ektemnein:* to cut out]. However, both procedures are difficult to perform when the IOP is extremely high. Laser iridotomy is hampered by the corneal edema that not only blurs and reduces the patient's vision, but also impairs the ability of the physician to look at the eye's inner structures (poor view out for patient = poor view in for doctor). In order to cut the desired hole into the iris, it is essential that the laser beam pass unimpeded through the cornea. With corneal edema, there is a risk of injuring other intraocular tissues. Surgical intervention on an eye with high pressure also involves risks: ocular tissue that has been pushed forward by high IOP can become clamped in the incision.

For these reasons, the usual procedure is to first lower the eye pressure using drugs, at least during the initial hours of an acute glaucoma attack. Eye drops that are used in standard treatment of chronic glaucoma are inadequate in angle-closure glaucoma because of the extremely elevated IOP. These drugs are only slightly absorbed because diffusion is impeded.

Strong systemic drugs must therefore be administered. These drugs are not applied locally (to the eye), but are given as a pill or an intravenous infusion, and they reach the area where they are effective by circulating in the body's bloodstream. These substances temporarily decrease aqueous humor production, such as acetazolamide, or exert an osmotic effect, as is the case with glycerol and mannitol (cf. Chapter 7.2.6). Similar to proteins that dehydrate tissues, described in Chapter 2.2.2, mannitol removes fluid from the eye and directs it into the bloodstream, thus lowering the IOP. When the pressure has been sufficiently decreased, "classical" IOP-reducing eye drops are given and laser therapy or – less frequently – surgical treatment is performed.

Naturally, if at all possible, acute glaucoma attacks should be prevented. Both an iridotomy and iridectomy can be performed prophylactically, meaning as a preventive measure. This might be considered if, after examining the eye, the ophthalmologist feels there is considerable risk that an attack might occur or if the other eye has already experienced acute angle closure.

3.5.1.2 Plateau Iris Mechanism

Plateau iris mechanism is another condition that can lead to a massive IOP increase. In contrast to pupillary block, a plateau iris results from a pre-existing anatomical situation where an anteriorly-positioned iris blocks the anterior chamber angle (Fig. 3.23). If the pupil dilates, the increase in thickness at the peripheral iris can completely occlude the iridocorneal angle (Fig. 3.24).

When the aqueous humor flow cannot enter the trabecular meshwork, the IOP rises sharply. The likelihood of such an attack increases with age. Once again, predisposition (an anatomical variant that is associated with a higher risk) must be differentiated from the attack itself. In order for such an attack to be initiated, the pupil has to undergo extreme dilation. Under normal circumstances, a mild spontaneous dilation or a slight pupil dilation (mydriasis) induced by drops during an eye exam will not result in an acute attack. However, if this anatomical variant is present, your doctor will be

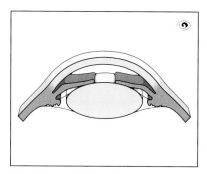

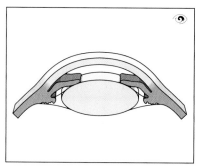

Fig. 3.23: A shallow chamber angle with a plateau-shaped iris.

Fig. 3.24: Angle-closure with a plateau iris mechanism.

most cautious with dilation. The plateau iris mechanism is much rarer than the pupillary block mechanism, but there are also combinations of both conditions or cases where distinguishing between the two is not easy.

Treatment. In an acute situation, the first step is to lower the IOP, as described with the pupillary block mechanism. To prevent another extreme IOP rise, a permanent and mild miosis (i.e. constricted pupil) has to be achieved. Administering a mild miotic drug each night is usually adequate (cf. 7.2.1). Because pupillary block mechanism may also develop, a laser iridotomy is also often performed.

Prophylaxis. It is important to prevent an extensive dilation of the pupil. Therefore, affected patients must be very cautious with drugs that cause mydriasis, such as some anti-depressants. In severe cases, just as is done in patients who have already had an attack, the pupil is slightly constricted with medication, especially at night. Since pupillary block mechanism and plateau iris mechanism can occur together, when there is some doubt present, a prophylactic peripheral iridotomy is performed. The peripheral parts of the iris can occasionally be tightened and thinned with laser treatment (iridoplasty), and the anterior chamber angle widened (gonioplasty).

3.5.2 Intermittent Angle-Closure Glaucoma

If the chamber angle is not completely blocked (meaning closure all the way around), the increase in the IOP is usually less extreme and does not last very long. The symptoms are accordingly less severe. In most cases, the patient notices dull aches in or around the eye and headaches. Depending on how high the pressure rises, the patient might also experience transient visual disturbances. Stronger generalized symptoms, such as nausea and vomiting, are rare. As long as the underlying cause has not been treated, these episodes might occur repeatedly (intermittently), and this form of the disease is thus termed "intermittent angle-closure glaucoma" [Lat. *intermittere:* to interrupt, to suspend]. Intermittent angle-closure glaucoma is a mild form of acute glaucoma. The symptoms are not as severe because the angle is not completely, circularly closed and episodes will continue to occur if the anatomical cause is not removed. In most cases, the partially closed chamber angle spontaneously opens again, the IOP returns to a normal level and relieves the patient of his symptoms. However, the trabecular meshwork becomes permanently damaged by the frequent contact with the iris. This eventually results in a moderately elevated IOP, even after the angle has reopened. This is termed a "simplex component." Just as in *glaucoma chronicum simplex* (also called primary open-angle glaucoma, POAG), the IOP is elevated although the anterior chamber angle is open; there is likewise an increase in the outflow resistance at the trabecular meshwork (cf. Chapter 3.4.1). These alterations are not visible to the ophthalmologist.

Therapy. Depending on the IOP level and the iris morphology, the ophthalmologist initially reduces the intraocular pressure with drugs. The next step is to create a situation that ensures a permanent opening of the chamber angle. This can be achieved by miotics (eye drops that constrict the pupil), laser iridotomy or both. Occasionally, the increase in lens size and thickness requires its surgical removal (cataract operation, cf. S 5). Should there still be a "simplex component," then treatment, described in Chapter 3.4.1, must be initiated.

3.5.3 Chronic Angle-Closure Glaucoma

The term, chronic angle-closure glaucoma, refers to an eye with a high IOP. The anterior chamber is narrow and closed in places by synechiae, as shown in Figure 3.25.

It is often not possible to identify what has caused the synechiae at the angle. Some patients suffer from intermittent occlusions. The iris does not completely free itself during "reopening." Chronic angle-closure glaucoma is sometimes the result of slight intraocular inflammations that may have gone totally unnoticed. In other cases, it is a side effect of certain medications. In addition to synechiae, there is often a "simplex component" as described under intermittent angle-closure glaucoma.

The first line of treatment is to attempt to open the angle with the procedures already described. However, some synechiae cannot be reopened and then the IOP has to be treated, just as in POAG. This means using medication to reduce the IOP and, if this is not sufficient, then surgery. The goal of any prophylaxis is to prevent further contact between the iris and the trabecular meshwork. If there is a risk of recurrence, either iridotomy is performed or drug-induced miosis is introduced.

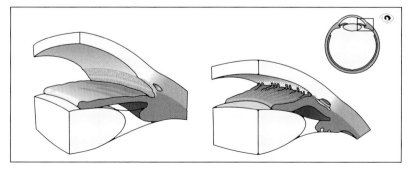

Fig. 3.25: Chronic angle-closure with synechiae and adhesions. On the left is a normal chamber angle for comparison.

3.5.4 Ciliary Block Glaucoma

In this very rare form of glaucoma, the ciliary body touches the lens. As a result, part of the aqueous humor is directed into the vitreous cavity instead of the space in front of the lens. This, in turn, pushes both the iris and lens in an anterior direction. As mentioned, this situation is rare and is mostly a consequence of an intraocular operation, a surgical procedure during which the eyeball has to be opened. Spontaneous cases are extremely rare; middle-aged women are most likely to be affected. The anatomical situation that predisposes to an attack is shown in Figure 3.26, and the acute attack itself in Figure 3.27.

In this case, treatment differs from acute angle-closure glaucoma. Eye drops are prescribed to dilate the pupil (mydriatics). These drugs exert an influence on both the iris and the ciliary body and, ideally, disrupt the contact between the ciliary body and lens. Nevertheless, surgery or a laser procedure is usually required. During such an operation, a connection must be made between the vitreous cavity and the posterior chamber (the space between iris and lens) and, if possible, with the anterior chamber as well. However, the lens must occasionally be removed.

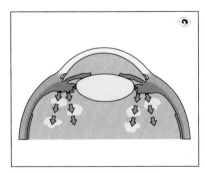

Fig. 3.26: With ciliary block glaucoma, the aqueous humor is directed into the vitreous chamber.

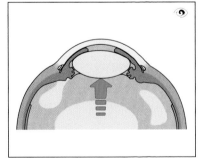

Fig. 3.27: The swelling of the vitreous chamber pushes the iris-lens-diaphragm forward and leads to the closure of the chamber angle.

3.6 Secondary Glaucoma

Numerous diseases, injuries, and operations of the eye, as well as even medical treatment, can lead to increased or, less frequently, low IOP. The focus now turns toward the most notable diseases that can result in an elevated intraocular pressure.

3.6.1 Secondary Open-Angle Glaucoma

Secondary open-angle glaucoma occurs when the increased IOP is due to a different eye disease, but the anterior chamber angle remains open.

3.6.1.1 Glaucoma Associated with Pseudoexfoliation Syndrome

Pseudoexfoliation [Lat. *folium:* leaf] glaucoma is a form of glaucoma that can develop in patients afflicted with pseudoexfoliation syndrome (PEX Syndrome). The term *pseudo*exfoliation has been introduced because, clinically, it appears as if the lens were peeling off. Should this indeed occur, it would be a *real* exfoliation syndrome, but this does not happen with PEX.

One must distinguish between the pseudoexfoliation syndrome and the glaucoma that is associated with PEX, also called pseudoexfoliation glaucoma. Not all individuals having a PEX syndrome necessarily develop glaucoma, but PEX certainly increases the likelihood. A POAG that would have occurred even without PEX could become worse if PEX were present, and the IOP increase might commence much earlier.

PEX syndrome describes the grayish-white deposits of abnormal proteins on all surfaces of the eye irrigated by the aqueous humor. PEX material is most easily visible on the anterior surface of the lens. There is a typical pattern for these deposits on the anterior lens capsule with a central disc and another band in the periphery (Fig. 3.28); they arise from the iris rubbing against the lens during pupil dilation and contraction, thus a "cleansing" of the PEX material from part of the lens surface. There are also deposits of PEX material inside the trabecular meshwork (Fig. 3.29). This increases

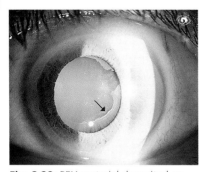

Fig. 3.28: PEX material deposited on the lens surface.

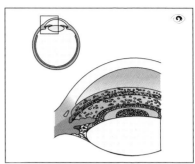

Fig. 3.29: PEX material on the lens, iris and in the chamber angle.

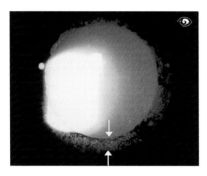

Fig. 3.30: Transillumination phenomenon of those segments of the iris close to the pupil in a patient suffering from PEX (→).

the outflow resistance and leads to glaucoma in some patients. PEX syndrome increases with age and is more frequent than previously believed. PEX is an age-related phenomenon of the body's fibrils that can develop in other organs as well and may lead to various eye alterations. Among these is an increased fragility of the zonules (also called zonular fibers) that hold the lens in place, thereby encumbering later cataract operations (cf. S 5).

The rubbing of the iris on the somewhat uneven lens surface leads to a loss of pigment in the posterior layer of the iris causing a transillumination phenomenon [Lat: *transilluminare:* to shine through]. When light enters the eye through the pupil, it is reflected by the fundus (technically, primarily back-scattered), and can usually only leave the eye through the pupil, but not through the iris because this structure acts as an optical diaphragm. This effect is lost in those areas where larger amounts of iris pigment have been lost.

These defects appear red because they are illuminated by the reflected light (Fig. 3.30).

By the way, light from the fundus appears red because these structures have a high blood perfusion; this color is even called "fundus red." This also explains why in some flash pictures, the pupils appear red. These "red eyes" can be avoided by either holding the flash at a slight distance from the side of the camera or by using a "pre-flash" that causes the pupils to constrict before the second (main) flash occurs.

The cause of the PEX syndrome is unknown. It is seen more frequently in certain geographic regions, such as Scandinavia, and slightly more often among women than men.

As mentioned above, patients having PEX syndrome have an increased likelihood of IOP elevation. Although there is no basic difference between "PEX glaucoma" and POAG, some distinquishing characteristics of PEX glaucoma are noteworthy.

The IOP usually rises within a rather short time and fluctuations are sometimes huge. Indeed, these steep up and down spikes are more damaging to the papilla than is an elevated, but stable, IOP. Another probable contributing factor for developing glaucomatous damage is reinforced by PEX-associated alterations of the blood vessels. Patients with PEX glaucoma require a particularly intensive treatment and surgery is usually inevitable.

3.6.1.2 Glaucoma with Pigment Dispersion Syndrome

Pigments are the dyes of the body [Lat. *pingere:* to paint], and the most important of these is melanin [Gr. *melas:* black]. It is responsible for skin coloring and also plays a crucial role in the eye; between the retina and choroid is a pigment layer rich in melanin. This pigment epithelium serves several purposes, including the absorption of those quantities of light not needed by the retina for vision.

The iris (cf. S 1) also contains quite a bit of pigment due to its function as a diaphragm for absorbing light. Except for those people who suffer from albinism (albinos), the posterior iris layer is rich in

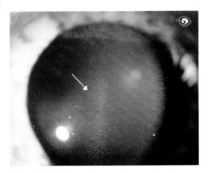

Fig. 3.31: Deposits on the posterior surface of the cornea (endothelium) in pigment dispersion syndrome (→).

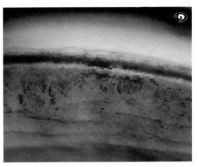

Fig. 3.32: Pigment deposits in the chamber angle in a patient suffering from pigment dispersion syndrome.

melanin. In front of this dark layer is the iris stroma that, being somewhat pigmented, determines eye color: Individuals with little or no pigment are blue-eyed, those with more melanin are darker eyed.

There is a distinction between pigment dispersion syndrome and glaucoma occurring with pigment dispersion syndrome (i.e. pigmentary glaucoma). While pigment dispersion syndrome significantly increases the risk of an increased IOP, not every person with pigment dispersion syndrome will automatically develop pigmentary glaucoma.

Pigment dispersion [Lat. *dispersio:* dispersion] syndrome is identified by melanin deposits on those surfaces of the eye that are in constant contact with the aqueous humor. The most characteristic finding is a deposit on the posterior surface of the cornea (the endothelium), called the Krukenberg spindle after the physician who first described it (Fig. 3.31). The deposits take the form of a spindle due to the constant rotation of the aqueous humor. The anterior surface of the cornea is exposed to air, which has a cooling effect. Therefore, the anterior part of the aqueous humor, being cooler than the posterior, tends to move down and the warm posterior fluid moves up, which induces fluid rotation.

Especially impressive is the pigment deposition on the trabecular meshwork (Fig. 3.32) that may lead to pigment glaucoma, discussed below.

These dispersed melanin deposits originate from the posterior iris surface. Patients with pigment dispersion syndrome are endowed with a different ocular architecture. They are usually moderately myopic, the anterior chamber is especially deep and the angle wide open. The iris is concave with a posterior bowing (Fig. 3.33). This brings the iris into contact with the zonules, and mechanical rubbing leads to pigment loss.

With each blink of the eye, a patient having pigment dispersion syndrome with the corresponding abnormal ocular anatomy presses aqueous humor from the posterior into the anterior chamber, and tension becomes temporarily higher in the anterior chamber. A back flow of the aqueous humor is impossible since the iris, pressed against the lens, acts as a valve. The tension gradient pushes the peripheral parts of the iris backwards, resulting in the described intermittent contact with the zonules (Fig. 3.34).

Due to rubbing with the zonules, the iris loses pigment and radial tissue defects occur. These defects are responsible for a transillumination phenomenon often compared to light passing through a "church window" (Fig. 3.35). Light entering the eye not only returns through the pupil, but also through these defects (comparable with the transillumination phenomenon in PEX syndrome, Figure

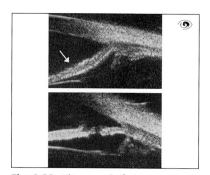

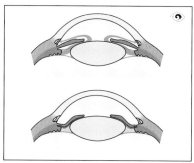

Fig. 3.33: Ultrasound of pigment dispersion syndrome: in the top picture, the iris is bent backwards (→); in the bottom picture, the iris is again in its normal position after an iridotomy has been performed.

Fig. 3.34: Iris configuration in pigment dispersion syndrome: a) regular position; b) after blinking.

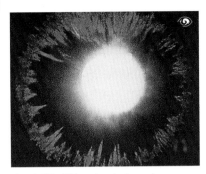

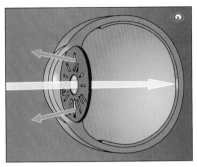

Fig. 3.35: "Church window phenomenon" in pigment dispersion syndrome.

Fig. 3.36: The church window phenomenon is created by light that is reflected from the red fundus which then leaves the eye through the iris defects.

3.36). Pigment dispersion syndrome is more common among men than women and most patients are moderately near-sighted (myopic). This syndrome often develops between the ages of 20 and 50 and, in older patients, it sometimes disappears or at least gets much better. The reason is that the lens, as it increases in thickness with age, pushes the iris away from the zonules, and because accommodation decreases and the melanin reservoir gets smaller. This syndrome, therefore, can be "outgrown" and is hardly ever seen in elderly patients.

Some pigment dispersion patients experience an IOP rise, termed "pigmentary glaucoma." It is not known why some patients have an elevated IOP while others do not. Patients suffering from pigmentary glaucoma often have a strongly pigmented chamber angle, strikingly wide open, similar to that seen in congenital glaucoma, and covered with additional deposits. This glaucoma can take a severe course, especially when there are pronounced IOP fluctuations. In some patients, there is occasionally an IOP rise after rigorous exercise.

Treatment resembles that for POAG. First, a medical IOP reduction is attempted. A transient IOP decrease might also be accomplished by an argon laser trabeculoplasty (cf. Chapter 7.3). Most patients, however, require surgical treatment.

There are additional treatment options: A peripheral laser iridotomy reduces the pressure difference between the anterior and posterior chambers and thus prevents the posterior bowing of the iris (Fig. 3.34). If there are IOP peaks during physical activity, prophylactic miosis is recommended (for instance, applying a drop of 1% pilocarpine one half hour before exercising).

3.6.1.3 Additional Causes

There are several other causes for secondary open-angle glaucoma. Most are rare and therefore won't be discussed in detail here. But just to list a few examples:

Lens protein in the aqueous humor originating from "hypermature" cataracts (cf. S 4) can occlude the trabecular meshwork. This is hardly ever seen in developed countries because lenses with advanced opacification are almost always surgically removed.

Blood can also obstruct the trabecular meshwork. The red blood cells from a fresh hemorrhage are flexible enough to pass through the meshwork. However, this flexibility is lost if blood remains inside the eye for a longer period, for example, in the vitreous cavity. Should these red blood cells later find their way into the aqueous humor, they will block the trabecular meshwork and can cause a rise in the IOP at a certain time after the original hemorrhage. A tumor can block these pathways, both directly through its growth and indirectly from tumor cells being carried with the aqueous humor. Retinal detachment usually results in low intraocular tension, but rarely it increases the IOP and it is not unusual that retinal surgical procedures are also associated with a transiently increased IOP. The trabecular meshwork can be involved in ocular trauma, and when scarred, may lead to outflow obstruction and long-term IOP elevation. During laser iridotomy, iris cells disperse out into the aqueous humor. This could cause an increased IOP during the first one or two days after treatment before it then returns to normal.

Argon laser trabeculoplasty (cf. Chapter 7.3.2) is used to lower the IOP in open-angle glaucoma. There is frequently a slight

IOP rise in the first few hours or days, but a severe long-term elevation is a very rare complication.

Aqueous humor flows into the venous circulation via the trabecular meshwork and Schlemm's canal. If pressure in the episcleral veins increases [Gr. *epi:* on top of], then outflow is impeded and the IOP rises. There are several diseases that can cause such an increase in venous pressure, but sometimes the cause remains unknown. Figure 3.37 shows a typical picture of severely dilated veins in a patient having elevated venous pressure.

Locally administered steroids (anti-inflammatory eye drops and ointments containing cortisone) can lead to a mild, but in some cases severe, IOP rise. Steroids induce the synthesis of materials (such as mucopolysaccharides and proteins) that can form deposits inside the trabecular meshwork. The IOP normally decreases after steroid therapy has ended. Whether or not someone will react to steroids with an IOP increase is genetically determined. People who show a reaction are called "responders." Other people do not have these genes and are called "non-responders." They can be treated for a long time with steroids without experiencing any rise in intraocular pressure. Systemic steroid therapy rarely leads to an IOP rise but, if it does, it is milder than in local (at the eye) treatment.

The increase in the IOP among responders occurs approximately 10 to 14 days after the treatment has started.

Acute inflammation, such as iritis, can temporarily reduce IOP or lead to a long-term increase (Fig. 3.38). In particular, a condition called heterochromic cyclitis, usually leads to unilateral intraocular inflammation associated with a light-colored iris and IOP increases. These patients typically have one iris that is slightly lighter than the other [Gr. *heteros:* being different/Gr. *chroma:* color].

In order to treat these special forms of secondary open-angle glaucoma, the underlying cause must be addressed. If this is not possible and the IOP still remains high, treatment similar to POAG (cf. Chapter 3.4) is undertaken.

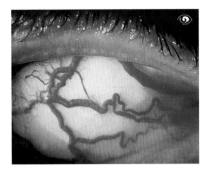

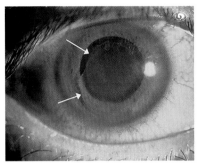

Fig. 3.37: Congested episcleral veins.

Fig. 3.38: Fibrin (→) in the anterior chamber of an eye afflicted with iritis.

3.6.2 Secondary Angle-Closure Glaucoma

In Chapter 3.5.1, several mechanisms that primarily lead to chamber angle obstruction were discussed. Here, secondary angle closures – those that result from other eye diseases – will be discussed.

Occlusion can either be rapid (acute) or slow (chronic). In acute closure, the iris usually blocks the trabecular meshwork in a circular fashion, a condition that is reversible. In the chronic form of the disease, the contact is not circular but the blockage of the trabecular meshwork is often irreversible. There are numerous diseases leading to secondary angle-closure glaucoma that won't be discussed in detail here. Secondary angle-closure can occur, for example, due to dislocation of the lens which might happen as a result of an accident, in various syndromes or post-operatively. Angle closure also occasionally occurs due to miotic therapy (cf. Chapter 7.2.1).

As with a primary angle-closure mechanism (cf. Chapter 3.5.1), in unfavorable conditions, the central parts of the iris can be strongly pushed towards the lens, thus resulting in a considerable pressure difference between the anterior and the posterior chamber. Such a gradient can also develop secondarily if the central part of the iris becomes permanently attached to the lens (Fig. 3.39). This con-

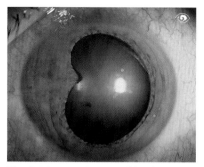

Fig. 3.39: Posterior synechia: the iris and the lens adhere to each other at one site.

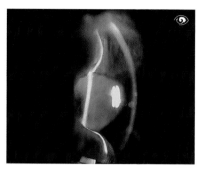

Fig. 3.40: Slit-lamp picture of an "iris bombé."

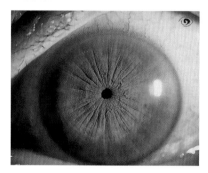

Fig. 3.41: Extremely small pupil as a result of treatment with miotics.

dition, called synechia, can result from long-term intraocular inflammation. Material from inflammation (cells and a substance called fibrin) acts like glue: the iris gets stuck onto the lens and the flow of aqueous humor from the posterior into the anterior chamber becomes hindered. The peripheral iris is pushed anteriorly and this causes the iris to "bow" out – called "iris bombé" (Fig. 3.40).

Fortunately, synechia formation is rare these days because treatment of chronic intraocular inflammations has become more effective and, as a means of preventing synechiae, the pupil is dilated when inflamed.

A similar, though not complete, synechia could develop as a side-effect of long-term (years) intensive therapy with miotics. This treatment causes a mild, inflammatory-like condition and, to make matters worse, keeps the pupil immobile (Fig. 3.41). If the iris could move, fresh synechiae would probably "burst open." This, however, has become a rare condition because current glaucoma medication is no longer associated with miosis as a major side-effect.

Neovascular Glaucoma. Neovascular glaucoma, meaning glaucoma associated with the formation of new blood vessels, is a special form of secondary angle closure. If these new vessels appear on the iris, the condition is termed "rubeosis iridis" [Lat. *ruber:* red] since these vessels make the iris appear slightly reddish (Fig. 3.42). When new blood vessels grow into the anterior chamber angle, it gradually becomes occluded – by the vessels themselves and by accompanying tissue, but especially by parts of the iris that become tented toward the trabecular meshwork from these neovascularizations (Fig. 3.43).

Neovascularization occurs when larger segments of the retina lack adequate perfusion. Those parts that still receive oxygen (though not enough) produce a substance that triggers the growth of new blood vessels on the retina. When these growth factors reach the anterior chamber (for example, when the lens has been removed after cataract surgery), new blood vessels form on the iris as well. This is a dreaded complication of diabetic retinopathy and of retinal venous occlusion, so-called central and branch retinal vein occlusion (Fig. 3.44).

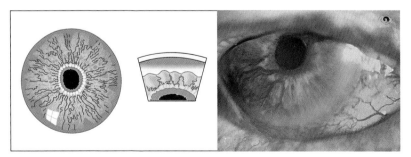

Fig. 3.42: Rubeosis iridis: Newly formed blood vessels block the chamber angle and evert the pupil's rim.

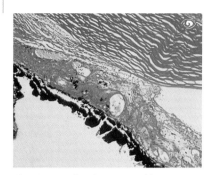

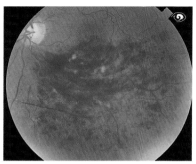

Fig. 3.43: Adhesions caused by rubeosis obstruct this chamber angle.

Fig. 3.44: Retinal vein occlusion: the red spots are retinal hemorrhages, the yellow-white areas are nerve fibers swollen due to a lack of oxygen.

Today, this complication from these two diseases can often be prevented by laser therapy of the retina. Diabetes and its complications will be discussed in Chapter S 7.

Treating secondary angle-closure glaucoma means first of all treating the underlying disease, however, the increased IOP may still be present. Should this occur, medical IOP lowering therapy is once again instituted. A peripheral iridotomy or iridectomy is performed with iris bombé. Nevertheless, as in neovascular glaucoma, additional surgical procedures are frequently necessary (cf. Chapter 7.4).

Summary

Many various causes lead to an increased IOP. In congenital glaucoma, the chamber angle is not developed completely. When the angle is more mature but still abnormal, the IOP will rise during infancy (infantile glaucoma) or adolescence (juvenile glaucoma). In primary, chronic open-angle glaucoma (POAG), the IOP is too high despite the chamber angle being mature and open, and with no associated eye disease. The increased IOP is caused by an increased outflow resistance through the trabecular meshwork. POAG is by far the most common form of glaucoma and is especially found among the elderly. The increase in the IOP progresses slowly and is not noticed by the patient. Especially in the early stages of the disease, the patient is not aware of the progressive visual field defects. In angle-closure glaucoma, there is a sharp and sudden increase in the IOP due to a rapid and complete obstruction of the chamber angle by the iris. Symptoms are most severe. IOP can also rise as a result of pseudoexfoliation syndrome or pigment dispersion syndrome. Secondary IOP elevations can be induced by certain drugs, inflammation and complications of diabetic retinopathy, retinal vein occlusion and other eye diseases.

4 Risk Factors

Glaucomatous damage was described in Chapter 2, where it was also explained that an increased IOP is an important, though not exclusive, risk factor. Chapter 3 then dealt with the causes of an increase in intraocular pressure, and in this chapter, other risk factors will be discussed. Again, it is important to make a clear distinction between risk factors that lead to a high IOP and risk factors that contribute to the glaucomatous optic nerve damage.

4.1 General Risk Factors for an Increase in IOP

Chapter 3 described several clinical pictures that cause an increased IOP. But there are a number of other factors that can have a more or less pronounced influence on the intraocular pressure, and these factors are discussed here.

4.1.1 Age

Age plays an important role in glaucoma, and particularly in primary open-angle glaucoma (POAG – cf. Chapter 3.4). Although children, even newborns, can suffer from glaucoma, it is very rare. Most patients having an elevated IOP are over the age of 40.

Throughout one's lifetime, even in healthy eyes, there is a gradual rise in the IOP. This is due to the aging of the trabecular meshwork. Because production of the aqueous humor decreases during the same period, the IOP rise is usually quite moderate.

Some people, however, experience a more significant IOP rise as they get older, but why this is so has yet to be completely explained. For most glaucoma patients, the IOP starts to rise between the ages of 40 and 50. In other patients, the IOP rises at a later age. Without treatment, the pressure continues to rise over the years. Indeed, the number of people with an IOP of 21 mmHg and above increases with age. This is particularly important because life expectancy is also on the rise.

4.1.2 Family Background

When glaucoma occurs more frequently within a certain family, then the "family background" is considered a risk factor. Genetics can certainly play a role, but it is also conceivable that family members (especially when they live together) are exposed to the same environmental influences. The genetics factor will be explained first.

It has long been known that children of glaucoma patients have a higher likelihood of developing glaucoma. This does not mean, however, that all children of a glaucoma parent will eventually suffer from the same disease. Glaucoma certainly can appear spontaneously, meaning it appears without an associated family history of the disease. Without a doubt, genetics does influence congenital, infantile and juvenile types of glaucoma. But even among these forms of glaucoma, there are "spontaneous" cases.

With glaucoma associated with aging, the situation is more complex. One must distinguish between the genetic tendency to develop a high intraocular pressure and the risk of developing optic nerve damage at a given IOP level, sometimes even with a normal IOP (cf. Chapter 4.2).

Genetics is of prime importance in modern medicine. Unraveling the human genetic code has only been possible because of molecular genetics (cf. S 3), and this science has also enabled researchers to identify pathological aberrations in the code. This then leads to a better understanding of how some diseases originate and develop (cf. S 3). With regard to glaucoma, current research in this field is rapidly forging ahead, but it is still too early to discuss findings here. What is certain is that there is not one single gene responsible for glaucoma, but rather there are several genes which, when pathologically altered, can lead to the disease. On the other hand, it is known that modification (mutation) of one gene alone does not necessarily lead to glaucoma. Apparently there are several factors that work together. A change in the genetic material just increases the likelihood of developing the disease. The disease actually appears only if there are other environmental factors present or if several genes are affected.

Many patients ask about the genetic risk. Unfortunately, the response is that there still isn't enough information available for a straightforward answer, but this will certainly change within the next few years. There is no doubt that regular eye examinations should be recommended for all family members of someone who has glaucoma. If the glaucoma developed during childhood, then all relatives – both young and old – should see an ophthalmologist. If the glaucoma occurred at a later age, then examination of adult relatives is sufficient. For individuals without an obvious genetic risk, an initial eye examination for glaucoma testing is recommended between 35 and 45 years of age. Those with a family history of glaucoma should have their eyes examined between the ages of 20 and 30, but certainly no later than 30 to 40.

4.1.3 Race

Ethnic origin plays a role although it is sometimes not easy to separate the influences of race from those of the prevailing socioeconomic conditions. But nevertheless, patients of African ancestry often have a higher intraocular pressure and develop elevated IOP at an earlier age. Caucasians, on the other hand, suffer more frequently from pseudoexfoliation glaucoma, particularly in northern European countries. Interestingly, pigment glaucoma is more common among light-skinned than among dark-skinned people. Angle-closure glaucomas are quite frequent in Asia. Studies have shown that the Japanese also frequently suffer from normal-tension glaucoma, explained in Chapter 4.2.4.

4.1.4 Gender

Although men and women have the same IOP levels, the different forms of glaucoma occur more often in one gender than in the other. For example, women suffer more frequently from angle-closure glaucoma, men more frequently from pigment dispersion glaucoma. Women are not only more commonly afflicted with normal-tension glaucoma but their optic nerve head is more sensitive to intraocular pressure, as described in Chapter 4.2.5.

4.1.5 Arteriosclerosis

Arteriosclerosis is one of the major health problems in today's society. It leads to heart attacks, cerebral ischemia and a host of other diseases. Because arteriosclerosis poses a significant problem in general medicine and, consequently, to the eye as well, there is a supplementary chapter dedicated to this topic (S 6). There various risk factors will be discussed, such as smoking, increased blood pressure and high lipid levels that lead to arteriosclerosis.

Just as is possible in any other artery, ocular blood vessels can also suffer from arteriosclerosis. Arteriosclerosis is therefore considered an important risk factor in a number of eye diseases, among which occlusions of retinal arteries and veins are the most important. It is interesting to note that patients having arteriosclerosis suffer more frequently, and at earlier ages, from cataracts (lens opacification, cf. S 5) and maculopathy (an age-related disease of the central retina, cf. S 9). Neither disease is probably the direct result of arteriosclerosis, but rather share the same pathogenetic mechanism. Therefore, the term "risk indicators" [Lat. *indicare:* indicate] might be more appropriate than "risk factors." Risk factors for arteriosclerosis are thus also important risk indicators for cataracts and maculopathy.

It actually appears that arteriosclerosis does not increase the chance of developing glaucomatous damage. This is quite surprising because it is now known that the average glaucoma patient suffers from a reduced ocular perfusion. The cause for circulatory problems in glaucoma is a dysregulation of the eye's perfusion rather than arteriosclerosis (as will be seen in Chapter 4.2.7). There is, however, a weak correlation between arteriosclerosis (and its accompanying risk factors) and increased intraocular pressure. This means that people suffering from arteriosclerosis are more likely to have an elevated IOP than healthy subjects of the same age without arteriosclerosis. But it should again be emphasized that this correlation is not strong.

Nota bene: Just because someone has an elevated IOP does not mean that there is also arteriosclerosis present. Interestingly, among healthy Japanese, the average IOP slightly decreases throughout life, and it is well known that arteriosclerosis is much less common in Japan than in Europe.

Occasionally, patients confuse intraocular pressure with blood pressure and start asking for a possible connection. Though both are regulated by independent mechanisms, someone having a higher-than-average blood pressure is just slightly more likely to have an increased IOP. But once again, this correlation is not strong. Many people with high blood pressure have a normal IOP and vice versa. The same applies for other risk factors of arteriosclerosis: Smokers and patients with high serum lipid levels have only a slightly higher risk for an increased IOP.

4.1.6 Near and Far-Sightedness

An eye may be normal-sighted (emmetropic), meaning no visual correction is required, far-sighted (hyperopic) or near-sighted (myopic). The refraction of the eye and its defects will be discussed in S 4.

Healthy hyperopic and myopic eyes have the same mean IOP as emmetropic eyes. But far-sighted eyes have an increased risk of developing angle-closure glaucoma (cf. Chapter 3.5), while near-sighted eyes are more frequently involved in pigmentary-dispersion glaucoma (cf. Chapter 3.6.1.2) and are more sensitive to the effects of increased intraocular pressure.

Since myopic eyes are, on average, larger than normal eyes, there is also a higher risk for eye diseases independent of glaucoma. For example, retinal detachment is much more common in myopic than in normal eyes.

4.2   Risk Factors for Glaucomatous Damage

Chapter 2.1 described glaucomatous damage in detail, and now the focus turns to those risk factors that can lead to glaucomatous damage, i.e. risk factors that make development and progression of such damage more likely. From a scientific stance, there are two methods for identifying these factors. For example, if one takes myopia as a potential risk factor for glaucomatous damage, then the first step is to find out if glaucomatous damage is more common among myopics than among emmetropics (no refractive error), or alternatively, one assesses whether the percentage of myopics among patients with optic nerve damage is higher than among the general population. The next step is to look for a quantitative correlation. In the case of myopia, one could determine whether the extent of myopia is statistically associated with the frequency or the severity of glaucomatous damage. But even when there is a statistical correlation, this does not necessarily mean that both factors are causally [Lat. *kausa:* reason] related. Two situations (A and B) can occur together without influencing each other if they are both the result of a third factor (C). A causal relationship can only be established after there is evidence (with the help of so-called intervention studies) that a disease becomes less common (or the disease has a better prognosis) after a risk factor has been eliminated.

A number of risk factors have been identified as being responsible for optic nerve damage. Some, but unfortunately not all, can be treated or at least influenced.

It has been known since the mid-19th century that an elevated IOP can lead to glaucomatous damage. Without a doubt, a high intraocular pressure is the most common and most important risk factor, and why an entire chapter (Chapter 3) was devoted to IOP. But other factors certainly play a role as well. Remember, about one-fourth of all patients with optic nerve damage do not have

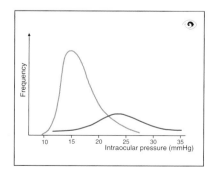

Fig. 4.1: IOP frequency distribution in healthy individuals (gray curve) and in glaucoma patients (red curve).

an elevated IOP (Fig. 4.1). And in some people, a moderate increase in pressure leads to damage while in most others, it does not. This then underscores the importance of the other risk factors. As was depicted in Chapter 2.2.1 with the example of a car accident, an event can be caused by several factors working together. The same applies to glaucoma: When strong enough, each factor alone can cause damage, but it is the exception that just one factor is present. What is usually seen is an interaction of several factors, and this will be described in Chapter 5.

4.2.1 Intraocular Pressure

The higher the IOP, the more likely the development, and progression, of glaucomatous damage (Fig. 4.2). A sudden (acute), high increase in the IOP (as in an acute angle-closure glaucoma) can be astonishingly well tolerated, and is indeed less damaging than a chronically elevated pressure. Interestingly, for glaucomatous damage, chronic rises and falls in the IOP level are more important than the average pressure. It has been demonstrated that patients having these major IOP fluctuations – and thus repeated pressure spikes – are most likely to experience damage and progression of the functional loss. The reason for this will be explained in Chapter 5. The

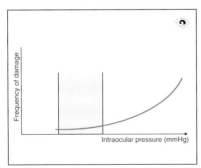

Fig. 4.2: The higher the IOP, the more frequently glaucomatous damage develops. The gray section represents normal pressure.

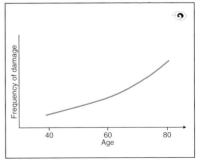

Fig. 4.3: Since glaucomatous damage is irreversible, its prevalence increases with age.

goal of therapy therefore is not only IOP reduction, but also protecting the eye from pressure fluctuations (cf. Chapter 7).

The following facts should be kept in mind: 80% of the people with an elevated IOP will never have optic nerve damage and 30% of glaucoma patients never experience increased IOP.

4.2.2 Age

In Chapter 4.1.1, the influence of age on intraocular pressure was discussed. The occurrence of glaucomatous damage is even more age dependent (Fig. 4.3). The reason for this is that not only an increase in the risk factors, but also – and this is particularly important – the loss of nerve fibers adds up throughout a lifetime. Nevertheless, there is no evidence that progression is more rapid in elderly patients or that senior citizens are more pressure sensitive. Because progression of the damage occurs slowly and over a long period, it is either not – or hardly – noticed by the patient. However, in the late phase of the damage, it becomes dramatically noticeable and the probability for a subjective worsening of sight is thus greater in old age. But again, this is not because glaucomatous damage rapidly progresses in old age, but rather because the slow deterioration has accumulated throughout the patient's life, and in an older patient, this means more time to acquire damage.

4.2.3 Family History

Chapter 4.1.2 discussed the influence of genetics on the intraocular pressure. To a certain degree, a patient's genetic code determines whether he can tolerate – without damage – a certain IOP level. A family cluster of glaucomatous damage provides the doctor with important indications about disease severity. When there is a history of family members having glaucomatous damage, then the chances for the onset or progression of already existing optic nerve damage increase. This means that someone from a family having numerous members with glaucomatous damage should receive particularly careful counseling and therapy, if necessary. Apparently there is a genetic predisposition that determines the IOP sensitivity, but specifics about this are not yet known. This is probably due to other risk factors for glaucomatous damage (such as vascular dysregulation) that can also be inherited (cf. S 8).

4.2.4 Race

Ethnic origin certainly influences both the IOP (cf. Chapter 4.1.3) as well as optic nerve damage. However, it should be reiterated that it is not easy to distinguish between a genetic predisposition and the influence of environmental conditions. Patients of African descent generally have a higher IOP and a greater likelihood of developing damage at a certain pressure level (Fig. 4.4), and thus require a particularly intensive treatment.

It is interesting to take a look at the distribution of IOP levels among patients with POAG: Normal-tension glaucoma is much more common in Japan than in Europe (Fig. 4.5). Japanese people also have a higher rate of vascular dysregulation (cf. Chapter 5). Besides a genetic predisposition, conditions of everyday life certainly play a crucial role. In Switzerland, for example, we have noted that normal-tension glaucoma is more frequent among urban than rural residents, among those that are ambitious perfectionists than among the tranquil and calm, among slim individuals than the obese, etc.

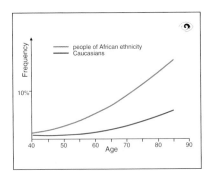

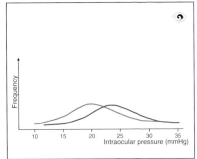

Fig. 4.4: Glaucomatous damage is more frequent among people of African ethnicity than among Caucasians.

Fig. 4.5: The mean IOP of patients with glaucomatous damage is higher in Europeans (blue curve) than in Japanese (green curve).

One reason for this difference could be the varying frequency of vascular dysregulation (cf. S 8).

4.2.5 Gender

Although there is no difference in the IOP between the sexes, women have normal-tension glaucoma more frequently than men. This is at least partly related to the fact that the vasospastic syndrome is more common in females (cf. S 8). But additionally, women with primary open-angle glaucoma and a high IOP have a slightly higher risk of developing glaucomatous damage at a certain pressure level than do men.

4.2.6 Near and Far-Sightedness

Even though hyperopic (far-sighted) individuals have a higher risk of developing acute angle-closure glaucoma, they do not have an increased sensitivity to intraocular pressure. Therefore, they do not develop optic nerve damage more frequently than someone with normal refraction and the same IOP. For near-sighted individuals, the situation is a bit different: the myopic eye has an increased sensitivity to pressure. This means that someone near-sighted is more likely to experience optic nerve damage than an emmetropic

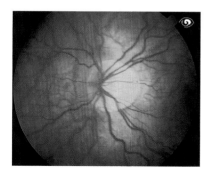 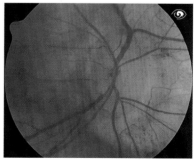

Fig. 4.6: Optic disc in a healthy myopic eye.

Fig. 4.7: Glaucomatous optic disc in a myopic eye.

individual with the same IOP. What makes matters worse is that the glaucomatous cupping of the optic disc in a myopic eye is much more difficult to evaluate than the excavation of an eye without refractive error (Figs. 4.6 and 4.7). Likewise, visual field defects are often harder to interpret. Indeed, it is sometimes difficult to distinguish whether the visual field defects are caused by the myopia or by glaucoma. All these factors contribute to myopic glaucoma patients requiring especially intensive monitoring and treatment.

4.2.7 Circulatory Problems

Since the discovery of glaucomatous damage in the mid-19th century, there has been the suspicion that not only intraocular pressure, but disturbances in blood perfusion as well, contribute to the pathogenesis of the disease. Unfortunately, though ocular perfusion is easy to see, it is tremendously difficult to measure (cf. S 11). This particularly applies to the perfusion of the choroid and optic disc – where perfusion data could be most helpful in following glaucoma. Therefore, the hypothesis that perfusion plays a crucial role in glaucoma has, to date, only been supported by indirect observations (cf. S 8). However, modern techniques, though far from perfect, increasingly allow the measurement of ocular perfusion and there are clear indications that ocular perfusion is indeed reduced in glaucoma patients. It was initially assumed that impaired perfusion was a secondary symptom and thus a consequence of glaucoma. However, the fact that the reduction in ocular blood flow usually comes first and glaucomatous defects second, evidence that glaucoma patients commonly have perfusion disturbances in other organs and a lower vessel density in parts of the tissue around the optic nerve head, clearly indicate that at least some of these problems are primary, causative agents, and not secondary results.

Some glaucoma patients show alterations in their circulation, even at rest, but especially following certain triggers, such as cold or emotional stress. For example, patients with normal-tension glaucoma often have an abnormal reaction in their fingertip perfusion when faced with a cold stimulus (cf. S 8). Although people with

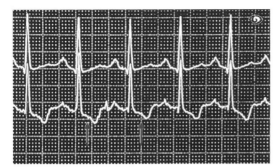

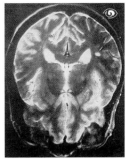

Fig. 4.8: Electrocardiogram showing an ST-depression (red arrows) indicating myocardial ischemia.

Fig. 4.9: Ischemic lesions (→) in a glaucoma patient's brain (MRI picture).

glaucomatous damage do not frequently have hearing problems or tinnitus (ringing in the ears), the incidence is clearly higher than among healthy individuals. The same applies to episodes of silent myocardial ischemia (Fig. 4.8) and occasionally ischemic changes in the brain (Fig. 4.9). There are various indications that this is caused by vascular dysregulation rather than by arteriosclerotic circulation problems.

It has been statistically proven that patients with glaucomatous changes have circulatory problems more frequently than healthy individuals of the same age. The lower the IOP level at which glaucomatous damage commences or progresses, the more likely that circulatory defects also participate (cf. Chapter 5). In extreme cases, an inadequate perfusion (and thus nutrition to the optic nerve) can lead to structural damage, even at very low IOP levels. In general, studies have shown that normal tension glaucoma patients demonstrate the most disturbed circulation, next to them are high tension glaucoma patients, then normal individuals, whereas ocular hypertensives are on the opposite side of the spectrum. This observation further underscores the dual influence of IOP and circulatory factors in the origin of glaucoma.

What produces disturbances in the blood flow? In general, arteriosclerosis is the most common cause of reduced perfusion. It can lead to narrowing of the blood vessels, thrombosis and emboli.

However, the main cause for perfusion problems in glaucoma is not arteriosclerosis (cf. S 6). Certainly a glaucoma patient can have arteriosclerosis and this condition could contribute to disease progression. But in the 1980s, we established that the main cause of reduced ocular blood flow in glaucoma is dysregulation of the blood vessels, including those of the eye (cf. S 8). It is not possible to go into great detail here describing these mechanisms and the chain of evidence, but the interested reader can take advantage of the literature mentioned (cf. A 3). Patients who are likely to suffer from vascular dysregulation tend to have blood pressure levels lower than normal (systemic hypotension), especially at night, and may experience vasospasms. Both factors will be explored in more detail.

Blood Pressure. It is widely known that elevated blood pressure poses a health risk. But until recently, it was long ignored that low blood pressure can also pose a health risk, especially in the development of glaucomatous damage. However, several recent studies have been published which have established a link between development and progression of glaucomatous damage and decreased blood pressure. There is no such thing as a constant blood pressure. Throughout the day, the blood pressure rises and falls depending on physical activity, whether one is lying down or standing upright, and on nutrition and drug use. Therefore, in order to obtain an accurate depiction of this important circulation parameter, the blood pressure must be monitored for 24 hours (Fig. 4.10).

Glaucoma patients often have quite normal blood pressure during the day, but at night, they experience a much stronger decrease than is noted in a healthy individual. This nighttime "dip" deserves special attention (Fig. 4.11). Some patients with a nighttime dip even experience an elevated blood pressure during the day, and might even be treated with blood pressure (BP) lowering medications.

For glaucoma patients, a strong orthostatic [Gr. *othos:* upright/Gr. *stasein:* standing] pressure drop when rising from a supine position can be potentially damaging.

When tissue damage cannot be adequately explained by the

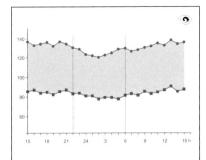

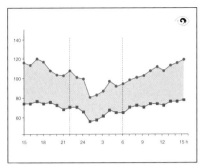

Fig. 4.10: 24-hour blood pressure graph of a healthy individual. Red: systolic pressure; blue: diastolic pressure (mmHg).

Fig. 4.11: 24-hour blood pressure of a glaucoma patient: marked dip at night (mmHg).

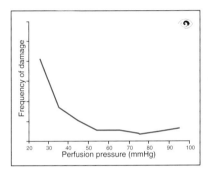

Fig. 4.12: The lower the perfusion pressure (blood pressure minus intraocular pressure), the more frequent glaucomatous damage arises.

elevated IOP alone, or if there is glaucoma progression after IOP has been brought under control, then a 24-hour BP monitoring is highly recommended (Fig. 4.11).

Some glaucomatous patients have abnormally low blood pressure when they are young, normal BP readings in middle age, and sometimes even an elevated BP when they are older. If there are no longer dips at the time glaucoma is diagnosed, the potential danger from a low BP is spontaneously eliminated and a therapy for arterial hypotension is not necessary.

On the other hand, increased blood pressure – as important as it is in the pathogenesis of other diseases – is of minimal importance in glaucoma (Fig. 4.12). Naturally, a chronic, increased BP will lead to arteriosclerosis, a condition that is generally unfavorable for the eye and may exert some negative influence on how the glaucoma develops.

Blood pressure dips are quite common among patients suffering from vasospastic syndrome. Unfortunately, the ocular perfusion specifically among these patients is quite sensitive to a decreased BP since their abnormal vascular regulation does not permit adequate adaptation to changes in blood pressure levels (cf. Chapter 5.3).

Interestingly, also the glaucoma patients that do not exhibit a nighttime BP decrease at all, the so-called non-dippers, are at the increased risk of glaucomatous damage.

Vasospasms. There are people whose vascular reaction to certain stimuli, such as cold and emotional stress, is more intense than those of normal individuals (Fig. 4.13), a condition termed vasospastic syndrome (cf. S 8). In these cases, the vessels of certain organs constrict in a more pronounced fashion; the hands are often involved and patients often complain about having cold hands. We have shown that these patients also suffer from ocular vascular dys-regulation.

The blood vessels of the eye are responsible for perfusion and, therefore, the nutrition of the different parts of the eyeball. The amount of blood transported in these anatomical structures is continually adapted to satisfy the tissue's actual demand. For example, when light falls into the eye of a healthy subject, blood flow into the retina and the optic nerve increases immediately. If the blood pressure decreases, the vessels dilate to prevent a circulatory deficit. Ocular blood flow is thus actively regulated.

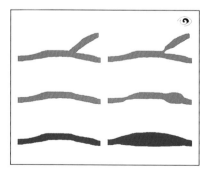

Fig. 4.13: Diagram of vascular dysregulations. Red: arteries; blue: veins.

These mechanisms for adapting to changing conditions are impaired in patients having vasospastic syndrome. This is why an ophthalmologist might ask about cold hands or low blood pressure. These symptoms provide an initial indication that someone could have a vasospastic syndrome. Examining the conjunctival vessels and the ocular fundus, but especially a monitoring of the blood flow under various conditions, provides more information that supports or refutes this suspicion (cf. S 11).

Sleep apnea. An apnea is clinically defined as a cessation of breathing that lasts at least ten seconds. Sleep apnea is a common sleep disorder characterized by brief interruptions of breathing during sleep [Gr. *apnea*: without breath]. There are three types of apnea: obstructive, central and mixed. Of the three, obstructive is the most common. Typically the soft tissue of the rear of the throat collapses and closes the airway, leading patients with sleep apnea to stop breathing repeatedly during their sleep.

The apnea induces transient hypoxia and thereby increases the risk for cardiovascular and neurological damage. To this regard, apnea is also a risk factor for glaucomatous damage.

4.2.8 Diabetes Mellitus

Diabetes is a major disease that can lead to severe ocular damage (cf. S 7). Here the focus is on the role diabetes plays in glaucomatous damage. As mentioned earlier, diabetic retinopathy can lead to dangerously increased IOP levels as a dreaded complication (cf. Chapter 3.6.2). However, it is not yet known whether, at the same intraocular pressure, diabetic patients face an increased risk for optic nerve damage than do normal subjects. In other words, the question, "Are diabetics more sensitive to the effects of IOP?" remains unanswered. It was previously assumed that diabetes was a major risk factor for glaucomatous damage. However, today, diabetes mellitus is regarded as being of lesser significance or as being even protective against glaucomatous damage.

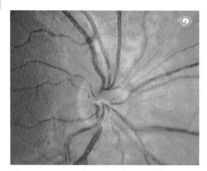

Fig. 4.14: Small, normal optic disc.

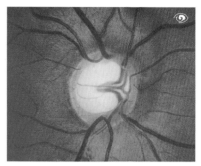

Fig. 4.15: Large, normal optic disc, with large physiological excavation.

4.2.9 The Appearance of the Optic Disc

The greater the tissue damage at the optic nerve head, the more likely a future progression of nerve fiber loss; but whether this is a genuine risk factor is still debated. Theoretically, it seems possible that an already damaged disc could be more susceptible to increased IOP. In this case, it would be a risk factor. But it is also possible that it is just a risk indicator. If the patient has suffered from previous damage, chances are high for a further deterioration if the causes have not been eliminated. Hemorrhages at or near the optic disc are clear risk factors. The appearance of these hemorrhages point almost with certainty to a progression of existing damage. However, what is not known is whether blood that has leaked from ocular vessels is just a sign of the damage, or if it actually causes further damage. The current view is that this blood leads to local vasospasms as a secondary effect.

The size of an optic disc does not seem to be a risk factor. A given IOP will cause the same degree of damage, regardless of whether the optic disc is large or small. However, for assessing the condition of the optic nerve, the disc size is important: Since the number of nerve fibers is about the same in all healthy people, there is some "empty space" in the center of those having a large papilla. This is called a normal (= physiological) excavation. For healthy individuals, the size of the neuroretinal rim is quite constant. The rim is that part of the optic disc that is filled with nerve fibers. Figure 4.14 shows a small normal optic disc, and Figure 4.15, a large but also normal optic disc. When one looks at the physiological excavation, it becomes clear why the disc size must always be considered when the disc appearance is interpreted.

4.2.10 Additional Factors

There are several other risk factors that will not be discussed here. Some are rare; others have yet to be fully investigated. Primary open-angle glaucoma (POAG), for example, is more common among patients with autoimmune diseases, a group of conditions characterized by a reaction of the immune system against certain parts of the patient's own body. Remarkably, many POAG patients have disturbances of the thyroid gland. Additionally, there are conditions where the blood vessels become inflamed and these also lead to glaucomatous damage. And finally, among glaucoma patients, there is occasionally a so-called empty sella – a void space on the x-ray where the hypophysis is usually seated.

Summary

A condition that increases the likelihood of a certain event is called a risk factor. We have to distinguish risk factors that lead to an IOP increase from risk factors that cause optic nerve damage.

Primary risk factors for an increased IOP are age, family history, race, and arteriosclerosis. Primary risk factors for glaucomatous damage are increased IOP, vascular dysregulation with systemic hypotension and vasospasm, female gender, short-sightedness, and race.

5 Pathogenesis of Glaucomatous Damage

Glaucomatous damage was discussed in Chapter 2, Chapter 3 was devoted to the causes of increased intraocular pressure, and Chapter 4 covered additional risk factors in the development of glaucomatous tissue loss. It is now time to explain the mechanisms by which these risk factors induce the damage that is so typical of glaucoma. This damage is primarily due to cell loss: retinal nerve cells (i.e. ganglion cells) and their axons die, as do other cells in the optic disc area. Cells die in either of two ways: by necrosis (Fig. 5.1) [Gr. *nekros:* death] or by a process called apoptosis (Fig. 5.2) [Gr. *apoptein:* to fall down].

In necrosis, the cell breaks up in a rather chaotic manner and this leads to a surrounding inflammatory reaction. Necrosis can be caused by mechanical trauma, burns, chemical injury or by a lack of oxygen. Because apoptosis is so crucial to understanding glaucoma, it will be discussed in some detail.

5.1 Apoptosis, "Programmed Cell Death"

This form of cell death is a fundamental biological process. It plays a pivotal role in the development of an organism but is also of importance for what is called tissue homeostasis (a form of dynamic equilibrium) and for the removal of pathologically altered cells. A cell can produce enzymes with which it can actually "digest" itself, leaving behind only tiny, membrane-wrapped globules which can then be ingested by other cells (Fig. 5.2).

5.1.1 Cells in Dialogue

A normally functioning cell can "sense" if it is still needed by the organism. The cell receives a constant stream of information from the environment that tells it what to do: continue living, divide in two (reproduce) or simply go away (apoptosis). For example, when you get slightly cut, the defect grows back together within a few days or weeks. But what happens at the cellular level is this: the

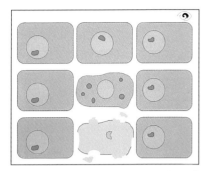

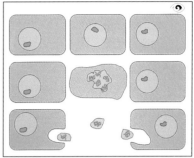

Fig. 5.1: Cell death by necrosis: the cell in the middle "disintegrates" and the contents are released into the surroundings.

Fig. 5.2: Cell death by apoptosis: the cell in the middle "digests itself." Its components, enclosed in membranes, are absorbed by surrounding cells.

cells surrounding the wound receive orders to reproduce. When the defect is completely covered by new tissue, the cells are then told to stop multiplying. Another example: When a white blood cell is no longer needed, it receives a signal to dissolve (apoptosis). These signals from the cell's surroundings are both physical (contact with other cells) and chemical. In the latter case, the cells receive messenger substances "delivered" by adjacent cells (Fig. 5.3).

Following these "orders to die," the cells resort to different mechanisms for self-destruction without affecting other parts of the organism.

Unfortunately, this process doesn't work in cancer cells. Although their surroundings have not reported any demand for cell

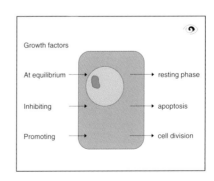

Fig. 5.3: The cell reacts to information received from its environment.

proliferation, these cells reproduce themselves, even if this isn't beneficial for the organism as a whole.

Just the opposite happens in degenerative diseases [Lat. *degeneratio:* to substitute a good material with another of lesser quality], such as Parkinson's disease: cells that are actually still needed erroneously die.

Molecular biology (cf. S 3) has enhanced the understanding of how cells exchange and process information among each other. For example, it has been shown that even several days after primary damage has occurred, such as with an arterial occlusion in the brain, there is prolonged secondary nerve cell loss in the same area that results from "erroneous information." The secrets to these secondary mechanisms of damage and how to prevent them are slowly unraveling.

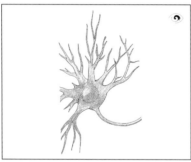

Fig. 5.4: Detail of a normal nerve cell (neuron).

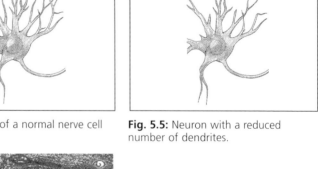

Fig. 5.5: Neuron with a reduced number of dendrites.

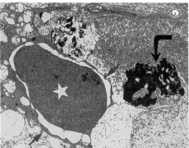

Fig. 5.6: Dying ganglion cell, on the left in an early stage (→) with a homogenous cell nucleus (*); on the right, in a terminal stage (bent arrow).

In glaucoma, at least some of the nerve cells (ganglion cells) die via apoptosis. The shape of these ganglion cells is extremely complex because they establish direct contact with numerous other cells (Fig. 5.4). Before these cells die, the number of contacts to other nerve cells is reduced. This is morphologically visible: the number of the cell's extensions, or dendrites [Gr. *dendron:* tree, the delicate extensions of a nerve cell resemble the branches of a tree], gradually decreases (Fig. 5.5). This reduction in contact results in discreet functional disturbances. And finally, the cell dies (Fig. 5.6). It is not yet known whether some ganglion cells also die by necrosis.

Why does a ganglion cell receive erroneous information that makes it believe it is no longer needed? This question is currently a major concern for researchers. Although many of the interactions are not yet completely understood, several possible mechanisms are discussed below.

5.1.2 Causes of Apoptosis

Lack of Information. Inside a nerve fiber, many different molecules continuously flow in both directions. This is called axoplasmic flow (Fig. 5.7) [Gr. *axon:* axis, the axis-shaped extension of a ganglion cell]. Some of these molecules provide the nerve cell with the information that the contact to the nerve cells located at the end of the axon (the nerve fiber) is intact. When this contact is lost, the cell loses its *"raison d'être."*

With very high intraocular pressure, the axoplasmic flow is halted. One of the consequences is that the "connection intact" information is no longer relayed to the retinal ganglion cell body from the nearest brain cell. This might be one reason why the cell death process starts. Axoplasmic flow can, on the one hand, be mechanically impaired by the pressure difference between the eye and optic nerve and, on the other, by a reduction in the region's blood flow (Fig. 5.8).

Erroneous Information. In glaucoma patients, the retinal level of certain chemical substances that serve as "messengers" is too

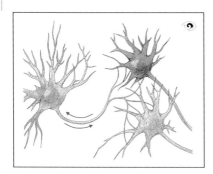

Fig. 5.7: Molecules and cell organelles are transported by the axoplasmic flow.

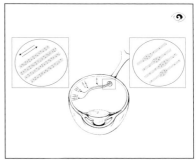

Fig. 5.8: Normal (left) and partly blocked (right) axoplasmic flow in the optic disc region.

high. One of these chemical messengers is glutamate. A normal concentration of glutamate stimulates nerve cells; a concentration too high virtually kills them. There is still no definitive explanation for the glutamate increase in glaucoma. It is probably a consequence of an insufficient oxygen supply related to inadequate perfusion (cf. below).

Lack of Oxygen. Another powerful stimulus for apoptosis is ischemia [Gr. *ischein:* to hold back/Gr. *haima:* blood], a term that means inadequate blood supply. We know that ischemia can lead to cell death in the brain. Glaucoma patients suffer permanently or episodically from decreased ocular perfusion.

5.2 The Importance of Ocular Perfusion

It has been shown that an elevated IOP, low systemic blood pressure and vascular dysregulation act as risk factors for the development of glaucomatous damage. But how do they interact?

5.2.1 The Role of Vascular Dysregulation

Vascular dysregulation can affect the eye as well as other organs (as will be described in detail in S 8). Vascular dysregulation interferes with normal autoregulation [Gr. *autos:* self]. Autoregula-

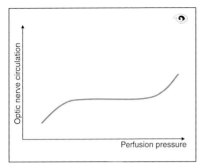

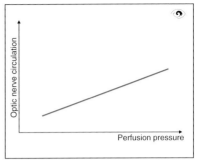

Fig. 5.9: In a healthy person, up to a certain point, the blood flow in the retina and optic nerve is independent of the perfusion pressure.

Fig. 5.10: If autoregulation is disturbed, blood flow is directly linked to perfusion pressure.

tion is defined as a tissue's ability to self adjust its perfusion to the current requirement and to do so independently of perfusion pressure. Perfusion pressure is the difference between the tension in arteries and the tension in veins. The pressure inside the ocular veins has to be at least as high as the IOP – or these vessels would collapse. This means that perfusion pressure in the eye is the difference between the arterial blood pressure and the IOP. When autoregulation works properly, there are no changes in retinal and optic disc perfusion when either the IOP or the blood pressure fluctuates within a certain range (Fig. 5.9).

When there is a disturbance of the autoregulation, ocular perfusion varies depending on the IOP and blood pressure, a condition that is unfavorable to the tissue (Fig. 5.10).

5.2.2 The Role of Intraocular Pressure

The IOP can induce damage in several ways. It can mechanically affect the weakest spot inside the eye, the optic disc. Here the sclera is thin and is perforated in an area called the lamina cribrosa [Lat. *cribrum:* strainer]. Some eyes are more sensitive than others to intraocular pressure; for example, this is the case with myopic eyes.

A sharp rise in the IOP can block the axoplasmic flow and thus diminish the exchange of information among the cells.

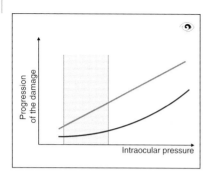

Fig. 5.11: As long as autoregulation functions properly, damage will occur only at significantly elevated IOP levels; if autoregulation is disturbed (green), low or normal IOP can cause damage.

Finally, the IOP can reduce ocular perfusion. A decrease in the ocular blood flow always occurs with extremely high intraocular pressure and occasionally with moderate increases as well. Decreased blood flow can even occur with a normal IOP when the autoregulation is disturbed (Fig. 5.11).

5.2.3 The Influence of Blood Pressure

The blood pressure measured in one individual can be quite different from that measured in another. Furthermore, the blood pressure fluctuates throughout the day and night, but this does not affect the eyes of a healthy person. A decrease in the BP results in a reduction of the ocular perfusion only when it is either excessive or there is a disturbance of the autoregulation. In these cases, ocular perfusion depends directly on the perfusion pressure, and a low BP exerts an influence similar to that of an elevated IOP.

5.2.4 Additional Factors

Perfusion depends on several other factors. Ocular perfusion, for instance, is poorer in people having severe myopia. There are many other anatomical differences that cause some individuals to develop perfusion problems earlier than others.

5.3   Reperfusion Damage

We have repeatedly emphasized that fluctuations in the IOP and blood pressure are more damaging than a stable, but increased, intraocular pressure or a stable, and decreased, blood pressure. This is even more pronounced in patients who suffer from disturbed autoregulation due to vascular dysregulation (Fig. 5.12). This means that a fluctuating ocular blood supply does more harm than a continuously reduced perfusion, as is seen in arteriosclerosis or e.g. multiple sclerosis.

But the blood flow is probably only rarely reduced to such an extent that severe ischemia resulting in cell death occurs; so-called reperfusion damage seems to be much more frequent. The return to a normal blood flow after a period of impaired circulation is called reperfusion. It is interesting – and certainly surprising to many – to learn that damage occurs in a phase when the blood flow is again normal. To explain: When perfusion decreases, there is a relative shortage of oxygen and other molecules. This causes a certain amount of damage inside the cell that affects, in particular, the mitochondria, one of the many cell components. Mitochondria have been described as the cell's power plants where glucose and fat are "burned." During this "burning" process, electrons migrate from one energy level to the next as they flow through the respiratory chain. This thereby provides the cell with the energy – or power – it needs. In reduced perfusion, electron transport is partly impaired. After the blood flow returns to normal, some of these electrons go astray and encounter oxygen molecules that are once again present. This leads to the creation of so-called free oxygen radicals. Hypoxanthine, a catabolic product of the energy transmitter, adenosine triphosphate (ATP), also contributes to the formation of these free radicals. This results in oxidative damage to various cell structures, but particularly to the mitochondria and the cell nucleus. The cell recognizes the damage and is able to repair most of it, but when the damage is too widespread, the cell "gives up" and decides to "commit suicide," i.e. undergo apoptosis. This explains why fluctuations in intraocular as well as systemic blood pressure can be more harmful with disturbed autoregulation than a high but stable IOP or a low but stable blood pressure. The mechanisms of reperfusion also explain why there is glaucomatous papillary atrophy and not bland papillary atrophy (cf. Chapter 2.1.2). The reason is the high susceptibility of the astrocytes (supporting cells) to free oxygen radicals. Instead of forming gliosis scars, they induce tissue remodeling and vanish later on.

5.4 Activation of glial cells

The optic nerve head, like the retina and the whole central nerve system, consists of both neural and glial cells. There are different glial cells. In the optic nerve head these are mostly so called astrocytes. These cells have many extensions connecting ganglion-cell axons with blood vessels. The extensions gave the name astrocytes (starlike cells). When stimulated, astrocytes change their appearance and produce molecules which are normally either not produced, or produced to a much lesser extent, which alters the micro-environ-

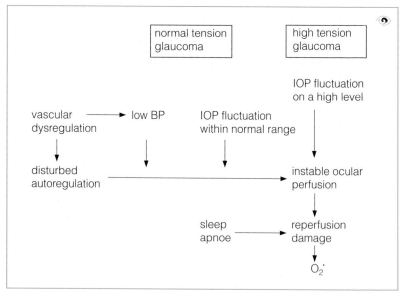

Fig. 5.12: Concept of pathogenesis as proposed by the authors: Both increased IOP as well as decreased blood pressure can lead to glaucomatous damage, especially when accompanied by vascular dysregulation.

ment of the cells. Activated astrocytes can migrate and ultimately disappear, contributing to the development of glaucomatous excavation (Fig. 5.13).

The glial cells of the retina can also get activated to some extent. The retina contains astrocytes and so called Müller cells. The activated astrocytes in the retina are morphologically altered, thus causing a slight increase of light scatter. A healthy retina is transparent, which is why the retina itself can hardly be made out in photographs. What we see on color photos is the light back scattered from the choroid and pigment epithelium as well as from the column of blood in the retinal vessels. An increased light scattering by activated astrocytes can be detected in red-free photographs (Fig 5.14b). The glinting areas do not show up on regular fundus photos (Fig 5.14a, see corresponding areas) and are easily overlooked by clinicians. They do not involve macula as there are no astrocytes in the macula, and they are few in the periphery as the number of astrocytes declines centrifugally.

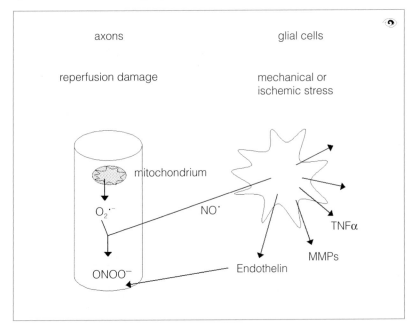

Fig. 5.13: The simultanous oxidative stress brought about by reperfusion and activation of astrocytes leads to the damaging peroxinitrate.

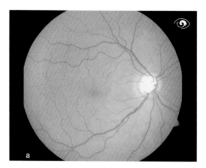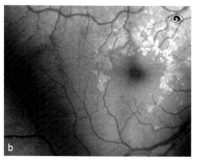

Fig. 5.14: Activated astrocytes scatter the light more than quiescent astrocytes. This can hardly be seen in the regular fundus photo a) but easily in the red free picture b).

5.5   Altered micro-environment

Activated astrocytes produce molecules like NOS-2, COX-2, TNFa, MHC II, MMPs, Endothelin, etc. As a consequence, both the nerve axons and the glial cells find themselves in an altered environment. For example, it is known that Endothelin not only reduces blood-flow in the ONH, but also directly affects the axoplasmatic transport. Increased metalloproteinases (MMPs), enzymes that digest extracellular matrix, lead to disappearance of components of extracellular matrix and their replacement by others. This in turn leads to tissue remodelling including changes of the lamina cribrosa and ultimately to the hallmark of glaucoma, the excavation of the optic nerve head.

An increased expression of some of these molecules, including MMP-9, has been observed not only locally in the optic nerve head, but also in the monocytes of circulating blood. Furthermore, the level of Endothelin-1 is increased. While this can be used for diagnostic purposes, it is not yet known how far these molecules in the circulating blood contribute to the damage. They may diffuse from the choroid -which has fenestrated vessels- into the optic nerve head and the surrounding retina, which could explain changes observed in glaucoma patients, e.g. peripapillary atrophy, local retinal vasoconstrictions and small haemorrhages (Fig 2.8 / 2.9 / 5.15). Although not specific for glaucoma, these changes occur more often in glaucoma than

Fig. 5.15: The retinal vessels in the peripapillar area are often constricted.

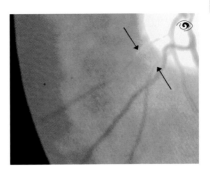

in normals. A change of an individual gene expression in circulating monocytes is also not specific for glaucoma. It is rather the pattern of change of several genes that is specific. Thus, new avenues for diagnosis, risk assessment and monitoring of treatment efficacy can be opened in the future. Note that we are dealing with changes in gene expression and not with changes of the genes themselves.

5.6 The pathogenetic concept

Glaucomatous damage implies loss of retinal ganglion cells and their axons, tissue remodelling leading to the excavation of the optic nerve head, thinning of the retina and of the optic nerve and cell loss in the lateral geniculate nucleus. All of the damage components can be explained by the alterations discussed above. A mild but recurrent reperfusion injury is present, leading to an oxidative stress and an increase of reactive oxidative species like $O_2^{\cdot-}$ especially in the mitochondria of the optic nerve head axons, thus decreasing the power supply. This is supplemented by a change in the micro-environment, mainly due to the activation of the glial-cells, which on one hand leads to a tissue remodelling, on the other reduces blood flow even further and interferes with the axoplasmatic transport. Moreover, activated astrocytes produce NOS-2 and thereby secret NO which diffuses easily in the surrounding tissue, including axons. If there is a simultaneous increase of $O_2^{\cdot-}$ in the axons, the damaging molecule peroxinitrite ($OONO^-$) is produced (Fig 5.13). Peroxinitrite is trapped within the axons and diffuses along the axons both towards the retina, inducing apoptosis of retinal ganglion cells, and in the direction of the brain inducing cell loss in the lateral geniculate ganglion.

It is important to stress, that both mechanical stimulus in the form of high intraocular pressure, as well as ischemia can lead to an activation of astrocytes, explaining how astrocytes can be activated both in high tension and in normal tension glaucoma. Reperfusion injury occurs either when the IOP fluctuation exceeds the capacity of autoregulation, as in high tension glaucoma, or if IOP fluctuates on a normal level in cases with a disturbed autoregulation, as in normal tension glaucoma (Fig 5.12). The proposed concept explains why there is no strict separation between high tension and normal tension glaucoma. The final damage is similar in high tension and in normal tension glaucoma, they are merely two ends of same continuum.

The lower the pressure at which a damage occurs or progresses, the higher the probability of a disturbed autoregulation of ocular blood flow. The main cause for a disturbed autoregulation in turn is the PVD (S8.2.1).

Summary

Glaucomatous damage implies the loss of retinal ganglion cells and their axons, and a major tissue remodelling causing, among other effects, the visible optic nerve head excavation. Two main elements contribute to the damage: a) the activation of the glial cells by ischemic or by mechanical stress, leading to a change in the micro-environment; b) a reperfusion injury and thus an oxidative stress, inducing free radical formation in the axons of the optic nerve head and thereby destroying various structures. If both mechanisms occur simultaneously, highly toxic molecule called peroxinitrite is produced in the axons. Peroxinitrite diffuses within the axons, both to the retina and to the brain, leading to the neural tissue apoptosis. The loss of neural cells, together with tissue remodelling, is termed the glaucomatous damage.

6 Diagnosing Glaucoma

Early detection of glaucoma is extremely important because treatment is much more likely to succeed when started early than when damage has already progressed to an advanced stage. Though this sounds simple enough, it actually isn't because: a) diagnosing glaucoma is possible only if the patient visits his ophthalmologist and b) changes in the early stage of the disease are sometimes not easily differentiated from variations that pose no threat. There is often a period of uncertainty as to whether or not the patient will develop glaucomatous damage.

6.1 Which Symptoms are Noticed by the Patient?

As already mentioned, the chronic glaucoma patient will not notice anything unusual for a long time. The ophthalmologist occasionally encounters someone who has his eyes examined for the first time but has already lost most of his visual fields. Glaucoma must therefore actively be sought out and diagnosis should not wait until the first symptoms appear.

In the rare case of acute glaucoma, things are quite different. Due to the sudden and extreme rise in intraocular pressure, there are obvious symptoms, such as headache, nausea, vomiting, visual disturbances, red eyes, etc. Acute glaucoma almost always brings the patient right into the doctor's office. Occasionally, however, these symptoms are so non-specific and without accompanying ocular pain that acute glaucoma is not immediately suspected.

6.2 When Should an Ophthalmologist be Consulted?

An eye exam is recommended whenever there are visual problems, no matter in which form they appear. Visual disturbances always deserve an evaluation. They can arise from many causes. A consultation with an ophthalmologist is even more critical when problems have developed within just a short time. The same applies with pain in or around the eye or if flashes of light appear, if the eye turns red or double vision occurs. When in doubt, it is always safer to consult your ophthalmologist once too often than not often enough.

Many people have absolutely no eye symptoms and feel they have no problems with their eyes. If there is no family history of glaucoma, it is recommended that the first eye examination take place around the age of 40. This is about the time when most people first require reading glasses and therefore might be more aware of their eyesight. When symptoms are present or there is a family history of glaucoma or other risk factors (cf. Chapter 4), then an eye examination even earlier is recommended.

The ophthalmologist can quickly and easily tell if glaucoma could possibly be present. If there is some indication that this might be the case, then other, slightly more involved tests will be made to support or refute the diagnosis and, if present, then determine the extent of the damage.

6.3　Examination by the Ophthalmologist

Today's ophthalmological practice is equipped with modern technology, but this should not frighten patients: The eye examination is neither painful nor dangerous.

The doctor first asks the patient a few questions. In particular, he will inquire about visual problems, any family history of eye problems, and whether certain diseases are present, such as diabetes. He will also ask questions about circulation, for instance, whether cold hands and feet are often experienced. Additionally, he will want to know about any medications currently being taken. It is a good idea for the patient to write down the names of these drugs, and if glasses are worn, these should also be brought along.

6.3.1 Routine Eye Examination

The ophthalmologist will first check visual acuity, a measure of the optical resolution or the eye's discernment, i.e. how well one can read and recognize things, people, traffic signs, etc. from a distance and up close. If the visual acuity is identical to that of the general (healthy) population, it is described as being 1.0, 100%, or 20/20. (The latter referring to testing with the well-known Snellen charts. With 20/20 vision, the "20 line" can be read at a distance of 20 feet.) A patient with a visual acuity of 0.5 (50% or 20/40) needs the chart letters to be twice the size of those that can easily be read by someone having 20/20 vision. If vision is impaired, the ophthalmologist will investigate the reason. In glaucoma, visual acuity stays normal for quite some time. However, many glaucoma patients suffer from a reduced visual acuity because they also have other eye diseases, such as cataracts. People who already wear glasses should bring either the glasses or the prescription to the eye exam. After measuring the visual acuity, the eyes are checked using the slit lamp (Fig. 6.1).

The slit lamp is a special ophthalmological microscope that swivels so that the eye and its interior parts can be viewed from various angles; it is equipped with a light source that is also movable. The eye can thus be examined from various directions using different intensities of light. The light beam usually takes the form of a slit (hence the instrument's name), thereby enabling the eye to be examined in different layers, i.e. in "optical sections" (Fig. 6.2).

To get a clear image of the eye's posterior segment, and in particular, of the retina and optic disc, a contact glass (Fig. 6.3) is placed on the (anesthetized) eye or it is examined through a magnifying lens (indirect ophthalmoscopy) that is held about an inch away from the eye (Fig. 6.4).

The contact glass is flat on the side facing the doctor, but concave on the patient's side; in this manner, the glass is adapted to follow the curvature of the cornea. This eliminates the strong refractive effect of the cornea and the ophthalmologist can examine the posterior segment with the microscope. Several mirrors are located inside the contact glass (Fig. 6.5), and these permit viewing of even the peripheral parts of the retina through the pupil. One of these mirrors provides a good view of the chamber angle.

The fundus and posterior eye sections can likewise be viewed

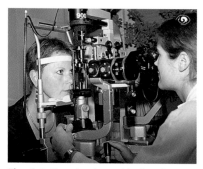

Fig. 6.1: Examination with the slit-lamp.

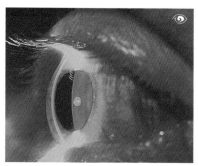

Fig. 6.2: With a slit-like beam of light, the different structures of the eye can be examined.

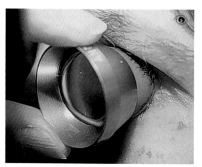

Fig. 6.3: Chamber angle and posterior segments are assessed using a contact glass.

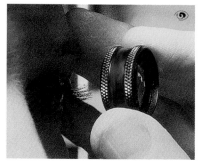

Fig. 6.4: A lens, such as that shown here, helps the ophthalmologist examine the posterior parts of the eye (inner eye or fundus).

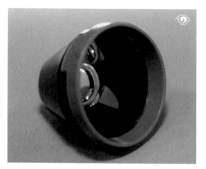

Fig. 6.5: Contact glass with built-in mirrors.

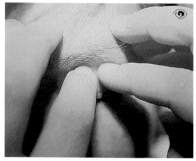

Fig. 6.6: The IOP can be estimated by pressing the eyeball through the closed eyelids with the fingertips.

with the slit lamp using a strong convex lens (Fig. 6.4). In contrast to the contact glass examination, the image seen is upside down and considerably smaller.

For a good stereoscopic view of the posterior segments, the pupil has to be dilated using medication. A few drops of a mydriatic (dilating drug) are administered into the patient's eye [Gr. *amydros:* dark]. It usually takes about 15 to 20 minutes before the pupil is sufficiently dilated to allow examination. Mydriasis impairs the patient's near vision and makes him more sensitive to light, but vision returns to normal within a few hours (in rare cases, it takes a few days).

6.3.2 Measuring the Intraocular Pressure

Tonometry [Gr. *tonos:* tension/Gr. *metrein:* to measure] is another term for measuring the IOP. Before instruments for tonometry became available, the IOP had to be "felt." The physician used pressure from his fingers to determine the quality of resistance by pushing on the eye alternately with both forefingers (Fig. 6.6). An experienced ophthalmologist is able to at least guess the IOP level using this method which is still used when information about the actual IOP is urgently needed and instruments are not readily available.

Today there are different devices available that measure the IOP, and these instruments include contact instruments that actually touch the surface of the eye during measurement and non-contact instruments. The international standard in ophthalmology is the Goldmann applanation tonometer, named for Hans Goldmann (1899–1991), an ophthalmologist from Bern (Switzerland) who developed this method (Fig. 6.7). Applanation tonometry measures the force that is necessary to flatten (i.e. to applanate) a defined part of the cornea (Fig. 6.8a). Since this force depends on the IOP, these instruments are calibrated so that the pressure can be read from a graduated dial.

To ensure that an area of identical size is applanated in each measurement, Goldmann developed a simple but effective tech-

Fig. 6.7: Goldmann
applanation tonometer.

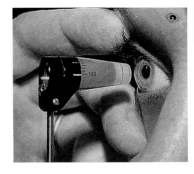
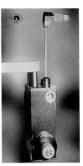

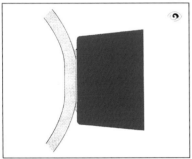
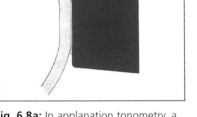

Fig. 6.8a: In applanation tonometry, a
defined area of the cornea is flattened.

Fig. 6.8b: What the ophthalmologist
sees when measuring IOP: on the left,
the applanated area is too small; on
the right, too large; and in the middle,
the desired size.

nique. The ophthalmologist observes the eye through a small plastic
cylinder that flattens the cornea. Immediately before the measurement, a yellow dye (fluorescein) is instilled into the eye. This dye is
pushed to the side when the plastic cylinder flattens the cornea, and
the ophthalmologist sees a colored ring that lights up at the periphery of the cylinder when the eye is illuminated with blue light (fluo-
rescence). This causes the dye to fluoresce green and thus becomes
easier to distinguish.

Goldmann also had the idea of inserting a bi-prism into this
plastic cylinder. This bi-prism induces a horizontal shift of the upper
half towards the lower half. Therefore, instead of seeing one round
circle, the ophthalmologist sees two semicircles. The shift of the image corresponds exactly to the diameter of the desired applanation.

Figure 6.8b illustrates how the ophthalmologist recognizes the correct diameter and thereby whether the correct pressure is applied. Applanation is insufficient on the left, appropriate in the middle, and too strong on the right. The tension dial on the tonometer is adjusted until the inner edge of the lower and upper semicircles are aligned. The IOP can then be read from a graduated dial (Fig. 6.9).

Since the eye is lightly touched with the plastic prism, the corneal surface is first anesthetized. A few seconds after a drop of local anesthetic is applied to the cornea, it becomes insensitive to discomfort. Immediately after the pressure measurement, the patient's vision might be slightly blurry, but this disappears within a few minutes.

Non-contact devices flatten the cornea using a jet of air (Fig. 6.10). An optic receiver detects when and how fast the cornea has been flattened to a predetermined degree. The unit then converts the amount of time it takes for applanation to occur into millimeters of mercury. This method's advantage lies in the fact that a local anesthetic is not required and potential contamination from a tonometry cylinder is prevented. However, the measurement is not as accurate as Goldmann's tonometry, particularly with high IOP levels. Levels should thus be confirmed with a Goldmann tonometer when data from a non-contact instrument is inconclusive.

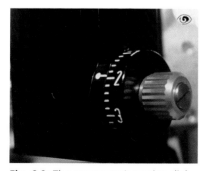

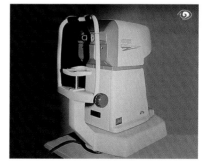

Fig. 6.9: The tonometer's tension dial.   **Fig. 6.10:** A non-contact tonometer.

Fig. 6.11: Dynamic Contour Tonometer (DCT).

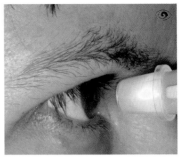
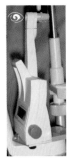

In addition, there are also other methods to measure the intraocular pressure. One can use a handheld device, named Tonopen, which uses the piezoelectric phenomen to measure the IOP. Recently, a new device for the continuous measurement of the IOP has been developed, a so called dynamic contour tonometer. Because of the continuous mode of measurement with a sampling rate of 100Hz it can capture the IOP changes during the heart cycle, und thus estimate the pulsatile component of the blood flow. Despite its special functioning principle (the surface of the tip is concave, so the cornea takes the contour as if the pressure on both sides of the cornea were the same, allowing the electronic pressure sensor to measure IOP

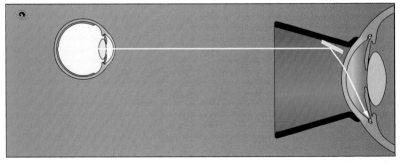

Fig. 6.12: Using a special contact glass, the ophthalmologist can look into the chamber angle.

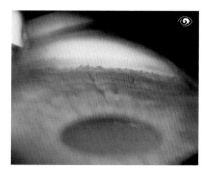
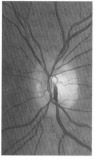
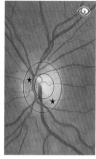

Fig. 6.13: Gonioscopic view of a normal chamber angle.

Fig. 6.14: The neuroretinal rim (*) where all the retinal nerve fibers come together to leave the eye (as the optic nerve) through the optic disc.

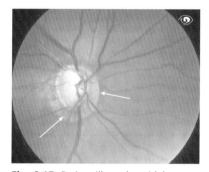
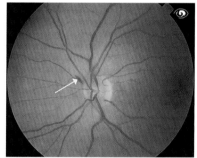

Fig. 6.15: Peripapillary choroidal atrophy (→).

Fig. 6.16: Disc hemorrhage (→).

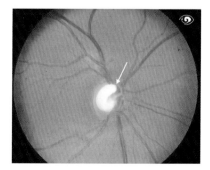

Fig. 6.17: Bayoneting of blood vessels at the rim of the excavation (→).

independent of corneal properties; fully automated, so the human bias is reduced to a minimum), so far it did not prove clearly advantageous to the classical Goldmann applanation tonometry, in particular regarding the effect of corneal thickness on the IOP measurements (Fig 6.11).

There are additional aspects of the IOP measurements worth addressing, in the first place the corneal thickness. At the given real IOP, the thicker the cornea, the higher are the measured IOP values, and vice versa. This can lead to the overestimation of IOP for example in ocular hypertensives, and to the wrong decision to initiate the antiglaucomatous therapy. More significant is the possible underestimation of IOP in persons with thin corneas. However, the following general rule puts this problem into perspective: an IOP at which a glaucomatous damage occurs or progresses is too high for the given eye. Corneal thickness can be measured with optical devices, nowadays with ultrasound and laser pachymeters. It is to date not clear whether thin cornea is in itself a risk factor for glaucomatous damage independent of IOP level.

6.3.3 Examining the Anterior Chamber Angle

The examination of the chamber angle is called gonioscopy [Gr. *gonios:* knee/Gr. *skopein:* to observe, to watch] because this angle slightly resembles a bent knee. The ophthalmologist always visualizes the chamber angle when investigating the cause for an IOP increase or when there is some indication that the angle could close, thereby triggering an acute glaucoma attack. Because the peripheral cornea is not transparent, the anterior chamber angle cannot be directly viewed. The physician thus uses a special contact glass, a goniolens, to perform gonioscopy.

After applying a local anesthetic, the goniolens is placed upon the eye. Using the mirror system inside the goniolens, the angle can be examined (Fig. 6.12). By turning the lens, the ophthalmologist gets a 360° view of this important anatomical structure.

Using this technique, the angle can be checked for material that should not be there (such as blood, cell debris or signs of inflammation) and even whether there are adhesions of the iris at any site. Evaluating the width of the angle helps assess the threat of angle-closure and whether there are congenital anomalies present inside the angle. Figure 6.13 shows a normal anterior chamber angle; Figure 3.32 depicts an angle covered by pigment due to pigment dispersion syndrome.

6.3.4 Evaluating the Optic Disc

The most important step in diagnosing glaucoma is the evaluation of the optic disc (also called the optic nerve head and the papilla), a task requiring much experience by the ophthalmologist. The ophthalmologist first assesses the size of the optic nerve head. As noted in Chapter 4.2.9, a large papilla has a more pronounced physiological excavation than a small one, but this is not a sign of disease (Fig. 4.15). One rule of thumb that applies: the larger the papilla, the larger the excavation (cupping) in a healthy person. This must be considered when a physician has to decide whether cupping is normal or pathological.

The ophthalmologist also interprets the shape of the excavation. It indicates whether cupping is congenital or if it has developed during the patient's lifetime as a result of a pathological process. The color of the neural rim area where the nerve fibers gather is also evaluated (Fig. 6.14).

Atrophy around the papilla (peripapillary atrophy) can indicate glaucomatous damage (Fig. 6.15), but it can also occur in other diseases and even in healthy eyes. However, a small hemorrhage at the rim of the optic disc is almost always a sign of glaucoma, especially when other eye diseases have been ruled out (Fig. 6.16). Disc hemorrhages are markers of progressing glaucomatous damage. Local vasoconstrictions of retinal vessels are another sign of glaucoma, but are also present in other diseases of the papilla. If the vessels make a sharp bend as they cross the cup margin ("bayoneting"), then there is even more reason to suspect glaucomatous excavation (Fig. 6.17).

Based on all these indications, the ophthalmologist can then decide whether glaucoma is present or not. Unfortunately, there are

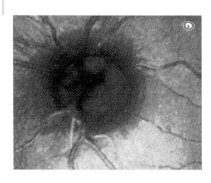

Fig. 6.18: HRT image of the optic disc.

borderline cases that are ambiguous. If visual field testing shows normal results, then one often must wait and see whether the changes remain the same or progress. Progression is then a sure sign of disease.

6.4 Documenting the Papilla and Nerve Fiber Layer

Several techniques have been developed in recent years that make the assessment of the optic disc more objective and even permit a certain quantification of the disc's alterations. However, none of the methods described below is completely satisfactory. The ophthalmologist's assessment of the optic disc still remains the most important decision criterion.

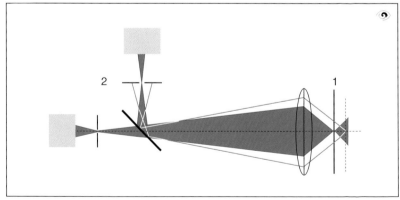

Fig. 6.19: The principle of confocal imaging: (1) Plane from which the light passes through, (2) Confocal diaphragm.

6.4.1 Papillary Photography

Taking a picture of the optic disc and its environment can prove helpful in assessing the early detection or progression of damage. When the patient returns to the ophthalmologist at a later date, the current state is examined with a slit lamp and then compared to past pictures. Another possibility is to take stereoscopic pictures for measuring the changes, such as the size of the neural rim. If the neural rim is smaller in later pictures, then this is a sure sign that glaucomatous damage has progressed.

Other procedures have been developed to facilitate comparisons between old and new pictures, for example, chronostereophotography. The slightest changes that would be invisible to the doctor's naked eye can now be better detected. These techniques are not widely used in a general ophthalmologic practice and are therefore not discussed here.

6.4.2 Laser Scanning Tomography

A laser scanner is a device that, in simple terms, sends out a laser beam which illuminates one spot on the retina, measures the amount of light reflected by that spot, and then proceeds to do the same with a large number of spots (cf. S 13). Several different scanners are available that function similarly. For example, the Heidelberg Retina Tomograph checks 65,536 spots (256 spots on each line with a total of 256 lines) in 32 milliseconds. The results are directly visible on a monitor. Figure 6.18 depicts the reflected intensity in reference to the evaluated retinal spot (designated as x/y). This mode of visualization is called a "reflectivity diagram." The measured reflectivity is transformed into certain colors: yellow means "high degree of reflectivity," dark brown indicates "low degree of reflectivity," and the areas in red are intermediate levels. The reflectivity diagram does not provide any information about the actual color of the papilla (as does a color photograph) because the laser beam is monochromatic, but it does supply valuable diagnostic information.

A simple laser scanner that produces reflectivity images does not permit quantification of the posterior eye's three-dimensional

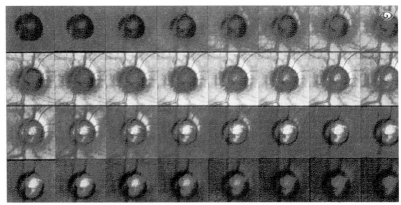

Fig. 6.20: Reflex images of different focal planes in the HRT.

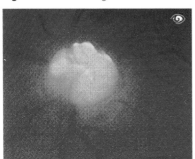

Fig. 6.21: Three-dimensional optic disc configuration, analyzed and decoded by HRT.

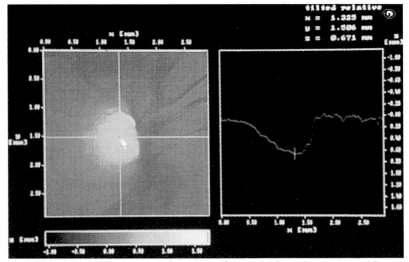

Fig. 6.22: Profile of a surface configuration of an optic disc using HRT, providing information about the excavation's shape and depth.

structures. To achieve a three-dimensional assessment, a so-called confocal technique is required. Such an instrument does not capture the entire amount of light reflected from a given spot (x/y) illuminated on the retina, but rather only measures the amount of light scattered from a certain plane, which is perpendicular to the z-axis. This is technically achieved by placing a confocal diaphragm in front of the detector [Lat. *detegere*: to uncover] (Fig. 6.19). Light that is reflected from a defined focal plane can pass through the diaphragm; light that is reflected either in front of – or behind – the focal plane becomes absorbed.

Confocal techniques thus provide reflected images from different focal planes (Fig. 6.20).

Because a series of these cross-sections from different planes resembles the series of pictures made with computer tomography, the term "laser scanning tomography" has come into use [Gr. *temnein*: to cut/Gr. *graphein*: to paint, to write]. The computer can reconstruct the three-dimensional configuration of a surface, in this case, the optic disc's surface, using these series of cross-sections and then print it out in a color code (Fig. 6.21). The results of the tomography can be visualized in different ways, such as in a profile of the papilla (Fig. 6.22) or along a circle surrounding the papilla. The computer is also able to quantify the size of certain areas, such as the neuroretinal rim. It is hoped that with this technique, glaucomatous damage can be detected at an earlier stage and changes at the papilla better followed over the years. However, this technology is not yet widely used and still cannot replace the optic disc assessment by an experienced ophthalmologist.

The pictures shown here have been taken with a HRT. Other instruments from different companies are also available.

6.4.3 Other Imaging Possibilities

The loss of nerve fibers (axons) that lead from the retinal surface to the optic disc is one component of glaucomatous atrophy. It would be helpful if these fibers or axons were directly visible, then the ophthalmologist could immediately determine whether – and to

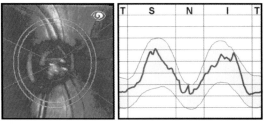

Fig. 6.23a: Nerve fibers shown as presented with a "Nerve Fiber Analyzer," which provides a color-coded image (left) and a graphic analysis (right).

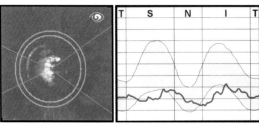

Fig. 6.23b: The same test done on an eye afflicted with glaucoma.

what extent – axonal loss had occurred. However, because the retina is transparent, this nerve fiber layer is difficult to identify. The retina must be transparent so that light can penetrate through it and reach the deeper layers where the photoreceptors (sensory cells) are located. Only the red-free light of the slit lamp permits the ophthalmologist to somewhat view the nerve fiber layer, but to assess it requires much experience.

Newer photographic techniques enable documentation of the nerve fiber layer. These pictures are taken in red-free (i.e. green) light with additional filters that enhance the contrast (cf. Figs. 2.2 and 2.3). However, these pictures are not easy to produce particularly when the patient has cataracts. But even under the best of circumstances, the interpretation of these pictures is challenging.

Another technique that employs the special features of polarized light has been introduced to assess the thickness of the nerve fiber layer. When polarized light hits a regularly structured surface (such as the nerve fiber layer), the light beam is split in two, thus causing the beams to oscillate perpendicularly to each other. The two light beams do not pass through the structure at the same velocity. The light passes through one polarization plane slower than the other ("retardation"). Since retardation is dependant on the thickness of the layer, a computer can estimate the thickness of the nerve fiber layer using the extent of retardation, and from this, produce a graphic image (once again using "artificial coloring"). The computer is also able to analyze cross-sections through the nerve layer. Figure 6.23a shows an image from a healthy 60-year-old person, and Figure 6.23b is from a 61-year-old glaucoma patient.

Because other tissues, primarily the cornea, have similar properties as the nerve fiber layer, the methods have been developed to automatically compensate the calculated nerve fiber layer thickness, thus rendering the measurement more precise.

There are also other available methods and instruments to measure the nerve fiber layer thickness. For example, projecting a green laser slit on the retina at an angle, and imaging of its intersection with the retina, yields the topographic thickness map of the retina. The distance between the vitreo-retinal and retina-retinal pigment reflections is directly proportional to the retinal thickness (the so called Retinal Thickness Analyzer). Another method, called optical coherence tomography (OCT), employs the basic imaging principle similar to the ultrasound B-Scan. Since, however, here the laser light is used instead of the ultrasound, the device compares and interferes the light backscattered from the retinal tissue with the reference light arm, and thus creates the picture based on the optical properties of the scanned tissue. Many such images combined yield a circumferential thickness of the retina adjacent to the optic nerve head (Fig 6.24).

6.5   Testing the Visual Field

Evaluation of the visual field is called perimetry [Gr. *peri*: about, around/Gr. *metrein*: to measure]. It is an important diagnostic tool in ophthalmology, not only for glaucoma, but also for a host of other diseases. There is thus an entire chapter (S 10) devoted to perimetry.

Perimetry plays a critical role in diagnosing glaucoma and in monitoring the disease's progression. Even though optic disc exami-

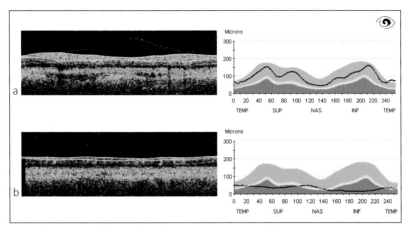

Fig. 6.24: Image of the peripapillary retina captured with ocular coherence tomography. The two white lines define the highly reflecting nerve fiber layer in a) healthy eye and b) glaucomatous eye. On the right, the graphic analysis of the nerve fiber layer thickness.

nation provides an indication of whether or not glaucoma is present, papillary assessment does not allow certain conclusions to be made about the patient's visual function. Only perimetry can provide this. Visual function is crucial for the patient: A defect in the visual field is annoying and (for example, when driving a car) even dangerous, but the size and shape of the papillary excavation, as such, is not. Furthermore, assessment of the optic disc often proves difficult and frequently only perimetry can render the actual diagnosis. Perimetry is of primary importance in analyzing the progression of changes. When a diagnosis is questionable, then the course the visual field takes over time is the only sure way to determine whether a visual field defect is due to glaucoma or whether it is a congenital anomaly. Because it is most difficult to follow the course of an advanced papillary excavation, perimetry is also quite useful here. Testing the visual field might strain the patient's time and energy but, nevertheless, it is well worth the effort. For example, it is essential to know whether a therapy has been able to stop further visual field loss or if the defects have progressed in spite of treatment. In the latter case, therapy must be changed.

Fig. 6.25: Glaucomatous visual field defect with loss of nerve fiber bundles.

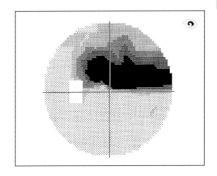

There are different programs that test the visual field and all have advantages and disadvantages. In general, the longer the examination, the more accurate the results. A slight degree of inaccuracy is not a problem in the diagnosis of many eye diseases. However, with glaucoma, where there is an urgency to detect even the slightest alterations over time, not being as precise as possible can have serious consequences. The most accurate perimetry possible is therefore recommended for the glaucoma patient. Naturally, there are exceptions to this rule: for patients who cannot cooperate for a certain amount of time due to old age or ailments, a shorter perimetry program for orientation purposes has to suffice.

How do typical glaucomatous visual field defects appear? There are defects that are quite specific (typical). When they are present, one can assume with a high degree of likelihood that glaucoma is present. This is the case with characteristic "nerve fiber bundle defects" (Fig. 6.25). These bundle-shaped defects are caused by the demise of one or several adjacent nerve fiber bundles.

Unfortunately, there are other non-specific defects in glaucoma that generally make it difficult to assess whether a visual field defect is due to glaucoma or to some other disease. Therefore, the optic disc and visual field have to be analyzed in relationship to each other. Examples of diffuse defects caused by glaucoma can be seen in Figure 6.26; and local, circumscribed defects (scotomata) in Figure 6.27. The results of a visual field test are depicted here on a "gray scale" and as a cumulative defect curve, also called a "Bebie curve," a graphic representation that allows easy recognition of diffuse versus

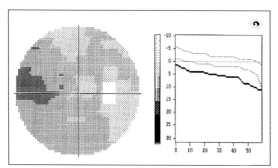

Fig. 6.26: Diffuse glaucomatous damage. On the left, shown in various shades of gray, and on the right, as a Bebie curve.

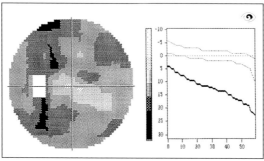

Fig. 6.27: Glaucomatous visual field defect with several scotomata.

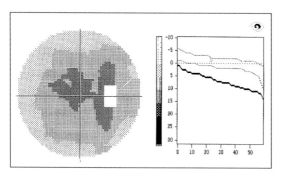

Fig. 6.28: Alterations of the visual field in a patient suffering from cataract.

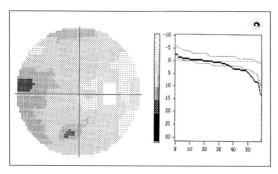

Fig. 6.29: Alterations of the visual field in an otherwise healthy person having a posterior-chamber lens.

local damage in relation to the age-adjusted normal values. Both will be described in detail in S 10.

In glaucoma, the type of the defect is less important than the total amount of tissue and functional loss. The latter is determined by a computer and designated as the "mean defect" (abbreviated MD). Nevertheless, the ophthalmologist will take a close look at the location and the extent of the defects as they appear on the computer's printout. The closer a defect is to the retina's center (the macula), the greater the threat to visual acuity. The patient subjectively perceives damage in this area as being particularly disturbing.

A glaucoma patient can, of course, have other eye diseases at the same time. In these cases, one important diagnostic objective is to distinguish between damage due to glaucoma and that related to other factors, such as cataracts, which cause diffuse visual field defects as well (Fig. 6.28).

Even after cataract surgery, the visual field is often slightly abnormal (Fig. 6.29), despite 20/20 visual acuity and without glaucoma. While the intraocular lens that is implanted during the procedure provides the patient with a clear and sharp macular vision, its optical capabilities with regard to the image projected onto the peripheral parts of the retina can't compare with those of the natural lens.

Some glaucoma patients also suffer from maculopathy (cf. S 9) that causes a central visual field defect. A patient afflicted with glaucoma and maculopathy at the same time is severely handicapped by this "dual attack." Glaucoma, in its initial stages, primarily affects the peripheral vision while the central vision is preserved. Maculopathy, on the other hand, reduces the central visual field. It is thus possible that the entire visual field of a patient having both diseases could be compromised.

It must be kept in mind that there can be considerable fluctuations in the outcome of the visual field tests of glaucoma patients. Repeating the test within a few hours or days might lead to very different results. One would suspect that this could be attributed to the patient, concentrating more on one occasion and less on the next. But this is rarely the case: good perimetry software analyzes the vis-

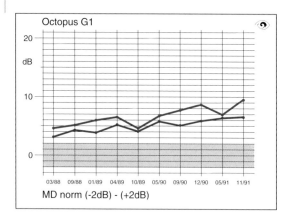

Fig. 6.30: Progression of the mean visual field defect (MD = Mean Defect). Right eye = red; left eye = blue.

ual fields relatively independently of the individual's capacity to co-operate (cf. S 10). The visual field variability is at least partly a result of changes in ocular blood flow. It is crucial to be aware of these fluctuations: one cannot just compare two test results and declare a definitive improvement or deterioration in the visual field. A complete series of tests is necessary to assess the long-term trend.

Figure 6.30 demonstrates such a trend using the mean defect index. A graphic representation such as is shown here explicitly depicts whether the visual field has stabilized or deteriorated over a longer period.

6.6   Assessing Ocular Perfusion

In Chapter 4, several factors were introduced that can contribute to glaucomatous damage. The most important risk factor is an increase in intraocular pressure. However, if the increased IOP does not explain the presence or the progression of glaucomatous damage, other risk factors must be investigated. Some risk factors can be influenced, others cannot. For example, age, gender and refractive error cannot be changed. But, at least to some degree, blood circulation, and thus ocular perfusion, can be influenced. This is why glaucoma research increasingly focuses on the latter.

The ophthalmologist asks questions whose answers provide

valuable information regarding the patient's blood circulation. For example, he might inquire as to whether the patient frequently suffers from cold hands and fingers (Fig. 6.31), or if he has low systemic blood pressure.

A look at the eye's conjunctival vessels provides additional information: alterations might be seen that are indicative, though not specific, for vascular dysregulation (Fig. 6.32). Of particular interest are also changes in retinal vessels, such as arterial constrictions or venous dilations. Shiny spots, also called gliosis-like alterations, on the retina are another sign of perfusion problems (Fig. 6.33).

However, a more precise measurement of ocular circulation is necessary as this provides parameters for following the disease progression and for ascertaining whether treatment has had a beneficial effect on the circulation.

Fig. 6.31: A warm hand (left) and a cold hand (right); the right picture shows a thermographic representation.

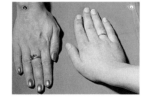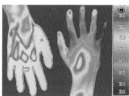

Fig. 6.32: Conjunctival blood vessels in a glaucoma patient having vascular dysregulations: vasodilations and vasoconstrictions are visible (→).

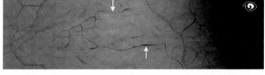

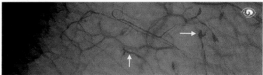

Fig. 6.33: Gliosis-like retinal changes (→): barely visible in a color picture (left), are easily seen in a picture taken with a laser scanner.

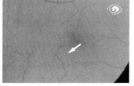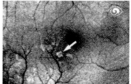

Several devices are currently available that measure different perfusion parameters. All these techniques have advantages and disadvantages, and these will be discussed in detail in Chapter S 11. For practical reasons, the presentation here is limited to four different methods that the authors, based on their clinical experience, consider particularly helpful in glaucoma. These include measuring the blood pressure, ultrasound assessment of ocular circulation, direct measurement of blood velocity in the capillaries (the smallest blood vessels) of the fingers, and finally, taking the corneal temperature.

6.6.1 Measuring Blood Pressure

Blood pressure plays an important role in medicine, but here the focus is on those aspects that are relevant for glaucoma.

As mentioned before, low blood pressure (arterial hypotension) is a crucial factor in the genesis of glaucomatous damage (cf. Chapter 4.2.7), while in most other fields of medicine, it is rather high blood pressure (hypertension) that is considered a problem. Since blood pressure depends on physical activity and shows circadian variations, one single measurement does not provide sufficient information. Added to this is the fact that people are often nervous and tend to have higher blood pressures when they go see the doctor. Under these circumstances, hypotension often remains undetected. A 24-hour monitoring has evolved as a helpful means in diagnosing low blood pressure and thus decreased ocular perfusion pressure (S 11).

Of special importance in glaucoma are:

a) A low blood pressure throughout the entire day. These patients have blood pressure – day and night – that is about 10–30 mmHg lower than a healthy person of the same age. A typical case is shown in Figure 6.34.

b) Fluctuations in the BP (Fig. 6.35). These are of even greater pathogenetic importance; this is especially true for nighttime "dips." Blood pressure levels can be normal or even increased at several points, but occasional abrupt dips occur, usually at night during deep sleep. Interestingly, also the glaucoma pa-

Fig. 6.34: Blood pressure curve of a glaucoma patient with a generally low BP, shown in red. For comparison, the blood pressure curve of a healthy person is shown in gray.

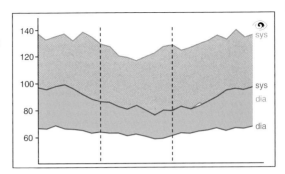

Fig. 6.35: Blood pressure curve of a glaucoma patient (red) with severe nightly dips (the gray shows the blood pressure curve in a healthy individual).

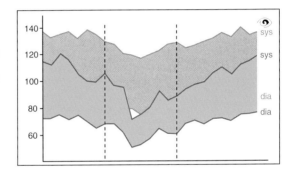

Fig. 6.36: Blood pressure when changing from a lying to a standing position. The curve of a healthy person (top) and of a patient with orthostatic hypotension (bottom).

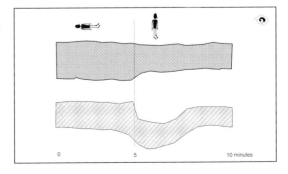

tients that do not exhibit a nighttime BP decrease at all, the so-called non-dippers, are at the increased risk of glaucomatous damage.

c) A severe drop in blood pressure when rising to an upright position after lying down (orthostatic hypotension). Figure 6.36 shows the different patterns of blood pressure adjustment during positional change in a healthy person and in a patient suffering from orthostatic hypotension.

Not every person with a low systemic blood pressure will necessarily develop glaucomatous damage. The likelihood increases, however, if low blood pressure is combined with an increased IOP and/or vascular dysregulation. Vascular dysregulation implies there is an impaired ability to adapt to low blood pressure values (cf. S 8). When blood pressure decreases, ocular vessels in a healthy individual react with vasodilation to ensure a constant perfusion (called autoregulation). This adjustment to changing circumstances does not function adequately in patients having vascular dysregulation. This leads to a transient decrease in the ocular perfusion and to those changes discussed in Chapter 5.

6.6.2 Capillary Microscopy

Many studies have contributed to the current knowledge that ocular perfusion is often impaired in glaucoma patients. Despite the availability of modern technology, measuring ocular perfusion still leaves many questions unanswered. However, there is ample evidence that certain similarities do exist between perfusion in the body's periphery – such as the fingertips – and ocular perfusion. These parallels are especially pronounced in patients having vascular dysregulation (cf. S 8). This is why a glaucoma patient's perfusion is also measured at the capillaries of the nailfold. If perfusion is reduced here, then there is a high probability that it is also reduced in the eye. As stated in Chapter 4.2.7, circulatory problems in glaucoma patients are rarely caused by arteriosclerotic alterations, but rather are usually the result of vascular dysregulation. To assess the degree of dysregulation, certain provocation tests are performed. For example, patients with vascular dysregulation react to stimuli, such as cold or emotional stress, with a constriction of the smallest blood vessels. This can be monitored with a technique called capillary microscopy that will be described in S 11. Unfortunately, it is extremely difficult to measure the effect of psychological stress that happens in daily life situations. In an emotional crisis, the patient is not available right then and there for immediate perfusion measurements. On the other hand, one can monitor the reaction to cold: If a patient has an interruption of capillary blood flow for more than 11 seconds following a cold stimulus, then this is considered proof that vascular dysregulation is present.

6.6.3 Color Doppler Sonography

Color Doppler sonography, described in S 11, is used in glaucoma patients to determine the blood velocity in several vessels leading to the eye. This enables a calculation of the resistance index, a parameter for downstream resistance to flow that is of particular importance in glaucoma. Figure 6.37 shows data from the ophthalmic artery of a healthy individual; Figure 6.38 the results from the same test in a glaucoma patient with reduced ocular perfusion.

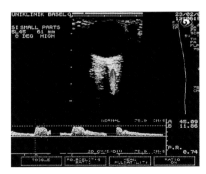

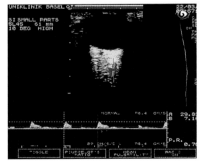

Fig. 6.37: Color duplex sonography of the ophthalmic artery of a healthy person.

Fig. 6.38: Color duplex sonography of the ophthalmic artery of a glaucoma patient.

6.6.4 Measuring Temperature

One of the oldest means of assessing perfusion in medicine is temperature measurement. For example, when there is decreased perfusion in one foot, it is considerably colder than the other. Temperature can thus serve as an indirect indicator of perfusion.

A simple instrument has been developed that measures the temperature of the eye without touching it (S 11). Initial studies indicate that the eye's temperature provides a quite reliable indication as to the quality of its perfusion. The value of this information can be further enhanced by a provocation test: Directing a cold stream of air towards the eye's surface leads to a short-term decrease in the temperature. This cooling down period and the time it takes to return to the original temperature provide another measure of ocular perfusion. It is not yet known whether this simple principle will prove valuable over the long term or will ever become routine in daily ophthalmological practice.

Not all glaucoma patients suffer from poor perfusion. Some patients vacillate between perfusion that is adequate and then decreased. Measuring normal blood flow at any given time is no guarantee that disturbance is not present and manifesting itself, at another time. Therefore, any test that evaluates blood flow and perfusion has to be repeated many times if data remain inconclusive. Blood flow parameters provide valuable indications about the origins of glaucomatous damage and which treatment possibilities would be prudent.

6.7 Special Examinations

Certain functional losses occur relatively frequently among glaucoma patients. These include problems with adaptation to darkness, color vision, and glare, etc.

These disturbances are seldom investigated in depth because they rarely affect the ophthalmologist's decision-making process. The critical decision – does the patient need therapy, and if so, which is best and how intense should it be – depends on the appearance of the optic disc, the visual field, the IOP situation and the circulatory parameters. It is nevertheless important to know that there are additional functional losses in glaucoma. If a patient is aware that these problems may appear, he is then better equipped to deal with them and perhaps will not be overly concerned. However, as mentioned above, they are not routinely investigated in depth.

6.7.1 Dark Adaptation

The ability of the eye to adjust to different levels of light is called adaptation, and this can be measured. There is both light adaptation and dark adaptation. With regard to glaucoma, dark adaptation is more important. On a moonlit night, the surrounding light is perceived as being about a hundred times less bright than on a sunny day. But, in reality, it is about 10,000,000 times darker. The impression that the intensity of light is reduced by "just" a factor of 100 is due to the eye's ability to adjust its sensitivity to the actual brightness. This adaptation requires a certain amount of time. This is easily observed whenever a dark room or a tunnel is entered. After a few minutes, the darkness seems less complete and objects are easier to discern than when the darkness was first entered.

During an adaptation test, patients sit in the dark and a barely visible light becomes brighter and brighter until the patient can recognize it – then the brightness is reduced until it seems to disappear. This test is then repeated within a half minute. As time goes by, the eye adapts (becomes more sensitive) and the patient is able to see increasingly weaker sources of light.

The sensitivity and the degree of light necessary for perception are graphically illustrated in Figure 6.39. Normal values are age-dependent. The ability to adapt to darkness gradually decreases after the third decade of life. There are patients whose dark adaptation is severely impaired, for instance, those suffering from retinitis pigmentosa (Fig. 6.39). In these cases, characterized by "night blindness," the evaluation of dark adaptation is particularly important. Dark adaptation can also be impaired in glaucoma patients and they should be aware of this. But, dark adaptation is rarely tested in glaucoma since the result does not influence the therapeutic approach.

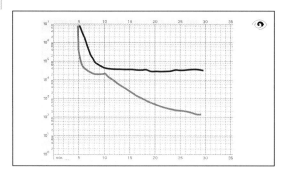

Fig. 6.39: Measuring dark adaptation: The deeper the curve dips, the higher the sensitivity to light. The green line is from a healthy individual, the blue from a patient with disturbed adaptation.

6.7.2 Color Vision

The human eye is not only able to distinguish between light and dark, it also differentiates between spots located close to each other, registers movement, and is also capable of perceiving a variety of colors. Color vision is a complex and intriguing process. For centuries, man has questioned the nature of colors and how they are perceived. Indeed, both Newton and Goethe conducted intensive research in color vision and each created his own theories to explain it. It is now known that there are two different kinds of retinal receptor cells, cones and rods. The cones are specialized in color vision. Three different subgroups of cones exist, each having a peak sensitivity at a certain wavelength. Based on the relation of these three basic colors to each other, the brain "reconstructs" the entire spectrum of colors. In congenital color blindness, one or even two of these specialized cone pigments are lacking. Because the retina can be considered as part of the brain (cf. S 1 and S 2), it is not surprising that incoming information is already processed here: the retina compares the signals that various receptors are receiving. The message that is finally delivered to the visual cortex has been adjusted to the intensity of these incoming signals. Several diseases that result in "acquired color vision defects" can disturb this complex system. These defects, which are quite common, can occur, for example, in diabetics but also in individuals suffering from glaucoma. They are of particular interest in glaucoma because they can precede the

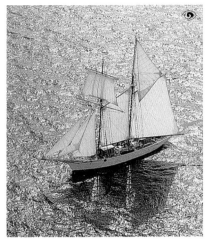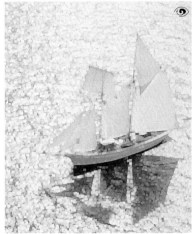

Fig. 6.40: A patient with reduced contrast sensitivity might see the boat in the left picture but not in the right.

"classical" visual field defects by several years. On the other hand, it is known that color vision defects in glaucoma are usually associated with diffuse visual field loss. Such diffuse visual field defects can be identified by modern automated perimetry (cf. S 10). This is why color vision is rarely tested in glaucoma. For the patient, however, it is essential to know that problems with color vision (in situations such as buying clothes, etc.) can be caused by glaucoma.

6.7.3 Contrast Sensitivity

When checking the visual acuity, one attempts to find out the smallest distance between two points or two lines that the eye can still distinguish as being separate. Contrast sensitivity is defined as the ability to discriminate between various shades of brightness. Imagine a sailboat on a foggy lake (Fig. 6.40). In order to discern the white sails from the surrounding mist, there must be a certain difference in brightness between the two objects, and this perception of the difference is called contrast sensitivity. There is much variation in contrast sensitivity among individuals. Certain diseases reduce this sensitivity, for example, diabetes mellitus and glaucoma. Just as with problems of color vision, these disturbances occur primarily in cases where there is a diffuse visual field loss. Correctly performed perimetry will identify these defects, and there is thus no need for additional testing of contrast sensitivity. But, once again, it is important that the glaucoma patient be aware of this change. Under certain circumstances, such as reading with insufficient illumination, the glaucoma patient will have more difficulties than a healthy person. This is why glaucoma patients prefer to read with all the lights turned on: there is an enhancement of the text's contrast.

6.7.4 Glare

Even healthy people are occasionally bothered by glare. For example, when driving a car with dirty windshields, oncoming headlights appear blinding. This phenomenon will be explained in S 5.

There is also a form of glare that is not caused by opacification, but rather is the result of disturbed information processing in the retina. The retina perceives light and is also specialized in identifying even slightly differing degrees of brightness (S 1). A nerve cell does not just report to the brain how bright its field of perception is, but rather how bright it is in relation to the surroundings. This information is the result of many enhancements and inhibitions. If this process is impaired and particularly when the mechanisms of inhibition are not adequately functioning, the subjective perception of light increases and the patient is blinded. Abnormal sensitivity to light is a symptom of several retinal diseases. This impression of being blinded is quite disturbing for the patient and may be due to advanced glaucomatous damage.

6.7.5 ERG

Both the retina and its underlying layer, the pigment epithelium, produce electrical fields. Short flashes of light can change these fields. A test known as electroretinography (ERG) documents these changes in the retina's electric fields. ERG is an important tool in diagnosing certain diseases of the retina, such as the previously men-

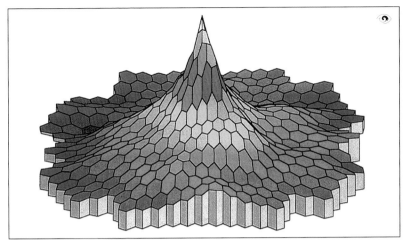

Fig. 6.41: Three-dimensional representation of the results of a multifocal ERG made in a healthy person.

tioned retinitis pigmentosa. In glaucoma, there can be ERG defects as well, but this procedure is not that useful in diagnosing glaucoma, thus explaining why this test is usually not performed.

Modern state-of-the-art instruments can perform an ERG on specific parts of the retina, thus providing a quantifiable and graphic representation of this area. Figure 6.41 depicts the results of such a measurement. In the center of this field is the macula, the "spot of the best vision."

6.7.6 VEP

Visually evoked potentials, abbreviated VEP, are electric potentials that can be measured above the visual cortex in the occipital part of the skull. Small electrodes register the fluctuations in the electric fields produced by the brain. When light falls onto the eye, there are changes in these potentials above the visual cortex, but with a delay of about 1/10 of a second. Deducing VEPs is helpful in diagnosing a host of diseases, including multiple sclerosis (MS). The arrival of these changes in potentials and thus the "reaction" of the visual cortex can be delayed, and this is termed latency extension.

This is not uncommon in glaucoma but, once again, it is not a critical factor in making the diagnosis and therefore not routinely evaluated. Nevertheless, VEPs are occasionally performed if, for some reason, the visual field cannot be tested.

Currently new types of ERG testing are in evaluation in the field of glaucoma, the so-called pattern ERG in which a checkerboard pattern is projected onto the retina and thus a predominantly ganglion cell response recorded and analyzed.

Utilizing similar principle as in multifocal ERG, a multifocal VEP can be recorded as a form of objective visual field testing. This method is also still in the experimental phase.

6.8   Blood Chemistry

Checking the patient's blood for parameters specific for glaucoma is a concept that is still in its infancy, but its importance will certainly increase in coming years.

The blood sedimentation rate has long been tested in cases of giant cell arteritis (also called temporal arteritis), an inflammatory vascular disease that also frequently involves the eye. In some rare cases, this has a limited significance for glaucoma because giant cell arteritis causes ocular damage that resembles the symptoms of classical glaucoma.

Blood of increased viscosity can occasionally lead to circulatory problems. Blood viscosity [Lat. *viscum*: mistletoe, a plant with a thick (viscous) juice] is measured when there is some suspicion. An increased hematocrit indirectly indicates an increased viscosity. The hematocrit is the percentage of cellular components in the whole blood (in contrast to the liquid or serum portion). In certain diseases where there is a high hematocrit, doctors occasionally resort to the ancient method of bloodletting. Through the loss of blood, the viscosity is lowered and the blood again flows more easily.

Determining the level of endothelin in the blood is helpful in glaucoma patients. Endothelin is a protein produced inside the blood vessels' endothelial cells and is a key factor in regulating vessel diameter. Slightly increased levels of endothelin point to primary vascular dysregulation, while very high levels indicate secondary vascular dysregulation as seen, for example, in certain autoimmune diseases [Gr. *autos*: self/Lat. *immunus*: not susceptible to].

Glaucomatous damage or perfusion problems may lead to somewhat characteristic changes in white blood cells (leukocytes). Leukocytes and a subspecies of leukocytes, lymphocytes, are activated whenever damage occurs inside the body. Our studies on the gene expression in lymphocytes provide fascinating information about cause and stage of the disease. However, this information is not yet applicable in a routine diagnostic procedure.

Summary

Particularly in the early stages of the disease, diagnosing glaucomatous damage is quite challenging. It is especially dependent on the analysis of the optic disc and the visual field. Perimetry (evaluation of the visual field) is most important for assessing the disease's progression. The ophthalmologist also investigates risk factors, for example, by measuring the intraocular pressure and monitoring the anterior chamber angle for gauging the risk of angle closure. If a perfusion problem is suspected of playing a role in the development of damage, the circulation will be thoroughly investigated and, if possible, quantified. Suitable methods are the measurement of blood pressure, color duplex sonography and capillary microscopy. Though other tests are interesting as they provide an indication of other impairments possible in glaucoma, they are not routinely performed because they do not contribute significantly to the diagnosis and evaluation of the actual disease progression. Additional loss of function can appear in the form of disturbed dark adaptation, color vision, contrast sensitivity, or as an increased glare; it may also show up in electrophysiological tests, such as ERG and VEP.

7 Therapy

This book has gone into quite some detail explaining glaucomatous damage, how it arises and methods for its detection. A precise diagnosis is a pre-requisite for an appropriate and goal-directed therapy. Fortunately, many effective therapeutic options are available for patients having glaucoma. Severe and progressive loss of vision due to this disease that could eventually lead to total blindness can almost always be prevented with timely and proper treatment plus the patient's cooperation.

7.1 General Remarks Regarding Treatment Options

As discussed in the introductory chapter (Chapter 1.3), glaucoma is characterized by nerve cell loss. When cells of the central nervous system die, nature does not provide a replacement; this is a fundamental difference to other types of cells, e.g. muscle, bone, and skin. Indeed, this means that glaucomatous damage, once present, cannot be healed or reversed.

However, with regard to visual field defects, there is a slight chance for a limited recovery. This could happen when certain nerve cells no longer function properly but are not yet dead. When conditions improve, it is possible that these nerve fibers can mend to some extent. In this case, part of the visual field loss can be recovered. There is intense research underway investigating ways to stimulate renewed growth in nerve cells. Perhaps in the distant future, a reversibility of damage will be possible but, for the moment, therapeutic endeavors center on the prevention of glaucomatous damage. If damage is already present, the effort is directed at stopping further progression. Preventing the development and deterioration of nerve fiber loss is largely possible when the risk factors are tightly controlled. The attempt to safeguard the nerve cells in spite of the risk factors is termed "neuroprotection," and it is well possible that a major research breakthrough in this area is just around the corner. However, for the moment, the focus is still on "fighting" the risk factors.

7.1.1 Avoiding Risk Factors

Modern medicine has identified the risk factors for a host of diseases, and in many cases, means to neutralize, counteract or offset them. In the introduction, the example of a heart attack was mentioned. It is known that a high level of serum lipids is a major risk factor for arteriosclerosis and thus for heart attacks, but specific measures can be taken to influence these lipids in a positive way, including a healthy diet and physical activity. If the lipid level cannot be satisfactorily lowered by these dietary and lifestyle changes, the physician will also prescribe medication.

Even though knowledge of the risk factors for glaucoma has increased during the past few years, only a few of these can currently be influenced by behavior modification. The main risk factor for glaucoma is an elevated intraocular pressure. To date, there are no known behavior changes that can be exploited to reduce or prevent an IOP rise. Patients frequently ask, "What have I done wrong?" or "What can I do to lower the eye pressure?" Perhaps in the future, a satisfactory answer can be provided but, for the moment, options are still limited. Severe psychological stress can increase the IOP. Even though stress is a part of daily life, if it becomes overwhelming, measures should be undertaken to reduce it. Drinking a large amount of fluid in just a short time can create an IOP spike. Glaucoma patients should drink adequate amounts of fluids, but these should be distributed throughout the day.

Some patients experience an IOP rise that is dependent upon the body's position. In these rare cases, sleeping in a slightly upright position is recommended. In patients having pigment dispersion glaucoma (cf. Chapter 3.6.1.2), physical activity can trigger an IOP rise. Even in these cases, there are preventive measures that can be discussed with the ophthalmologist.

Naturally, it would be wonderful if certain ways of life could be recognized as being helpful in preventing an IOP increase, but this is not yet possible. Nevertheless, the following recommendations are made because they lead to a healthier lifestyle that is, in general, beneficial: get plenty of sleep, adequate exercise, a diet rich in vitamins and low in fat, avoid too much animal fat, eat fruits and vegetables daily, eat fish at least once a week, don't smoke and keep weight under control. Trying to lead a personal and professional life that is free from major psychological stress is also healthy. Individuals who can't achieve this on their own should contact a professional counselor for help in stress management.

Some factors, such as age, race and gender, cannot be counteracted. For other factors, such as the vasospastic syndrome, treatments are available. Vasospastic individuals frequently suffer from cold hands and low blood pressure. Both are signs of vascular dysregulation that can, to a certain degree, be influenced by changes in one's daily lifestyle (cf. S 8), including: increasing physical activity, eating a healthy diet, drinking plenty of water, using adequate amounts of salt, etc.

Fortunately, there are proven methods to prevent glaucomatous damage. The most important of these is seeing an ophthalmologist in time: Starting at the age of 40, eye examinations should take place at least once every five years. If there is a suspicion of incipient glaucoma, these intervals must be shorter. An even earlier initial visit (younger than 40) to the ophthalmologist is recommended if there is a family history of glaucoma or if other risk factors exist. Treatment will be initiated when the ophthalmologist discovers signs of glaucomatous damage or when the IOP rises above 25 mmHg.

7.1.2 The Therapy Spectrum

In theory, there are three different, but complementary, strategies for preventing damage. First, there is the lowering and stabilization of the IOP; second, improvement and stabilization of ocular perfusion; and third, neuroprotection, i.e. protecting the nerve cells from damaging mechanisms. All ophthalmologists agree that decreasing IOP is crucial, however, not all acknowledge the importance of ocular perfusion and its treatment. Neuroprotection has been investigated in animal experiments and the results are most interesting, but only time will tell whether this will eventually lead to treatment options in humans.

> Intraocular pressure can be reduced by:
> a) medication; b) laser treatment; and c) surgery.

The order in which these options are used may differ among treating physicians. Among ophthalmologists, there are various opinions about therapeutic strategies and which of these options should act as a "first line of defense." In most cases, drugs are initially employed to try to bring the IOP back to normal. If this does not prove effective, most patients will undergo surgery. But there are other schools of thought that recommend surgery first and then resorting to medical therapy if the operation has been unsuccessful. Another group of ophthalmologists even prefers laser treatment as a first step. Statistical data indicate that the prognosis for the visual field is slightly better with a surgically lowered IOP than with a purely conservative (drug) treatment. Nevertheless, in most cases, a pharmacological IOP reduction is first tried because of the inherent risk associated with any operation. Correspondingly, the question arises, "Are there any disadvantages to waiting with the surgery?" As long as the drugs are well-tolerated, medical therapy can continue if it sufficiently reduces the IOP and the damage present is neither extensive nor shows signs of progression. Nevertheless, after long-term medication, there is an increased risk of fibrosis and scarring after filtration surgery (cf. Chapter 7.4). This, in turn, means a higher risk for a recurrence of an increased IOP after surgery. But this danger is fortunately no longer a major concern in modern glaucoma surgery; scarring can now usually be prevented by administering certain drugs (e.g. mitomycin C) during the operation.

7.1.3 Glaucoma Therapy and the Quality of Life

The fundamental goal of each medical procedure is to provide an improvement in the quality of the patient's life. For many diseases, the link between quality of life and therapy is quite obvious. A patient suffering from painful rheumatoid arthritis relies on drugs to ease the pain and thus enhance the quality of life. At the same time, the doctors will try to change the course of the disease in such a way that, in the long term, fewer joint deformations occur.

From a psychological point of view, the situation with glaucoma is more difficult. A glaucoma patient does not suffer (the exception to this rule being the acute attack), either from the risk factors or from damage in its early stages. The objective of therapy, therefore, is not so much melioration of the current quality of life but rather to maintain this quality of life for the coming years or decades. A slight decrease in the current quality of life must occasionally be accepted to achieve this long-term goal.

Diagnosis and commencement of therapy can affect the current quality of life in different ways: Even the diagnosis itself can be stressful for some patients, as can the frequent appointments required and the time-consuming tests. A newly initiated therapy might have side effects. Additionally, it is possible that the visual acuity is poorer for some time after surgery (Fig. 7.1).

In close collaboration, the physician and the patient must evaluate the advantages and disadvantages of the various treatment options. However, the ultimate decision rests with the patient. In the final analysis, the patient must assess the weight of today's burdens for preserving tomorrow's vision. Such a decision depends on several factors, one of which is certainly life expectancy. If chances are small that the damage will play a significant role in the patient's life, both physician and patient are less willing to accept major incon-

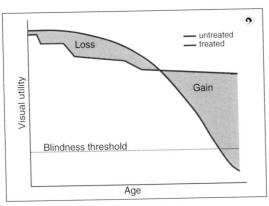

Fig. 7.1: Glaucoma surgery might reduce the vision for a short period, but enhances the long-term prognosis.

veniences. Hence, glaucoma therapy in elderly patients with a mild and slowly progressing damage has to be less aggressive than in a younger individual with a pronounced or rapidly progressing damage. A type of effort-to-benefit analysis must be made.

There are no general rules that universally apply as to when is the right time to start therapy or how intense its level should be. Ophthalmologist and patient must together seek the practical solution for each individual case. During the course of the disease, it might become necessary to reassess or even change the treatment goals.

7.1.4 Treatment Goals

The ophthalmologist's main goal is, of course, to preserve the patient's sight throughout life. To achieve this primary goal, secondary goals must be identified and targeted; in a glaucoma patient, these include the stabilization of the visual field. In this context, the term "target pressure" can be defined as that IOP level where it is least likely that pressure-related damage either occurs or progresses. There is not just one rigid target pressure that applies to everyone, but rather it is assessed specifically for each individual. The lower the IOP level where damage occurs, the lower the target pressure has to be. This is likewise the case when there is already advanced glaucomatous damage or if damage is progressing rapidly [Lat. *progredere*: advance]. There are several other factors that also must be considered so that, in the final analysis, the defining of target pressure is always a judgment call.

Once again, it should be emphasized that major IOP fluctuations are at least as damaging as an elevated mean pressure. Thus, the stabilization of intraocular pressure is an equally essential goal.

7.2 IOP-Lowering Medication

One fundamental rule that applies to this topic specifies that, when a medical therapy is initiated, it is imperative that the patient regularly use the eyedrops. If there are any questions about a drug or

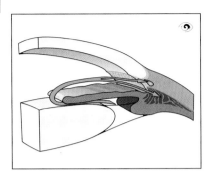

Fig. 7.2: Drugs lower the IOP by reducing aqueous humor production or by facilitating the outflow.

its application, the patient should not hesitate to ask his physician or pharmacist. Other physicians involved in a patient's care (such as the family practitioner) should also be informed about the glaucoma medication prescribed. If a hospital stay is planned, the patient should take the eye medication with him. However, some hospitals insist on administering all drugs; in this case, the staff must be informed of the glaucoma treatment.

Several new glaucoma medications have been introduced during the past few years, but options still remain rather limited. There are several classes of drugs that lower the IOP, but only a few are suitable for long-term treatment. This is explained in more detail in S 12. The drugs currently available decrease intraocular pressure by reducing aqueous humor production or by facilitating its outflow (Fig. 7.2).

Some of these drugs improve trabecular meshwork outflow, others primarily affect the uveoscleral outflow (cf. S 1).

Intraocular pressure is partly regulated by the autonomic nervous system. Drugs that either mimic or inhibit the effect of these nerves can influence the IOP. Within the autonomic nervous system, there is a parasympathetic and a sympathetic nervous system. Stimulation of the parasympathetic nervous system by so-called cholinergic drugs leads to an IOP reduction. In the sympathetic nervous system, things are a bit more complicated: both stimulating and inhibiting substances can decrease intraocular pressure [Gr. *sympathein*: to sympathize with/Gr. *para*: next to, beside].

7.2.1 Parasympathomimetic Agents/ Cholinergic Agents

The messenger substance (neurotransmitter) released by the nerve cell endings is called acetylcholine. Drugs that mimic the effect of acetylcholine are called cholinergic [Gr. *ergon*: action] agents or parasympathomimetics [Gr. *mimetein*: to mimic]. In theory, one could apply acetylcholine directly into the eye. But acetylcholine is rapidly hydrolyzed (inactivated) by the body, forcing scientists to search for other substances that have the same effect but exert their influence over a longer period. These parasympathomimetic agents are the oldest anti-glaucoma drugs, and one, pilocarpine, was used in glaucoma therapy as early as 1876.

7.2.1.1 Pilocarpine

Pilocarpine is the most important drug from among the cholinergic agents. It is a so-called alkaloid, that is, a basic component produced by plants. Other well-known alkaloids include morphine and codeine. Pilocarpine is an alkaloid harvested from the leaves of *Pilocarpus tennatifolius*, a type of fig that grows in South America (cf. Fig. 7.3).

It is available as eyedrops and ointment, administered in concentrations ranging from 0.5% to 3%, and easily penetrates into the eye. About half an hour after application, the IOP starts to drop, and the lowering effect lasts between four to eight hours. The medication must thus be administered at least three – but often four – times a day.

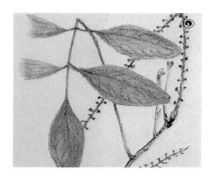

Fig. 7.3: Branch of a pilocarpine bush.

There are several ways to reduce the need for frequent administrations. With a small device called Ocusert®, the pilocarpine is enclosed within a polymer from which it is gradually, but continuously, released during a period of a few days. The pilocarpine polymer is an emulsion of a polymeric (i.e. composed of numerous molecules) substance that binds the drug. The polymer is slowly hydrolyzed, i.e. water is taken up by the substance and pilocarpine gradually released.

With pilocarpine gel, the agent is bound to a gel of high viscosity. Even though only once-a-day administration is required, this form has gained little popular acceptance.

Pilocarpine – usually in a low concentration – is a component of the standard therapy when there is a risk of angle-closure glaucoma due to the plateau iris mechanism (cf. Chapter 3.5.1.2). If the anterior chamber angle is occluded by a pupillary block mechanism, however, pilocarpine can be counterproductive and – though rare – can trigger an acute glaucoma attack. Pilocarpine has long been the treatment of choice in open-angle glaucoma, but today, it is relegated to a second-line drug status.

Ophthalmologists have considerable experience with pilocarpine; it rarely causes allergies and is quite inexpensive. It reduces the IOP by facilitating aqueous humor outflow. Cholinergic agents induce a contraction of the inner eye muscles that are innervated by the parasympathetic system (cf. S 1). This leads to ciliary muscle contraction and to pupillary miosis [Gr. *miosis*: diminution]. While the constricted pupil can be regarded as an undesirable side effect, the ciliary muscle contraction leads to an opening of the trabecular meshwork. The fundamental improvement takes place precisely where the main problem lies with open-angle glaucoma, i.e. at the reduced trabecular outflow. Unfortunately, the cholinergic agents do have quite a few significant adverse effects. The miosis that is evoked can be quite bothersome to the patient, especially when going from a light environment to a dark. Furthermore, the contraction of the ciliary muscles results in an undesired accommodation (the eye sees only near objects clearly), which is particularly disturbing to young people with intact accommodation functioning (accommodation decreases with age due to many causes; elderly people thus tolerate treatment with miotics much better than younger patients). At the start of therapy or when administered in higher concentrations, cholinergic agents, due to the muscle contractions they trigger, may cause pain.

A higher frequency of retinal detachment among myopics following pilocarpine therapy has been reported. This is not supported by the authors' observations; indeed, it must be kept in mind that myopia itself is a risk factor for retinal detachment. One additional caveat: Caution is recommended for asthmatic patients because, in rare cases, pilocarpine can trigger an asthmatic attack.

7.2.1.2 Aceclidine

Aceclidine, which is available in a 2% solution, has a similar effect to pilocarpine but has a weaker influence on accommodation.

7.2.1.3 Carbachol

Carbachol, available in concentrations ranging between 1.5% and 3%, is similar to pilocarpine, but is a bit more effective in reducing the IOP. Unfortunately, it does have more pronounced adverse reactions, and thus pilocarpine is preferred to carbachol.

7.2.2 Sympathomimetic Agents

As explained, the autonomic nervous system consists of a sympathetic and a parasympathetic system. Substances that mimic or enhance the effects of the sympathetic nervous system are called sympathomimetic agents. Adrenaline (also known as epinephrine), which circulates in the body's bloodstream, is just such an agent. Therefore, another name for this group of drugs is adrenergic agents.

Sympathetic nerve fibers end on signal receptors located on the various target organs that they innervate. There are both alpha and beta receptors (Fig. 7.4). Non-specific sympathomimetic agents, such as epinephrine or adrenaline, stimulate alpha and beta receptors. There are also other drugs (such as clonidine) that stimulate only alpha receptors and, in particular, one specific subtype, namely, alpha-2 receptors.

7.2.2.1 Epinephrine (Adrenaline)

Epinephrine, also called adrenaline, is a hormone that circulates in the blood. It is produced in the medulla (core) of the adrenal gland [Lat. *ren*: kidney/Lat. *adreno*: belonging to the kidney/Gr. *nephros*: kidney/Gr. *epinephron*: above the kidney, i.e. meaning the adrenal gland]. One hundred years ago, this substance was first used to reduce the IOP by subconjunctival injection. Since 1920, epinephrine eyedrops have been available for glaucoma therapy. Because epinephrine quickly oxidizes upon exposure to light, it gained widespread use as a drug only after it could be stabilized with antioxidants.

Despite years of research, the exact mechanism by which epinephrine works is still unknown. It is presumed that epinephrine facilitates aqueous humor outflow by stimulating alpha-receptors. Aqueous humor production is probably not reduced but rather is temporarily increased due to a stimulation of beta-receptors. But because this latter effect is much less significant than the outflow enhancement, the final result of epinephrine administration is an IOP reduction. Epinephrine is administered in concentrations ranging between 0.25% and 2.0%, and must be instilled three times a day. Because it can cause acute angle-closure in patients with plateau iris (cf. Chapter 3.5.1.2), its use is restricted to open-angle glaucoma.

Epinephrine acts as a vasoconstrictor, i.e. it leads to a constriction of blood vessels. Immediately after the eyedrops are instilled, the conjunctiva looks pale; some time later, due to some counteracting mechanism, the conjunctiva turns red. Some patients complain of recurrent "red eyes." Rarely, it even leads to chronic conjunctivitis. In patients who have had a cataract operation which removes the natural lens, macular edema can develop because local drugs diffuse more easily to the back of the eye. Therefore, adrenaline can induce macular edema.

Since epinephrine is a vasoconstrictor, it is not administered to patients who suffer from primary perfusion problems of the eye.

If circulation is normal and the lens is still in place, epinephrine might be used to lower the IOP. Nevertheless, it is a second-line drug because other medications are now available that are associated with fewer side effects. Among its systemic adverse effects are tachycardia (i.e. rapid heart rate), disturbances of the heart rhythm and an increase in systemic blood pressure.

7.2.2.2 Dipivefrin

Dipivefrin, a pro-drug [Lat. *pro*: pre, for] of epinephrine (or adrenaline), has been developed because the clinical usefulness of epinephrine is limited by local side effects. A pro-drug is an agent, in this case epinephrine, that is coupled with another molecule and which exerts its pharmacological effect only after the two components have been "de-coupled." With dipivefrin, epinephrine enters the eye as a pro-drug. Inside the eye, the accompanying molecule is removed and the drug is released. This mode of penetration has the advantage of bringing the epinephrine to the site where it is needed and thus reduces the frequency of side effects as well as conjunctival redness. Nevertheless, the intraocular adverse effects, such as macular edema, remain the same. Dipivefrin is administered twice daily in a 0.1% concentration. Just like epinephrine, it is a "reserve" drug.

Alpha-Selective Adrenergic Agents (i.e. Agonists). As already explained, fibers of the sympathetic nervous system terminate on alpha and beta-receptors, both of which can be further differentiated into subtypes. There are alpha-1 and alpha-2 receptors, as shown in Figure 7.4. Alpha-1 receptors are located on the target organ that the nerve innervates, such as a muscle cell. This is called a post-synaptic location, a synapse being the point of contact between two nerve cells or between a nerve cell and an "effector." Alpha-2 receptors are located both pre- and post-synaptically, i.e. both on the end of nerves and on the adjoining effector cell. Stimulation of pre-synaptic alpha receptors inhibit the release of noradrenaline, a messenger of the sympathetic nervous system. These receptors act to ultimately weaken the sympathetic activity.

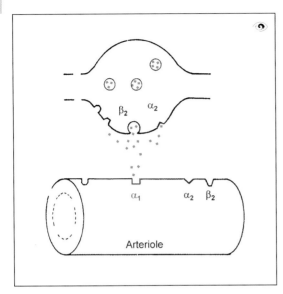

Fig. 7.4: Norepinephrine (green) is released at the sympathetic synapse. Stimulation of alpha-1 receptors leads to vasoconstriction, while stimulation of the presynaptic alpha-2 receptors results in reduced adrenaline release.

There are drugs that primarily stimulate alpha-2 receptors, while having only a minor effect on alpha-1 receptors. Depending on which effect is stronger, these drugs act as sympathomimetic (promoting the sympathetic system) or as sympatholytic (inhibiting the sympathetic system) agents. In glaucoma therapy, alpha-2 selective medications are generally used, including drugs such as clonidine, apraclonidine and brimonidine.

A contraindication for the administration of all alpha-type agonists is anti-depressant treatment with orally administered MAO-inhibitors.

7.2.2.3 Clonidine

Clonidine was originally developed as a decongestant due to its ability to cause vasoconstriction of the nasal mucosa, but its blood pressure lowering effect was soon recognized. In 1962, it was introduced onto the market as an anti-hypertensive drug (i.e. an agent that lowers systemic blood pressure). It was later noted that clonidine was also capable of reducing intraocular pressure. Since

1972, clonidine drops have been available in a limited number of countries for topical administration. Clonidine is applied three or four times a day in concentrations ranging from 0.125% to 0.5%. The mechanism of action (how it works) has not yet been precisely defined. It seems to reduce aqueous humor production and probably also facilitates its outflow. Especially when used in higher concentrations, clonidine leads to blood pressure reduction and also acts as a vasoconstrictor; these side effects relegate its use to a second-line drug.

7.2.2.4 Apraclonidine

Apraclonidine was developed by adding an amide group (-NH_2) to the clonidine molecule. This addition makes it less lipophilic, and thereby reduces its ability to penetrate the blood-brain barrier compared with clonidine. Clonidine exerts an influence on the blood pressure by stimulating the central (brainstem) alpha-2 receptors. Therefore, apraclonidine has fewer adverse blood pressure-lowering effects. Its IOP-reducing effect, however, is similar to clonidine and, like this drug, it probably also facilitates the trabecular outflow. Also like clonidine, it exerts a certain alpha-1 agonistic (stimulating) effect and thereby leads to vasoconstriction, at least in the anterior segments of the eye.

Apraclonidine is given twice or three times daily in a concentration of 0.5%. It is almost always used only for short-term treatment. Administering the drug just for a limited time rarely causes allergic reactions, but during long-term therapy, allergic reactions frequently occur. Applied one hour before and immediately after laser treatment of the anterior parts of the eye, apraclonidine is used to reduce inflammation and to prevent IOP increases.

7.2.2.5 Brimonidine

Brimonidine has only recently been introduced onto the market. Its alpha-2 selectivity is much more pronounced than that observed with clonidine or apraclonidine. This means that it stimulates alpha-2 receptors to a stronger degree and alpha-1 receptors to a lesser degree. It thus exerts no significant vasoconstrictive effect but it does have the same IOP-lowering potential. Besides curbing the aqueous humor production, it also seems to facilitate uveoscleral outflow. In addition, animal experiments have led to the assumption that the drug might act as a neuroprotective agent (Chapter 7.1.2).

Unfortunately, about 10% of the patients experience local adverse reactions after two to six months of treatment, but these disappear after therapy has been discontinued. Other side effects that have been reported after brimonidine therapy include a mild, though probably not significant, lowering of the blood pressure, drowsiness and a dry mouth.

Combination with the beta-blocker timolol has been recently introduced.

7.2.3 Sympatholytic Agents

It may seem strange that sympathomimetic as well as sympatholytic drugs can be used to decrease intraocular pressure for they are drugs that, respectively, promote and inhibit the sympathetic part of the nervous system. This can be explained by the fact that there are many different types of receptors present in various segments of the eye.

Beta-blockers. Beta-blockers are substances that block part of the sympathetic activity regulated by beta-receptors. They play a major role in internal medicine: in low dosages, they are used to treat alterations of the heart rhythm; in higher dosages, to treat systemic hypertension (i.e. high blood pressure).

Beta-blockers have been a constant feature in glaucoma therapy for the past 25 years. Since their introduction, they have achieved a leading position within a relatively short period of time and have replaced the older medications. They have a good IOP-lowering effect, are generally well tolerated, and are applied only once or twice daily. They work by reducing aqueous humor production.

Many beta-blockers are currently available, including timolol, betaxolol, carteolol, metipranolol, levobunolol, etc. They all basically share the same mechanism of action and the same adverse effects. The differences among them will be discussed below.

There are almost no ocular side effects that arise with beta-blocker therapy. They do not affect the pupil size; some rare, though harmless, side effects are: dry eyes, a slight burning sensation and a somewhat reduced corneal sensitivity.

Allergic reactions occur only rarely. But since all topically administered eye drugs can enter the body's circulation via the bloodstream (cf. S 12), locally applied beta-blockers have a range of side-effects similar to those observed with systemic administration. Although these cases are rare, they might lead to depression and phobias; in asthmatic patients, they can initiate severe attacks of bronchospasm. There is also a contraindication for using beta-blockers in patients having certain arrhythmias or cardiac insufficiency.

As mentioned above, though the various beta-blockers resemble each another there are some differences and these will be discussed.

7.2.3.1 Timolol

Timolol was the first topical beta-blocker approved for the treatment of glaucoma and, therefore, the drug with which ophthalmologists have had the most experience. Among the beta-blockers, its IOP-lowering effect reigns supreme. Timolol is given twice daily in concentrations of 0.1% to 0.5%. However, with a special gel-solution (XE) and a newly introduced 0.1% gel, once daily administration is sufficient.

7.2.3.2 Betaxolol

Betaxolol's IOP-lowering effect is slightly weaker than timolol's. Betaxolol preferentially blocks beta-1 receptors, while only slightly blocking beta-2 receptors. This causes fewer problems in asthmatic patients than does timolol, which tends to block bronchial beta-2 receptors and can cause brochospasms in predisposed patients. It is assumed that betaxolol might facilitate the ocular microcirculation and could exert a certain neuroprotective effect. This would explain why the prognosis for the visual field with betaxolol treatment is at least as good as that with a beta-blocker that reduces IOP to a level lower than betaxolol. Betaxolol is applied twice daily in a concentration of 0.25%.

7.2.3.3 Levobunolol

Levobunolol has effects similar to timolol, and is administered twice daily in concentrations of 0.1% to 0.5%.

7.2.3.4 Carteolol

Unlike other beta-blockers, carteolol has "intrinsic sympathomimetic activity," which means it not only blocks, but also slightly stimulates, the sympathetic system. This activity might result in fewer cardiovascular side effects. Compared to other beta-blockers, carteolol seems to have a favorable influence on the lipid level which is advantageous for hyperlipidemic patients. The drug is administered twice daily in dosages of 0.5%, 1.0% or 2.0%.

7.2.3.5 Metipranolol

Metipranolol is similar in its clinical effect to timolol and levobunolol. It is applied twice daily in 0.3% concentration. This drug's advantage is that, in most countries, it is less expensive than other beta-blockers.

7.2.4 Carbonic Anhydrase Inhibitors

Carbonic anhydrase is an enzyme that catalyzes the chemical reaction $CO_2 + H_2O = H_2CO_3 = H^+ + HCO_3^-$, which is the transformation of carbon dioxide and water into bicarbonate and vice versa. Several types of carbonic anhydrase (types 1, 2, 3, etc.) are present within the body. They are quite ubiquitous but are particularly active in the eyes, kidneys and erythrocytes. The activity of these enzymes can be blocked by substances called carbonic anhydrase inhibitors. Chemically, these inhibiting agents are sulfonamides, previously used as mild diuretics (i.e. drugs that facilitate urine production), but which have been gradually replaced by better and more effective diuretics. However, it was noted that carbonic anhydrase inhibitors were quite effective in lowering intraocular (and intracerebral) pressure.

Carbonic anhydrase inhibitors have quite a positive side effect: They lead to vasodilation in ocular as well as cerebral blood vessels. This feature has been exploited in neurology and neurosurgery to measure the reserve capacity, that is, the percentage by which perfusion can be increased when blood vessels are dilated as wide as possible. As some initial studies suggest, this vasodilative effect of carbonic anhydrase inhibitors might be quite advantageous in the treatment of glaucoma.

Carbonic anhydrase inhibitors also affect liquid transport in some organs. Acetazolamide, for instance, is given to patients suffering from increased intracerebral pressure; in ophthalmology, it is applied in cases of macular edema. Further studies are necessary to better define its clinical value in this context.

Carbonic anhydrase inhibitors have been available as antiglaucomatous drugs since 1954. Unfortunately, they are associated with such a host of systemic adverse reactions that scientists spent years searching for a topical version, which finally became available in 1995. First, the systemic carbonic anhydrase inhibitors (in pill form or as an i.v. infusion) will be discussed:

7.2.4.1 Acetazolamide

Acetazolamide is usually given in tablet form. The daily dosage required for maximal efficacy is about 1000 mg. It can be taken as four tablets, each containing 250 mg, or as two sustained-release capsules (a special form of tablet that slowly releases the drug inside the intestinal tract), each containing 500 mg. The effects of the sustained-release capsules last for a longer duration.

As with all carbonic anhydrase inhibitors, acetazolamide reduces the intraocular pressure by decreasing aqueous humor production. It can be given for all forms of glaucoma. The major disadvantages are the side effects: these are bothersome and numerous, but usually harmless and reversible after therapy has been discontinued. Side effects include paresthesias (unpleasant sensations, such as a feeling of "pins and needles" in the extremities), hearing problems, tinnitus (ringing in the ears), loss of appetite and libido, a bitter taste (particularly after drinking carbonated beverages), nausea, etc. The drug decreases the potassium level in the patient's blood, stressing the need for a potassium-rich diet or even taking supplemental potassium pills. A dreaded and extremely painful complication is urolithiasis (kidney stones). To prevent their formation, patients undergoing acetazolamide treatment should drink as much water as possible. There are other, more serious complications, but these are so rare that they are not mentioned here.

In emergency situations, for example, when the IOP reaches extremely high levels, the drug can be given intravenously. Depending on the situation, between 500 and 1000 mg are administered daily.

Since this drug lowers IOP exceedingly well and is indicated for all forms of glaucoma, it is still the most important emergency medication in glaucoma therapy. It can even be given to children – but of course, the dosage has to be adjusted.

7.2.4.2 Methazolamide

Methazolamide is comparable to acetazolamide in its pressure-lowering capability, and is given twice or three times daily in doses ranging from 50 to 100 mg. It can lead to severe fatigue and, in some cases, depression.

7.2.4.3 Dichlorfenamide

A 50 mg dose of dichlorfenamide is taken between one and three times daily. It results in a more marked loss of potassium and is generally associated with more side effects than acetazolamide.

Due to the considerable adverse reactions of systemic carbonic anhydrase inhibitors, there has been a need to develop substances of this class that can be applied topically. Though most of the systemic side effects have been alleviated, the number of local reactions has increased.

7.2.4.4 Dorzolamide

Dorzolamide is administered twice daily in a 2% eyedrop solution. It leads to a moderate IOP reduction. Just as with acetazolamide, there are indications that dorzolamide exerts a positive influence on ocular perfusion. It is therefore of special benefit for patients who suffer from a disturbed blood flow. After application, a slight burning sensation may appear and the eyes are occasionally a bit red. Patients with corneal problems may experience a temporary accentuation of their condition. Certain patients experience a transient bitter taste because some of the drug leaves the eye via the lacrimal (tear) duct, drains into the nose and then into the mouth. Here dorzolamide also exerts its effect of inhibiting carbonic anhydrase. Less CO_2 is converted to H_2CO_3, causing a relative increase in the level of CO_2, and thus the appearance of the bitter taste in the mouth. Unfortunately, allergic reactions are not rare.

7.2.4.5 Brinzolamide

Brinzolamide is administered twice daily in a 1% local concentration. It seems to lower the IOP as effectively as dorzolamide but fewer side effects are reported. Whether it has a similar beneficial influence on ocular circulation as noted with dorzolamide remains to be seen.

7.2.5 Prostaglandin Analogs

Prostaglandins, biologically active substances, belong to the eicosanoid hormones. The latter have their name due to their 20-carbon chain [Gr. *eicos*: twenty]. These compounds are released from phospholipids located in the cell membrane. Eicosanoids are important local regulators for a number of different biological processes.

Similar to other eicosanoids, prostaglandins are made of 20 carbon atoms but this subgroup is characterized by a 5-carbon ring structure. They were discovered in 1930 in secretions from the prostate gland – hence their name. However, today it is known that there are many prostaglandins present in basically all body tissues where they are active in a host of different biochemical reactions. Each prostaglandin is described using a capital letter and a small number, such as prostaglandin E_2 (PGE_2). The letter describes the substitution in the 5-carbon ring by oxy- or hydroxy- molecules. The number refers to the number of double bonds in the molecular side chains. Prostaglandins play an important role in inflammatory reactions; they increase the human body's sensitivity to pain and body temperature. For this reason, drugs that inhibit the synthesis of prostaglandins, called "prostaglandin synthetase inhibitors," are used to treat pain as well as inflammation [Gr. *synthesis*: composition, putting together]. Indomethacin, for example, is included among this group. Prostaglandins are also important for the proper functioning of thrombocytes (platelets). Therefore, prostaglandin synthetase inhibitors, such as acetylsalicylic acid (ASA, commonly known as aspirin), are administered in low dosages to prevent thrombosis. Since prostaglandins are also responsible for a well-working gastric mucosa, treatment with prostaglandin synthetase inhibitors can cause stomach and intestinal problems. Cox-2 inhibitors, a class of drugs developed in recent years, specifically suppresses those groups of prostaglandin synthetases crucial for inflammatory reactions, while barely influencing the other groups of prostaglandin synthetases vital for normal gastric mucosa.

While prostaglandin inhibition has been a focus of modern medicine for many years, prostaglandin analogues (i.e. substances chemically related to prostaglandins) have only recently been introduced into ophthalmology [Gr. *ana*: according to/Gr. *logos*: word, thought]. Although it has been known for decades that certain prostaglandins decrease the IOP, it has taken elaborate research to develop a molecule that sufficiently lowers IOP without simultaneously evoking intolerably severe local adverse reactions.

7.2.5.1 Latanoprost

Latanoprost is a phenyl-substituted $PGF_{2\alpha}$-isopropylester, which means two molecules have been added to the original $PGF_{2\alpha}$ structure; this alteration makes the side effects tolerable. The drug exerts its effects in the eye only after hydrolysis, i.e. after part of the molecule has been split off by absorbing water (Fig. 7.5).

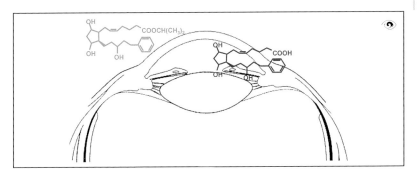

Fig. 7.5: The pharmacological effects of latanoprost (green) only become active inside the eye after part of the molecule (blue) has been split off.

The drug reduces the IOP by facilitating aqueous humor outflow. Unlike other anti-glaucomatous agents, it is the uveoscleral pathway (rather than the trabecular outflow) that is affected by latanoprost (cf. S 1). During the daytime without treatment, most of the aqueous humor drains by the trabecular meshwork, while only a slight amount exits via the uveoscleral pathway. At night, the uveoscleral route plays the major role. Even in very small doses, latanoprost increases uveoscleral outflow for an extended period of time and requires just one single daily application. The most appropriate time for administering the 0.005% concentration eye drops is in the evening. The IOP-lowering effect is at least as strong, or even stronger, than the effect of the other topically applied medications.

Latanoprost's major local side effects are conjunctival hyperemia ("pink eye"), stinging and a feeling that a foreign body is in the eye. Furthermore, in about 10%–20% of all patients, it produces an increase in iris pigmentation. This change of eye color most often occurs in eyes with a green-brown or a blue-green-brown iris. The pigmentation change is due to an increase of melanin inside the melanocytes. The change of color persists even after latanoprost therapy has been discontinued. To date, these side effects have caused no significant consequences, however, long-term studies of this phenomenon are still lacking. The drug can also lead to longer and darker eyelashes, and in some rare cases macular edema has been observed.

The latter complication is more likely to occur if the patient has previously experienced intraocular inflammation or eye surgery. The edema appears to be reversible in all cases thus far studied. It seems that patients with a history of inflammation in the posterior segments of the eye are susceptible to a reactivation of that process. The effect that latanoprost has on ocular perfusion is still not completely known.

7.2.5.2 Travoprost

Travoprost is a PGF_{2a} analog (a full agonist) that exerts its IOP-lowering effect via enhancement of the uveoscleral outflow (cf. Chapter S1) like latanoprost. Its effect on IOP is at least as strong as latanoprost. It is applied once daily in a 0.004% concentration. Its local side effects are comparable to those of latanoprost. Patients not responding to latanoprost might respond to travoprost.

7.2.5.3 Bimatoprost

Bimatoprost is also called a prostamide. Its effect on IOP is at least as strong as latanoprost by increasing outflow via the trabecular meshwork and uveoscleral outflow. Bimatoprost is administered once daily in a 0.03% concentration, preferably in the evening. Mild conjunctival hyperemia has been observed in some patients at the beginning of therapy.

7.2.6 Osmotic Agents

Osmosis is defined as the result of a one-sided diffusion difference through a membrane [Gr. *osmos*: stimulus, drive]. Figure 7.6 illustrates this phenomenon: A container is divided by a semi-permeable (meaning some substances are allowed through, others aren't; permeability depends on molecular size) membrane. For example, when glucose, a molecule that cannot penetrate the membrane, is added to one section, nature attempts to achieve a concentration equilibrium by transferring water from the other side into the compartment containing glucose. Since the membrane does not allow glucose molecules to pass through, a flow in the other direction is not possible. Therefore, the water level on the "glucose side" rises; the resulting difference in pressure between the two compartments is called osmotic tension.

Hyperosmotic drugs are administered to treat massive IOP-increases in cases of acute angle-closure glaucoma. In this emergency situation, the IOP has reached such an extremely high level that, due to physical reasons, it is almost impossible for tension-reducing eye drops to penetrate in the eye. When this occurs, systemic agents have to be given which can reach the eye through the bloodstream. The carbonic anhydrase inhibitor, acetazolamide, discussed earlier, is often not sufficiently effective in cases of acute glaucoma and has to be bolstered by hyperosmotic agents. These agents pull water from the eye into the bloodstream, just as glucose did in Figure 7.6, and by this mechanism, the IOP is temporarily reduced. During the resulting period of (relatively) decreased IOP, topical anti-glaucomatous drugs should be administered.

The side affects associated with hyperosmotic drugs include nausea, vomiting, headaches and confusion. Though these symptoms are indeed a nuisance, they are transient and relatively harmless. A more severe adverse reaction is a circulatory overload that could lead to congestive heart failure and a resulting pulmonary edema. Some hyperosmotic agents can be taken orally, such as glycerol, while others are taken intravenously, e.g. mannitol.

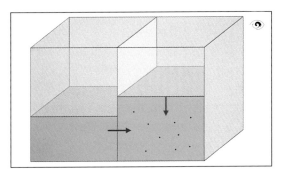

Fig. 7.6: Water flows through a semi-permeable membrane towards the side with the larger number of molecules in solution (blue arrow). The resulting difference in pressure is equivalent to the osmotic pressure (red arrow).

7.2.7 Combination Therapies

Glaucoma therapy usually begins as a monotherapy, i.e. with the administration of a single agent. The choice of this medication depends on the form of glaucoma, the patient's age and other factors. If the IOP reduction is not sufficient, another medication from a different class of substances is given. If treatment with a single drug (monotherapy) is not effective, a combination of two or even three agents is tried. There are many different ways to combine anti-glaucomatous drugs and the choice depends upon the patient's individual situation. However, as mentioned, in combination therapies, medications from various classes are usually combined. Some of these combinations proved so successful that drug companies began manufacturing them in a fixed form. An example is the combination of timolol and dorzolamide. The advantage for the patient is that he only has one bottle of eyedrops instead of two or three; moreover, the number of drops instilled is smaller and correspondingly, also the quantity of preservatives applied to the eye (cf. S 12).

7.3 IOP-reducing Laser Treatment

In the supplementary chapter, S 13, lasers and the way this special light beam is produced are discussed, as are the principles that define its use in ophthalmology. However, here attention is directed to the potential of laser treatment in glaucoma therapy. Several different laser procedures are possible, but three are of practical importance: iridotomy, trabeculoplasty and transscleral cyclophotocoagulation.

7.3.1 Laser Iridotomy

Aqueous humor is produced by the ciliary body and flows from the posterior chamber through the pupil into the anterior chamber from where it drains through the trabecular meshwork and Schlemm's canal into the venous bloodstream (cf. S 1). The pupil provides the connection between the anterior and posterior chambers; any disturbance of the transpupillary flow will lead to a tension difference between the chambers.

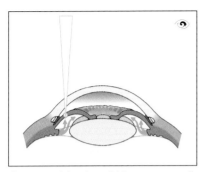

Fig. 7.7: With a laser iridotomy, a small hole is made in the iris.

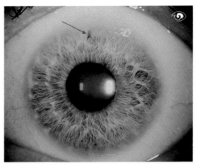

Fig. 7.8: An eye shortly after laser iridotomy. A small opening (→) is visible.

In angle-closure glaucoma, the pressure in the posterior chamber rises, thereby pushing the iris forward and leading to an obstruction of the trabecular meshwork (cf. Chapter 3.5.1). Just the opposite takes place in pigmentary glaucoma (glaucoma associated with pigment dispersion syndrome): the iris is pushed backwards and comes into contact with the lens' supporting structures, the zonules (cf. Chapter 3.6.1.2). Both of these situations require a reduction in the tension gradient between the anterior and posterior chambers, and then the iris can again assume its normal position.

For years, an iridectomy (the surgical excision of a piece of iris tissue) was the procedure of choice. This meant the eye had to be opened up with an eye incision that went through either the cornea or conjunctiva and sclera. Today, using a neodymium: YAG laser, a very fine and small hole can be cut into the iris without having to make any surgical incision onto the eye's surface. Figure 7.7 is a drawing showing how the laser light enters the eye and is focused on the iris. Figure 7.8 is a picture of a patient shortly after having undergone laser iridotomy, a tiny hole in the peripheral iris is visible.

The procedure includes the following steps: The patient is given a drop or two of a topical anesthetic; a contact lens is then placed on the eye. The aiming beam can now be focused on the iris, and when in focus, a hole is "shot" into the iris by one or several laser burns. During this very short treatment, the patient is aware of a sharp sound (like the firing of a toy gun) but does not feel any pain.

Following this procedure, visual acuity can be temporarily reduced for some time due to the effect of the contact lens and also to the dispersion of iris pigment. This mild blurred vision disappears within a few hours or, at most, a couple of days. Since immediately after treatment, there could be a transient IOP rise caused by deposits of iris pigment in the trabecular meshwork, it is recommended that on the day following the procedure, the patient see his medical ophthalmologist who will treat this condition, if necessary.

In acute angle-closure glaucoma, corneal edema can obscure the doctor's view into the anterior chamber. In these cases, the IOP is first lowered conservatively (using anti-glaucomatous drugs), and the laser iridotomy has to wait until the cornea is clear and the iris structures can be better seen. In rare cases, if the edema persists, a surgical iridectomy has to be performed.

After laser treatment, it is sometimes necessary to administer anti-inflammatory eyedrops for a few days. Some authors have reported that up to five percent of all iridotomies might undergo spontaneous closure. However, the authors have never observed such an incident.

7.3.2 Laser Trabeculoplasty

In the 1970s, some ophthalmologists used a laser to "shoot" tiny openings into the trabecular meshwork for enhancing trabecular outflow, but these holes inevitably closed up. However, during this evaluation period, it was noted that the small areas of scarring that arose due to the collagen shrinking inside the trabecular meshwork nevertheless did evoke a reduction in the intraocular pressure. This observation led to the development of argon laser trabeculoplasty (ALT) [Gr. *plastein*: to form]. As the name indicates, this procedure is performed using an argon laser (cf. S 13).

During this procedure, which takes place in either one or two sessions, 50 to 100 laser spots of comparatively low energy are applied circularly into the trabecular meshwork (Fig. 7.9). The spot size is approximately 50 µm (i.e. 1/20 mm) (Fig. 7.10). Within days, but sometimes taking weeks or months, the IOP starts to drop.

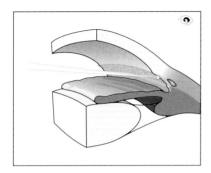

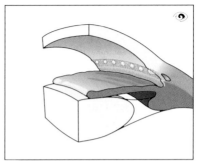

Fig. 7.9: With argon laser trabeculo-plasty (ALT), laser energy is beamed into the trabecular meshwork.

Fig. 7.10: After ALT, small laser spots are visible for some time.

This method is indicated in primary open-angle glaucoma, pseudoexfoliation glaucoma and pigment dispersion glaucoma. There might be a marked IOP increase within a few hours after treatment. This requires IOP measurements a few hours after laser trabeculoplasty and also on the following day and, if necessary, medical treatment for the high IOP. This is especially important for patients having advanced glaucomatous damage who require this post-laser treatment.

The procedure for laser trabeculoplasty is as follows: After application of a topical anesthetic, a contact lens is placed upon the eye while the patient sits at the slit-lamp. The laser treatment itself takes just a few minutes and is painless. When it is finished, the patient's vision might be temporarily blurred, an effect that disappears within minutes or hours.

The method's disadvantages include: a) only about 60% of all patients respond to the therapy; b) even when a patient does respond, the positive effect usually wears off after about three years; and c) even while the mean IOP may be reduced, fluctuations of intraocular tension are usually not affected.

For these reasons, the method is no longer frequently used. If glaucomatous damage progresses in spite of medical therapy, surgical intervention can be anticipated. Argon laser trabeculoplasty is sometimes performed with the hope that surgery can be avoided. Nevertheless, because it sometimes takes months before the success or failure of laser treatment becomes obvious, precious time can be lost with such a strategy.

Whereas argon laser trabeculoplasty induces coagulative damage to the trabecular meshwork, a new technigue has been proposed and named selective laser trabeculoplasty. In this method, by using another type of laser, only pigmented trabecular meshwork cells are targeted, thus sparing structural architecture of the collagen beams in the trabecular meshwork.

7.3.3 Transscleral Cyclophotocoagulation

There are situations where an IOP-lowering operation is not possible or where the chances for surgical success are slim. In these cases, the IOP is treated by reducing the number of cells inside the ciliary processes through coagulation [Lat. *coagulatio*: clotting, destruction], meaning that part of the tissue which produces the aqueous humor is destroyed. There are several ways to destroy tissue: heat (thermocoagulation), cold (cryocoagulation) or a laser beam (photocoagulation). When the ciliary body (cf. S 1) is coagulated, the procedure is called cyclophotocoagulation [Gr. *kyklos*: circle]; transscleral indicates that the laser beam is focused through the conjunctiva and sclera onto the ciliary body (Fig. 7.11). Although both conjunctiva and sclera are not transparent, the laser can nevertheless pass through these tissues because: a) the conjunctiva undergoes blanching due to the pressure exerted by the contact lens, making it relatively devoid of blood; and b) light of a long wavelength can pass through the sclera and an almost bloodless conjunctiva. Figure 7.12 shows ciliary processes that have been partially coagulated. The picture, however, is the result of cryotherapy, not of laser treatment. The scars resulting from cyclophotocoagulation are much smaller.

The ciliary body is quite sensitive to pain and, without certain precautions, the procedure would be quite uncomfortable. Therefore, numbing procedures are instituted: either retrobulbar anesthesia (numbing the eye's nerves by injection of an anesthetic behind the eyeball, cf. Chapter 7.4.2) or repeated administration of a strong topical anesthetic, such as Tetracaine eyedrops. Post-operatively, the

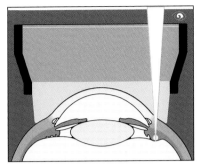
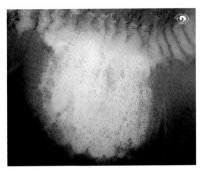

Fig. 7.11: In transscleral cyclophoto-coagulation, a part of the ciliary body is destroyed.

Fig. 7.12: Large scar and partly destroyed ciliary processes after cryocoagulation.

eye can be inflamed. Anti-inflammatory eyedrops and pills to ease the pain are thus administered on the first and possibly second day after the laser treatment. While the IOP decreases over the first several days, it can rise again within months or years. This is an indication that the treatment has to be repeated. It is recommended that only part of the tissue be destroyed in one session in order to minimize the threat of permanent ocular hypotension.

7.3.4 Argon Laser Iridoplasty

In some types of glaucoma, like with the plateau iris mechanism, or in narrow angles, moderate laser coagulation of the peripheral iris tissue achives shrinkage of the tissue and thus pulling the iris out of the chamber angle. The preparation and the type of laser are similar to the argon laser trabeculoplasty, only here the spots are larger, the laser exposition time is longer and the energy levels are lower.

7.4 IOP-Lowering Operations

In the field of surgical medicine, glaucoma surgery is something rather unique. Normally, a patient undergoing surgery seeks relief from pain, tumors, stones or other problems that are surgically correctable; he expects to be better off rather directly after the operation. A cataract patient, for instance, can be quite confident of gaining a better visual acuity following the lens removal.

In glaucoma, the situation is completely different: A glaucoma patient is usually not disturbed by his condition. Either his visual field defects are small or he has not noticed them at all. Nevertheless, he is expected to undergo an operation that will not result in better, but perhaps even in poorer vision. In particular, visual acuity might be mildly reduced for a short or perhaps even longer period. This situation requires a much more thorough patient education than other surgical procedures. It has to be made clear that the goal of the operation is not to improve the current visual function but rather to preserve vision and especially the visual field.

7.4.1 General Aspects

Education. The patient requires a thorough explanation of the benefits and the risks of the operation. Some aspects discussed here are the same topics covered in such an education. However, it should be stressed that this book is in no way a substitute for a personal discussion between the physician and patient. Each individual patient has unique concerns and each physician has his own methods and experiences. This book is meant to provide needed and tangible support for this crucial interchange, and to assist the patient in asking those questions that are of particular importance to him.

During this consultation, a decision has to be made regarding the appropriate time for the operation or whether it will be an out-patient or an in-patient procedure. Other points of discussion are the type of anesthesia that is recommended by the physician and acceptable to the patient. Compromises here are often possible. Other concerns include how the glaucoma should be treated until the day of surgery, and how frequently the patient should undergo post-operative examinations and who should perform them.

A Second Opinion. It is not uncommon for a patient to consult with another expert before consenting to an operation. Physicians completely understand this. Getting a second opinion is not considered a "vote of no confidence" to the treating ophthalmologist, but rather it may help both the patient and treating physician feel comfortable with the anticipated therapy.

The Goal of the Surgery. Unfortunately, it is not possible to remove glaucomatous damage, therefore, the operation's goal is "only" the reduction and stabilization of intraocular pressure. If this goal is achieved, the likelihood for progression of visual field damage is considerably reduced. Following any procedure performed, frequent and constant examinations evaluating IOP, optic disc morphology and visual field remain crucial because progression is still possible, even when the IOP is normal. Other risk factors (cf. Chapter 4.2) must also be considered.

Indications for Surgery. As a general rule, operations are performed whenever the IOP is markedly increased even though medical treatment is administered, or when glaucomatous damage progresses in spite of conservative therapy. Another reason to consider surgery is intolerance to medical therapy. There are exceptions to these general rules: the patient's age, his general health, the condition of the other eye and the individual form of glaucoma have to be considered when making a decision about surgery. As has been seen (cf. Chapter 3.6.1.1), an eye suffering from pseudoexfoliation syndrome is more likely to be operated on at an earlier stage than an eye afflicted with POAG. It is crucial that the patient accept the possible disadvantages associated with the surgery because of the accompanying long-term benefits.

Advantages of Surgery. If the operation is successful and leads to a decrease and stabilization of the IOP to an acceptably low level, the patient no longer needs medical therapy. Unfortunately, such an ideal situation does not always occur after an initial operation. Additional operations are occasionally necessary and always a possibility. Lowering and stabilizing the IOP significantly enhances the long-term prognosis for the visual field.

Disadvantages of Surgery. The patient has to invest a considerable amount of time in preoperative examinations, the operation itself and in those check-ups that are necessary after surgery. A transient, but sometimes even a permanent, slight reduction in visual acuity is possible. In rare cases, a lens opacity (cataract) can develop more rapidly after glaucoma surgery than in a healthy eye. Cataracts, however, can be removed without creating any major problems for the patient (cf. S 5).

By far the most common problem is a renewed increase in the intraocular pressure. A rise in the IOP, often slow to develop, can occur after months or even years. Since the introduction of mitomycin C (see below), this problem has become increasingly rare. The patient has to be aware, however, that sometimes IOP-reducing medications or another operation might become necessary. There is usually a relatively good prognosis after a second or even third operation. The IOP could also be too low after surgery; the corrective measures that have to be taken in this case are discussed below.

Out-Patient or In-Patient. If he feels well enough, the patient can get up immediately after the procedure. This leads to the question of whether the operation should be performed on an out-patient or in-patient basis. Out-patient procedures are safe and effective for a number of indications in ophthalmology, such as cataract surgery. In glaucoma surgery, the out-patient approach is possible, though the authors feel that it should not be recommended. Caring for the patient immediately after the procedure is as crucial for the long-term prognosis as the operation itself. Therefore, a hybrid protocol is recommended: The patient stays in the hospital but is free to go home on the first or second post-operative day if there are no complications. If problems do arise, the patient stays in the hospital for a few extra days; fortunately, this is a rare event.

Preparing for Surgery. The patient is requested to contact his primary care physician, who is asked to send the ophthalmologist a report on the patient's general health, including results from blood tests taken in the past and any special conditions that the patient has. The patient takes his glaucoma medication as well as any other drugs prescribed by his treating physician until the day of the operation. Whether or not these other drugs should be taken on this day is determined by the anesthesiologist. The administration of blood thinners (anti-coagulants) should be stopped, if possible, ten days before the operation. Sometimes this is not possible and requires a discussion between the surgeon and the treating physician to decide the best course. An operation while the patient is still under the influence of these drugs is basically possible, but requires certain precautions.

7.4.2 Anesthesia

In many hospitals, an anesthesiologist is always present during the operation, even though the procedure is usually performed under local anesthesia [Gr. *aisthäsis*: sensitivity/Gr. *anaisthäsis*: insensitivity]. Before the operation, this specialist discusses anesthesia and general medical aspects with the patient.

The authors usually operate under local anesthesia. General anesthesia is usually only required for children. Some patients express an initial preference for general anesthesia, but after discussing the advantages and disadvantages, they usually decide on local anesthesia. Even though both provide a pain-free operation, the local anesthesia is less cumbersome for the patient as a whole. Taking a sedative shortly before the procedure helps many patients.

After the operation is finished, patients often report that they had expected the procedure to be more painful and that they would no longer be afraid should a second operation become necessary. In uncomplicated cases, retrobulbar anesthesia is performed (Fig 7.13); if glaucomatous damage is advanced, subconjunctival anesthesia is preferred (Fig. 7.14). During the procedure, the patient is able, and even requested, to relate if and when he suffers discomfort. The surgeon or the anesthesiologist can easily inject or instill additional anesthetic.

Depending on the individual situation, the patient may receive a preoperative sedative from the anesthesiologist. Immediately before administering the local anesthetic, the specialist will give a drug intravenously which will reduce anxiety and discomfort within seconds for a few minutes. This makes the injection of the local anesthetic less unpleasant.

Figure 7.13 shows the principle of retrobulbar anesthesia; and Figure 7.14, the principle of subconjunctival anesthesia. In retobulbar anesthesia, the eye muscles are immobilized, the optic nerve is numbed (the patient no longer sees anything) and, most importantly of all, the fibers transmitting pain are switched off for a while: they no longer transmit their signals to the brain.

Subconjunctival anesthesia renders the area of operation completely painless. Some of the anesthetic diffuses backwards through the tissue and partially incapacitates the muscles. The patient is still able to see but will not be disturbed since the eye is ro-

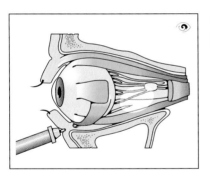

Fig. 7.13: In retrobulbar anesthesia, a drug is injected into the orbit, bypassing the eyeball.

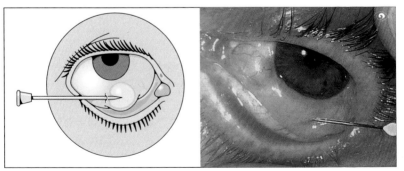

Fig. 7.14: In subconjunctival anesthesia, the drug (local anesthetic) is injected beneath the conjunctiva.

tated and fixated in a downward looking position. The patient is not blinded by the bright lights from the operating microscope.

It was once assumed that the use of general anesthesia might be the best way to protect the optic nerve during the operation; however, subconjunctival anesthesia is now considered the safest method.

Patients often worry that they won't be able to keep the eye still during the operation; this is not a problem. The chance of an unintentional eye movement is small due to the effect of the anesthetic and the fact that the eye will be fixed by a suture. Even if the patient does move a bit during the procedure, this hardly constitutes a threat to the operation. When the patient feels the urge to move – such as before sneezing – he should tell the surgeon who will simply remove his instruments from the eye for a moment.

7.4.3 Surgical Procedure

The goal of all IOP-lowering operations is to enhance the aqueous humor outflow. There are numerous techniques that cannot be discussed in detail here. What is important is to know that these are not techniques that are either intrinsically good or bad; but rather the technique is chosen and adapted to the needs of the individual eye, while at the same time, corresponds to the personal experience, skill and training of the surgeon. The procedure, so to speak, is a surgeon's trademark signature. The authors' method of choice for an IOP-lowering procedure is a modified trabeculectomy, a procedure discussed more elaborately below. Figure 7.15 shows the principle of trabeculectomy. The aqueous humor is directed through an artificial opening beneath the conjunctiva; this leads to the formation of a "bleb," depicted in Fig. 7.16.

Trabeculectomy. For this procedure, the skin surrounding the eye is first sterilized and draped with sterile cloths; next, a lid retractor is put in place (Fig. 7.17). This keeps the eye open throughout the entire procedure. The eye is then fixed to the retractor by two sutures (so-called bridle sutures), which are placed at the lim-

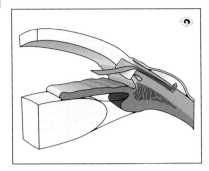

Fig. 7.15: In trabeculectomy, a new outflow (under the conjunctiva) is created for the aqueous humor.

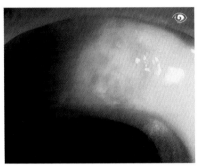
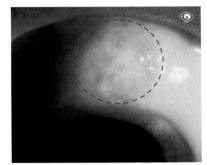

Fig. 7.16: The bleb is usually covered by the upper lid. On the picture at the right, the conjunctiva, which has been soaked with aqueous humor (bleb), is indicated by the circle.

bus, the transition zone between the cornea and sclera (Fig. 7.18). By rotating the eye downward, the patient is not disturbed by the bright light of the operating lamp and the surgeon has a perfect view of the surgical field.

Both the conjunctiva and the underlying Tenon's capsule are lifted with a forceps and incised with scissors. (Tenon's capsule is a slightly movable and extensible connective tissue layer between the conjunctiva and sclera.) Both layers are gently pulled back, which exposes the sclera (Fig. 7.19). Should a second operation become necessary, this is the area where the surgeon will encounter adhesions that will have to be dissected with scissors. Next a small plastic sponge is soaked with mitomycin C and placed between Tenon's capsule and the sclera (Fig. 7.20). The duration of this application depends upon a host of factors, as discussed later in this chapter.

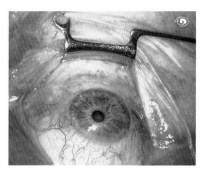

Fig. 7.17: A lid opener keeps the eye from closing …

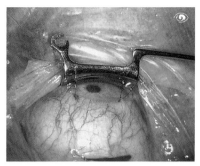

Fig. 7.18: … the eyeball is then rotated downward and fixed to the lid opener with two sutures.

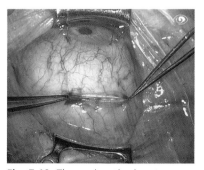

Fig. 7.19: The conjunctiva is cut open and separated from the sclera …

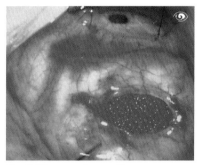

Fig. 7.20: … and a small sponge soaked with mitomycin is placed between the sclera and Tenon's capsule for a few seconds.

After the sponge's removal, the involved area is thoroughly irrigated, ensuring that the mitomycin C has been completely removed.

The conjunctiva is then fixed with the bridle suture, thus exposing the sclera (Fig. 7.21). In case of bleeding, the small vessels are coagulated by diathermy, an instrument at whose tip electricity is transformed into heat. The hemorrhages are not at all dangerous; they just make the surgeon's job a bit more difficult.

Next a corneoscleral tunnel is prepared using a special diamond scalpel; the sclera and cornea are split into two different layers (Fig. 7.22). The inner wall of this tunnel is opened with a punch instrument (Fig. 7.23).

A tunnel is thus created which provides direct access to the

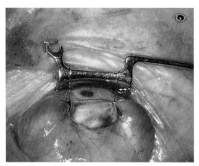

Fig. 7.21: The conjunctiva is then pulled in the anterior direction and held in place by sutures.

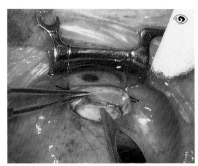

Fig. 7.22: A tunnel is cut through the sclera and cornea (the opening is visible here).

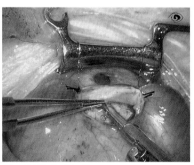

Fig. 7.23: Inside the corneoscleral tunnel, an opening is created in the anterior chamber using a punch instrument.

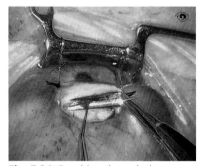

Fig. 7.24: Reaching through the tunnel, the iris is grasped and a small part is cut off.

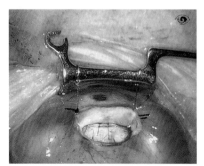

Fig. 7.25: The tunnel is closed with sutures to prevent a rapid drop in the IOP.

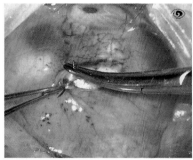

Fig. 7.26: The conjunctiva is brought back into its normal position and closed with a resorbable suture.

anterior chamber and whose outside remains covered by a scleral layer. Pushing a small forceps gently though this tunnel, the iris is held in place and a small part is cut off with scissors (Fig. 7.24). This is called an iridectomy (cf. Chapter 3.5.1).

Then the outward opening, the scleral flap, is closed with sutures (Fig. 7.25). This suture is necessary to keep the IOP from going down to zero immediately after the operation (before the wound has started healing), sometimes even keeping it rather high. This is meant to prevent the numerous complications that come with a sharply reduced intraocular pressure, also called ocular hypotony (cf. Chapter 2.2.2). The sutures generally used are made of resorbable [Lat. *sorbere*: to swallow] material (meaning they are broken down and gradually digested by the body). After 10–15 days, these sutures gradually resorb, thereby spontaneously further opening the tunnel. Two or three sutures using material that is not resorbable are also made. These keep the tunnel relatively closed after the other sutures have dissolved, thus preventing the IOP from dropping to extreme lows. If, on the other hand, the IOP remains elevated after weeks or months, the non-resorbing sutures are cut with the tip of a needle or with a laser, thereby evoking a reduction in the intraocular pressure.

Following these steps, Tenon's capsule and the conjunctiva are separately closed with a resorbing suture in a continuous fashion (Fig. 7.26). The bridle sutures are then removed. The patient is given local steroids to prevent post-operative inflammation, antibiotics to minimize the risk of infection and atropine, an effective preventive measure against ciliary block, which works by relaxing the ciliary muscle (cf. Chapter 3.5.4). If a bandage is placed on the eye, this is only done on the first day.

Alternative Approaches. As mentioned, there are many different types of filtering surgery, and these differ to varying degrees from the method just described. All these approaches have their merits but describing them here is not within the scope of this book. Many surgeons prefer, for instance, the classic trabeculectomy where a scleral flap is created. Under this scleral flap, an opening through the trabecular meshwork is cut with a scalpel or scissors (Fig. 7.27). The authors do not perform this procedure because of the higher incidence of extremely low IOP experienced during the initial post-operative days, and the increased corneal astigmatism encountered long-term. Another approach is to remove the inner layer including the trabecular meshwork with a trepan, a procedure called goniotrepanation [Gr. *trypanon*: drill].

Deep Sclerectomy and Viscocanalostomy. There are other ophthalmic surgeons who prefer the deep sclerectomy. During this procedure, there are no penetrations into the anterior chamber [Lat. *penetrare*: to penetrate] and part of Schlemm's canal and the inner layer, the trabecular meshwork, remain in place. Some surgeons implant a piece of collagen between the scleral flap and the inner scleral

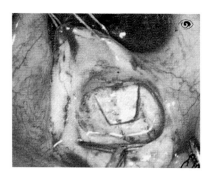

Fig. 7.27: Classical trabeculectomy with a scleral flap.

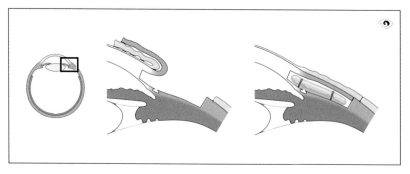

Fig. 7.28: The principle of deep sclerectomy: a small collagen implant (yellow) helps keep the sclera open.

wall (Fig. 7.28). The advantage is seen in the fact that a deep sclerectomy (with or without a collagen implant) rarely leads to very low IOP levels, and that post-operative visual function is quickly restored. This makes the operation more acceptable to the patients. The disadvantage is a relatively small pressure reduction. Therefore, the post-operative IOP might be too high for many patients.

When performing viscocanalostomy, Schlemm's canal is "washed out" with a substance of high viscosity. This mechanical opening of the canal likewise lowers the IOP in some patient, but not in all.

Since the goal in most patients is to achieve a relatively low IOP level that will remain low for years to come, the authors rarely use these latter methods.

New techniques are continuously being developed. A high percentage of these variations disappear within a few years, and only a few find a lasting place in glaucoma surgery.

Complications of IOP-reducing Operations. One must distinguish between complications that occur: a) during the operation, b) in the first few post-operative days, and c) some time after the procedure.

a) Intraoperative complications: In extremely rare cases, a pronounced arterial hemorrhage within the choroid occurs which is a potential threat to the entire eye. Fortunately, the authors have not seen this type of dramatic complication within the past 10–15 years. Other complications are less dangerous, although they do render the operation more difficult and time-consuming and, being of a technical nature, are not discussed here.

b) Complications during the first few post-operative days: There is sometimes bleeding into the anterior chamber. While this temporarily reduces the visual function for some time, it is basically harmless. There might be an increase in the IOP or even a drop to 0 mmHg. The IOP rise is no problem if diagnosed and treated in time with medication. The initial IOP gives no indication about how the pressure will develop in the years to come. A drop to zero itself is no catastrophe but requires intense supervision by the ophthalmologist. A shallowing of the anterior chamber must be identified in time since any contact between the lens and the posterior (inward) layer of the cornea has to be prevented.

A much-dreaded complication is "malignant" glaucoma, caused by the ciliary block discussed in Chapter 3.5.4. Since the ophthalmologist can anticipate which eyes are more likely to develop ciliary block, precautions can be taken. In most cases, a ciliary block can be prevented by administering a few drops of atropine post-operatively. During the past ten years, this group has seen malignant glaucoma develop only after one single trabeculectomy, and this problem was immediately solved by quick intervention.

c) Complications within the first three post-operative months:
In the first few weeks and months, the IOP can still fluctuate or remain too high or too low. If, after resorption of the resorbable sutures, the IOP is still dangerously high, the physician will temporarily prescribe IOP-lowering drugs and refer the patient to the surgeon who, in most cases, will cut the non-resorbable sutures in order to open the tunnel. Other groups that use the scleral flap technique seek to achieve immediate filtration; they try to avoid any IOP-lowering drugs in the immediate post-operative period. If the IOP is too high, they resort to massage of the eyeball with the desired goal of opening the trabeculectomy.

If there is a tendency to scar, a low concentration of mitomycin C is injected into the bleb. Some other ophthalmologists prefer to inject 5-FU under the conjunctiva far from the bleb. If, on the other hand, the IOP remains too low after two or three months and the patient suffers from this condition, either the patient's blood or an agent of high viscosity is injected into the bleb to initiate the process of scarring. Injections into the bleb are possible at any stage.

Infections of the bleb are always a dreaded consequence, but fortunately, are quite rare. If the eye turns red or when ocular pain is present, the patient should immediately consult his doctor to rule out an infection.

Mitomycin C. Mitomycin C was originally developed as an antibiotic. Today it is primarily used by oncologists (doctors specializing in tumor treatment) because of its cytostatic effect in cancer therapy. A cytostatic is a drug that is capable of inhibiting cell division (i.e. the multiplication of tumor cells).

In ophthalmology, diluted mitomycin solution is applied to the operation field. In the short-term it reduces inflammation and intraoperative bleeding, and has antibiotic properties. Even more important, in the long-term, it prevents or at least greatly reduces the chance that the bleb will scar and therefore the IOP will rise.

Even though the use of mitomycin C is extremely effective, it is not without its own dangers. When this drug was first used in ophthalmology, severe complications were reported. However, it was soon shown that these complications occurred especially when the medication concentration employed was too high or it was used for a prolonged period of time. Another danger arises when the drug is not adequately rinsed out after its application. Nevertheless, with the correct dosage and duration, it has proven quite useful. The authors have been using mitomycin C for the past 10 years in very low, but constant, concentrations; the application time is adjusted to the particular situation which, in itself, depends upon the patient's age, the duration and type of the antecedent pressure-reducing local therapy, etc. Especially long application times are required, for example, with neovascularization glaucoma (cf. Chapter 3.6.2); medium-long application is undertaken with, say, inflammatory secondary glaucoma; while very short administration times are used in initial operations on older patients.

Before the era of mitomycin, a long-term increase in the intraocular pressure was observed in about 50% or even more of the operated patients. Indeed, after re-operation, or in special cases, such as young patients or patients of African decent, the long-term prognosis was even poorer. Since the introduction of mitomycin, the pressure prognosis after an operation has significantly improved.

7.4.4 Post-operative Treatment

Because post-operative monitoring is crucial to the outcome of the operation, it is advantageous if the surgeon himself can perform the first and even second post-operative check-ups.

At the authors' clinic, the operation is usually performed in the morning; the first check-up takes place on the same afternoon, and then, as needed, once again in the same evening. The intraocular pressure is measured; if it is increased, this is not dangerous in light of the operation just performed. However, to prevent damage to the optic nerve from occurring, the pressure is normalized using medications. On the other hand, if the pressure is too low, frequent eye examinations are necessary. If the anterior chamber has flattened and the iris and lens are tending toward the cornea, special procedures must be undertaken because the lens should never come into contact with the posterior corneal surface.

After the operation, local antibiotics are prescribed. Additionally, in the first two to three days, atropine is also administered, and during the first weeks, drugs to reduce inflammation are also given, the doses depending upon the degree of eye inflammation. One must consider that locally administered steroids can reversibly increase the IOP, even after an operation (cf. Chapter 3.6.1.3). Therefore, we often use non-steroidal anti-inflammatory agents.

If the eye pressure is still too high several weeks after the operation or if it is normal but only with concomitant use of pressure-reducing medications, then the non-resorbable sutures on the corneoscleral tunnel are cut. If the pressure still remains high or again increases after weeks or months, then the conjunctiva is injected with a highly diluted mitomycin C solution. The authors have had good results with this procedure. Occasionally adhesions can form that require readministration of IOP-lowering medication or another operation. If the pressure remains too low for a longer period, then the bleb is injected with either the patient's own blood or a highly viscous gel. As long as the pressure remains low, vision can be significantly impaired, however, after pressure has returned to normal, in almost all cases the sight soon follows.

Activities After the Operation. There used to be strict guidelines that the patient had to follow after a glaucoma operation. However, with today's advanced techniques, the risks have become much smaller. The patient is usually told that he can go back to leading a normal life a few days after the operation. Depending on the visual function, a patient might not yet be able to drive a car (this should be discussed with the ophthalmologist). Showering and hair washing are permitted after about the 2nd or 3rd post-operative day. For those patients who work, when they can return to work is naturally a primary concern. This can only be decided by assessing the individual's particular case and depends not only on how well the operation went, but also on the patient's profession. Because both eyes are never operated on simultaneously, many activities (e.g. office work) can soon be taken up again. Naturally, there is the prerequisite that the non-operated eye have a satisfactory visual function. Caution is recommended with activities that require stereoscopic vision.

7.4.5 Other Pressure-reducing Operations

Trabeculotomy and goniotomy, performed for congenital glaucoma, are described in Chapter 3.1.

Iridectomy. In describing laser iridotomy (cf. Chapter 7.3.1), it was noted that there are cases (even though they are very rare) when the iris can no longer be opened with a laser beam. In these cases, surgery is required. Even here, many variations are possible. The authors prefer entry via the cornea. The iris is held with forceps, and a small piece is cut off with scissors. Then the cornea is sutured.

Cyclodialysis. Cyclodialysis is an operation that used to be performed quite frequently. Using a scoop, a connection is fashioned between the anterior chamber and the choroid. This enables the aqueous humor to flow directly into the subscleral space. The reason that this technique is only rarely used today is that the effect can only be poorly controlled: the pressure is frequently very low right after the operation, but then it suddenly spikes to high levels.

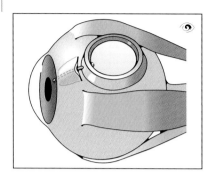

Fig. 7.29: The plastic implant directs the outflow of aqueous humor from the anterior chamber over the sclera.

Plastic Implants. Because there is a natural tendency for scar tissue to form, the intraocular pressure often rises again after operations where fistulae [Lat. *fistula*: tube-shaped connection] are formed. For decades, attempts have been made to implant "pressure valves" in the eye. There are now numerous implants available for this purpose, of which Figure 7.29 is an example. We very rarely apply these techniques as experience has shown that a reoperation with mitomycin C is, in most cases, a safer alternative than inserting a plastic implant. However, this is another area where many views are possible, and in some countries, these plastic valves are implanted quite frequently [Lat. *implantatio*: implantation].

7.4.6 Combined Cataract/Glaucoma Operation

If both glaucoma and a cataract are present at the same time, then a cataract operation (S 5) can be combined with an IOP-reducing operation. The advantage is that only one surgical procedure per eye is required for both diseases. However, the disadvantage is that the long-term prognosis for the pressure reducing effect is significantly poorer than with a pure trabeculectomy. If there is a large degree of glaucomatous damage present or if the damage occurs with only a moderate pressure rise, then the goal of the operation becomes achieving as low an IOP as possible. Each individual case must be uniquely assessed as to whether a combined operation or two individual operations would be better for that particular patient. If a patient has a cataract with an IOP that is only slightly increased and no glaucomatous damage, then usually only a cataract operation is performed. If the glaucoma is the primary problem and the lens is only slightly clouded, then usually only a trabeculectomy is performed. If both must eventually be performed, sometimes a combined operation will be considered. If the glaucoma problem is by far the more serious of the two, either because the pressure is very high or the damage is advanced, then a glaucoma operation is performed first and a cataract procedure is then done at a later time (cf. S 5). The reason that the sequence of operations is glaucoma first, cataract second, is that with glaucoma, the damage is continuously progressing, and once present, cannot be alleviated. A glaucoma operation should therefore not be postponed for too long. However, a cataract operation can successfully be performed at any time, even after the glaucoma operation. For this reason, the primary focus is to avoid progression of glaucomatous damage.

7.5 Enhancing Ocular Perfusion

For more than one hundred years, scientists researching glaucoma kept continually returning to the hypothesis that glaucoma patients suffer from a disturbed circulation. However, proving this was not possible because, until recently, there were no reliable methods available for measuring ocular perfusion.

In the early 1980s, we were able to prove that, compared to healthy individuals, a number of glaucoma patients have a markedly diminished perfusion in the fingertip, specifically, in the nailfold. Since nailfold perfusion changed parallel to alterations in the visual fields, it was suspected that perfusion problems occurring in the nailfold might be associated with reduced ocular perfusion.

Just a few years ago, it became possible to measure ocular perfusion directly and the author's hypothesis was proven: Glaucoma patients suffer much more frequently from reduced perfusion than healthy individuals, both in the eye as well as in the nailfold. The lower the IOP level at which there is a development – or progression – of glaucomatous damage, then the more probable that circulatory problems are also present.

In a subsequent step, we could prove that reduced perfusion in glaucoma is either not, or only rarely, due to arteriosclerosis, but rather is caused by vascular dysregulation (cf. S 8). Glaucoma patients often suffer from a disturbed circulation in other organs as well, but this is rarely associated with any symptoms, such as silent myocardial ischemia, in which there is a reduced perfusion of the heart muscle normally lasting just a few seconds or minutes. The patient does not notice it at all – thus the term "silent" ischemia. While patients with arteriosclerosis of the coronary arteries usually experience ischemia when exercising (such as riding the EKG bicycle ergometer), glaucoma patients usually suffer attacks of ischemia when at rest and under emotional stress. The ischemia present in glaucoma patients is almost always due to vascular dysregulation and not to arteriosclerosis. The fact that the heart and some other organs are involved in some patients proves that: a) this is not only a secondary phenomenon of glaucoma, but rather a primary circulatory condition; b) this circulatory disturbance can occur throughout the body in different organs; and c) it usually occurs in episodes.

Is it possible, or even necessary, that the vascular dysregulation also be treated? And if the answer is yes, then is the therapy prudent? If only glaucoma as an ocular disease is considered, there is some logic to the argument that underscores the importance of lowering the IOP – which, in fact, frequently stops the disease or slows its progression. One basic tenet that is assumed here is that vascular dysregulation increases the eye's susceptibility to the effects of intraocular pressure (cf. Chapter 5.2). When the IOP has been reduced to a safe level, the damage will not progress in many patients. Nevertheless, in others, one opts to treat vascular dysregulation for several reasons:

a) It is not possible to reduce the IOP in every patient to a long-term level low enough to prevent any further progression of damage;

b) The damage in some will progress in spite of a massive IOP reduction;

c) Vascular dysregulation is not restricted to the eye; the risk of developing other diseases cannot be ignored.

However, treatment of vascular dysregulation is far from easy. Because the associations and connections have only recently been made, there has not yet been enough time to develop appropriate medications. At this point, one must remember that for the past 150 years, it has been known that an elevated IOP can lead to glaucomatous damage. Nevertheless, excluding pilocarpine, effective tension-lowering drugs have only become available within the past few years or decades. There is good reason to believe that in a few years or decades, reliable drugs for treating vascular dysregulation will be available.

But what can patients do in the meantime? Patients cannot simply be told to come back in twenty years when these studies have been concluded. What they will be told is this: Medicine, as a scientific discipline, is obligated to study all feasible forms of therapy and thoroughly evaluate their possible efficacy (as well as their potential side effects). Often, however, physicians must act based on their clinical experiences and the results of preliminary studies before definitive proof has become available.

With regard to the following list of possible therapies, which is neither complete nor 100% guaranteed, the authors' experiences have been quite positive.

How does one concretely proceed? If a patient's blood pressure is very low and vasospasms are present, the blood pressure is first increased. Experience gathered in the authors' clinic indicates that low blood pressure can trigger vasospasms. Most importantly, night-time dips in the BP should be avoided. If the patient remains vasospastic despite an improvement in the blood pressure, antispastic therapy will be initiated.

7.5.1 Treating Low Blood Pressure

As a first step, daily physical exercise is recommended for patients. While extreme activities should be avoided, some degree of "light" sport is beneficial, such as jogging or bike riding. Additionally, it is imperative that the patient drink enough water and ingest sufficient quantities of salt. Since a salt-free diet is recommended for patients suffering from high blood pressure, many people believe that reducing the salt intake is beneficial for everyone's health. This does not apply to patients with low blood pressure, even more so if they suffer from glaucoma! Depending on the blood pressure situation, taking an additional 2 to 5 grams of salt each day is recommended by the authors. The additional salt should be ingested with plenty of liquids and in the evening, if possible.

Some drugs, for example, sleeping pills, frequently taken by patients have a side effect of lowering the blood pressure, particularly at night. Taking these medications should be stopped or substituted with drugs that exert no influence on the blood pressure. Other patients suffering from systemic hypertension need drugs that lower the BP during the day. If they experience nightly dips in the blood pressure, the dosage should be reduced or administered on a different schedule.

Even general supportive measures can be beneficial. Some patients benefit from a Kneipp therapy. Sebastian Kneipp, a German clergyman, lived from 1821 until 1887. The cure he developed is based on the following: 1) a water cure treatment; 2) medicinal herbs; 3) natural food nutrition; 4) taking a positive view of life; 5) exercise.

Patients who experience a major blood pressure drop when changing from a lying to a standing position or after longer periods of standing should undergo a test to determine whether wearing support hose would be beneficial.

If these general measures prove unsuccessful, medical therapy should be instituted. Many drugs that increase blood pressure are not suitable for glaucoma patients. Drugs that increase blood pressure by vasoconstriction should be avoided. For more than 10 years, we have been using fludrocortisone, a mineralocorticoid. Mineralocorticoids have fewer side effects than glucocorticoids, with which they should not be confused. Nevertheless, any therapy with mineralocorticoids deserves the supervision of an experienced physician; uncontrolled intake of drugs must be avoided! On the other hand, a patient who needs medication and uses the correct dosage should not be frightened or confused by the possible side effects listed on the package insert.

7.5.2 Treating Vasospasms

If vasospasms are prevalent or if vasospastic reactions continue despite a normalization of blood pressure, these should be treated as well. A therapy has to be initiated only if spasms really exist. In cases of doubt, the diagnosis can usually be made or refuted at a specialized medical center.

Once again, general health enhancing procedures are recommended. Since both cold and emotional stress can trigger spasms in predisposed patients, these should be avoided as much as possible.

If spasms continue to occur despite general precautions in a glaucoma patient, drugs will be administered. Some have proven to be quite useful. Usually one starts – in particular if glaucomatous damage has not progressed too far – with magnesium. Magnesium should be taken in granulate form because this ensures good and constant absorption. To be effective, a relatively high dosage is required, such as 10 mmol 1 to 2 times/day. The main adverse reaction of magnesium therapy is diarrhea, but this usually stops after reducing the dosage a bit. If magnesium therapy alone is insufficient or if severe damage is present, calcium antagonists are the next line of defense. This is a group of drugs that blocks the inflow of calcium into the smooth muscle cells and thus leads to a dilation, especially of those branches of vessels that suffer from spasms. There are many different calcium antagonists, each having its own profile of efficacy. Included among these drugs are, for example, nifedipine or nilvadipine. Both the diagnosis and the initiation of such a therapy should take place at a specialized institution. This book cannot go into the advantages or disadvantages of each calcium antagonist (cf. App. 3).

It is, however, important to know that calcium antagonists should be given in very low dosages to treat vascular dysregulations (for example, 5 mg nifidepine or 2 mg nilvadipine 1–2 times/day). The low dosages are associated with only few side effects and in most cases will not lead to a further blood pressure reduction. Nevertheless, blood pressure should be monitored immediately after such treatment is started. Only delayed-release forms of calcium antagonists should be used to avoid activation of the sympathetic nervous system. We do not prescribe calcium channel blockers to patients with diabetes mellitus or patients with severe arteriosclerosis.

Patients are often confused when they realize that they are supposed to take a drug that is usually used to lower blood pressure, even though their own BP is already quite low. They should be aware that: a) the drug they are taking is administered in an unusually low dosage; and b) that a drop in the blood pressure induced by calcium antagonists does not lead to an undesirable counter-regulation of ocular perfusion, as is the case with spontaneous BP dips (cf. Chapter 5.2.3).

We have been quite successful in treating vasospastic children with low dosages of propanolol. Propanolol is a beta-blocker that has, as a side effect, a calcium antagonist action. Hope is placed in the so-called endothelin blockers, however, long-term experience with these drugs is still lacking.

7.6 Alternative Forms of Therapy

Alternative medicine, within the framework of medical treatment, might also be of benefit in ophthalmology. However, both experience and scientific data regarding these alternative forms of treatment are still so scarce that caution is needed in assessing their possible role. Alternative therapies should only be tried under strict supervision by an ophthalmologist, and a change in medication should only occur after he has been consulted. Some forms of treatment which are sometimes used – or tried – in glaucoma will be discussed below.

7.6.1 Autogenic Training

Autogenic training (AT) was developed around 1920 as a form of self-relaxation by Johannes Heinrich Schultz, a Berlin psychiatrist and neurologist. Today autogenic training is the most common and widely used technique for physical and mental relaxation in the western world. It has proven its usefulness as a supportive therapy for several psychosomatic, somatic [Gr. *soma:* body] and psychological diseases as well as a means of enhancing general health.

In patients suffering from chronic open-angle glaucoma, autogenic training sometimes increases the sense of well-being and lowers intraocular pressure. A positive effect on ocular perfusion is also possible, however, current knowledge about this field is still severely limited. It is important to know that autogenic training can only lead to IOP reductions if practiced regularly. Reducing or even stopping medical IOP-lowering therapy should only be tried under constant supervision of an ophthalmologist. If autogenic training is practiced regularly, it might be considered a valuable supportive therapy in patients with chronic open-angle glaucoma. Besides reducing IOP and improving circulation, it can contribute to feeling at ease with oneself and ameliorating conditions such as depression or phobias.

7.6.2 Acupuncture

Acupuncture is a mode of treatment originating from ancient China. It should be kept in mind, however, that even in China, acupuncture – as well as massage and herbal medicine – is only applied in only about 20% of all cases of illness as the sole therapy. It is mainly used as supportive treatment and makes up only one sixth of all medical procedures in China today. In acupuncture, needles are inserted at specific acupuncture points of the body in different skin layers. This is meant to provide a harmonic balance between two opposing forces (Yin and Yang) which circulate throughout the body in different spheres. There has never been a scientific explanation for the mechanism of action of acupuncture. Some controlled studies documenting an effect have been published recently, but much more research is needed to prove an efficacy and the mechanisms by which this might be achieved. A placebo effect could possibly be involved [Lat. *placere*: to please].

Acupuncture is used in ophthalmology for certain chronic diseases. While it seems to exert almost no influence on the IOP, in some cases ocular blood flow could be enhanced. The therapeutic potential of acupuncture could therefore play a role in glaucoma treatment. The authors are currently carrying out related studies. Even though it is not currently in widespread use in ophthalmology, this does not mean that it will not play a larger role in the future. But once again, this form of treatment always requires supervision by an ophthalmologist.

7.6.3 Homeopathy

Homeopathy was founded by Samuel Hahnemann (1755–1843). Basically, this describes the search for a drug that evokes exactly the same symptoms that the patient suffers, but in a healthy individual. Homeopathy strives to gain a precise and complete – called holistic – account of the patient. A constant cause of debate between homeopaths and physicians anchored in science-oriented medicine is "potency." Hahnemann started applying drugs in dosages that were regarded as "normal" for his time. He soon learned that diluting those substances might enhance their healing effects while reducing any poisonous side effects. This led him to repeatedly dilute, in a step-wise fashion, the original medications by a factor of 10,000 or even up to 50,000. In theory, a drug diluted by the factor 10^{24} should have no effect at all since there are hardly any molecules of the medication present in the solution. Nevertheless, these substances seem to show an effect – if the patients can be believed.

Homeopathy has been used in ophthalmology and seems to work in certain diseases. There are no controlled studies available with respect to glaucoma, making it prudent to try any homeopathic approach only under strict guidance and supervision of an ophthalmologist.

7.6.4 Anthroposophic Medicine

Modern anthroposophy was founded by Rudolf Steiner (1861–1925) as a philosophical and human science. It deals with the immaterial in nature and humans just as natural science does with the physical world. Anthroposophy does not regard health, disease and therapy as the sole result of molecular reactions but rather as an expression of the complex interactions of processes taking place within the physical, spiritual and mental make-up of an individual. Anthroposophic medicine strives to enlarge traditional scientific-based medicine with a philosophical school of thought.

Physicians who are oriented toward anthroposophy offer treatments in glaucoma such as eye drops and injections beneath the conjunctiva, but the efficacy of this has not been scientifically proven. As in homeopathy, any attempt to treat glaucoma this way should be closely supervised by an ophthalmologist.

7.6.5 Eye Training

William H. Bates (1860–1931) invented a concept he called visual training. He felt that cramps of the ocular muscles, faulty perception and thinking were responsible for eye disease. He "created" a type of ocular gymnastics that was supposed to cure the eye from myopia, strabismus, cataracts, glaucoma and a variety of retinal diseases.

Although still referring to Bates, his theories no longer take a center stage. Teachers working with the method offer a combination of visual training and techniques for relaxation for the entire body, such as special breathing patterns, autogenic training, yoga, meditation, catathymic image perception, psychodrama, Feldenkrais method and bioenergetics.

The efficacy of visual training has to be evaluated from two different points of view. For the patient, it can lead to a subjective feeling of improved vision; for the ophthalmologist, there has never been solid proof of a positive effect on any eye disease. Therefore, a final appreciation (or condemnation) cannot be made at this time.

7.6.6 Dietary Treatment

Nutrition plays a critical role in an individual's health. Much has been learned about this subject during the past few years. Today, one knows, for example, that a diet low in animal fat is associated with a lower incidence cardiovascular diseases as well as cancer. Unfortunately, specific knowledge concerning nutrition's effect on glaucoma is still lacking (for more information on this topic, cf. Chapter 7.5).

In the strictest sense of the term, there is no genuine dietary treatment for glaucoma. But there are several indications that the type of nutrition that reduces the risk of arteriosclerosis is also likely to decrease the chance of an IOP rise. Furthermore, substances like poliunsaturated fatty acids, especially omega-3, flavonoids (in the dark chocolate) and red wine, if consumed moderately, may prove useful for glaucoma patients as well.

7.6.7 Phytotherapy

Treating a disease using plants or plant extracts is called phytotherapy [Gr. *phython*: plant/Lat. *extrahere*: to pull out, to extract]. Many patients prefer drugs made from plants instead of "chemicals." Here it should be mentioned that the oldest anti-glaucoma medication, pilocarpine, is derived from a plant. One must remember that plants contain many potent substances, including some that are extremely poisonous (such as certain mushrooms). Other substances are very potent and have to be given in exact dosages, such as digoxin, which comes from digitalis, and morphine, which is made from opium poppies. During the past few years, a host of plant remedies have been proven to have some positive effect, such as green tea, garlic, gingko, etc. Not enough is known to indicate whether their potential use in glaucoma therapy would be beneficial. Since free radicals are regarded as pivotal in causing glaucomatous damage, the intake of substances capable of binding these free radicals would seem to make sense. Food rich in vitamin C, vitamin E and selenium are therefore deemed helpful; the same applies to green tea, fruits and vegetables such as tomatoes.

Summary

Most glaucoma patients do not suffer from any symptoms at the time of diagnosis. Nevertheless, they have to be treated with methods that can be associated with potential side effects. These adverse reactions can be the result of medical therapy or surgery. A glaucoma patient sometimes has to accept a decrease in his current quality of life in order to ensure stabilization of his future visual function.

The spectrum of therapeutic options has greatly broadened during the past few years. Many IOP-reducing drugs are available; each has its advantages as well as disadvantages. According to the patient's unique situation and needs, an individual therapy is chosen from among this spectrum of drugs.

Laser treatment is of minor importance in glaucoma therapy. The laser (iridotomy) is predominantly used for the prevention of acute angle-closure glaucoma. In most cases where glaucomatous damage progresses despite medical treatment, IOP-lowering surgery becomes necessary. A number of different techniques are available. Here, too, each has positive and negative aspects. Post-operative care of the patient is just as important as the operation itself.

For some patients, one must do more than just lower the IOP; the intraocular perfusion must also be improved. This primarily means avoiding sharp drops in blood pressure. If this cannot be achieved with general methods, medical treatment of the blood pressure becomes inevitable. Several drugs are available that can reduce vascular dysregulation. How effective they are and how well they are tolerated depends on the individual patient and his situation. Furthermore, though alternative methods of therapy are available, experience in using them to treat glaucoma has been very limited to date.

8 Living with Glaucoma

Even though glaucoma is a serious disease that, in the worst case, may lead to blindness if not treated, a glaucoma patient can lead a normal life. As long as there are no severe visual field defects that prohibit driving, the patient's life hardly differs from someone without glaucoma. However, once again, it should be emphasized that a glaucoma patient must strictly adhere to his treatment schedule and have regular consultations with his ophthalmologist.

Some questions frequently asked by glaucoma patients are addressed here.

8.1 Lifestyle and Nutrition

Someone with glaucoma can certainly enjoy "the good things in life" just as anyone else, but moderation is the key word.

Coffee/Tea. Within the first hour after consumption, coffee and tea can lead to a moderate increase in the intraocular pressure, but this effect is so small that no glaucoma patient has ever had to abstain from drinking these beverages. Basically, the glaucoma patient should not restrict his fluid intake, but rather consumption should be distributed throughout the day. Glaucoma patients who drink a lot within a very short time – say, one liter in just a few minutes – will experience a short-term increase in the IOP. The recommendation is thus to drink adequate amounts of fluids, but not large quantities in a very short time.

Alcohol. A small amount of alcohol, especially wine, is well tolerated and even exerts a protective influence on the heart and circulation. A glaucoma patient can enjoy a drink, even daily, without having to worry about the consequences to his eyes. In cases of acute angle-closure, a large quantity of strong alcohol can lower the IOP for a few hours. Administering alcohol as a "therapy" only makes sense, of course, if there is no other way to lower the pressure in an emergency situation.

Smoking. Smoking is the most important preventable risk factor that threatens human health. Smoking leads to cancer as well as to arteriosclerosis. Several eye diseases (obstruction of retinal vessels, maculopathy, cataracts, etc.) are much more common in smokers and occur at an earlier age than in non-smokers. Older smokers also have a higher risk of developing increased intraocular pressure as compared to non-smokers, but there is no evidence that smoking is an independent (i.e. unrelated to the IOP) risk factor for glaucomatous damage.

Marijuana. Even though marijuana does decrease the intraocular pressure, its medical use has not yet been investigated to the extent that it can be recommended as a therapeutic drug. Very few controlled studies have been performed to date; the advantages and disadvantages of long-term treatment with this agent still need to be fundamentally weighed against each other.

8.2   Leisure and Sports

Regular physical activity is just as important to the glaucoma patient as is proper relaxation and adequate amounts of sleep.

Physical activity tends to cause a decrease, rather than an increase, in the IOP. However, patients with pigmentary-dispersion glaucoma are sometimes the exception to this rule: they can experience a significant rise in the IOP following physical activity (cf. Chapter 3.6.1.2). But even a patient with this special form of glaucoma should be able to participate in sports. Preventive measures, such as a laser iridotomy or administering pilocarpine before exercise, can avert an IOP rise. Sports are also recommended for patients with very low systemic blood pressure to help stabilize the body's circulation.

Patients who already suffer from a visual field defect should be made aware of their condition. For example, these defects could result in a ball not being seen in time when playing tennis or an approaching danger going unnoticed when bike riding.

Scuba Diving. When swimming or snorkeling in relatively shallow water, there are only minor changes in the IOP. Glaucoma patients who plan to scuba dive should first consult their ophthalmologist. Someone having advanced optic nerve damage should probably refrain from diving.

Saunas. Saunas can also be enjoyed without concern. The IOP reacts just the same in glaucoma patients as in healthy subjects: it decreases in the sauna and then returns to original levels within about an hour. However, there is no proof that saunas are beneficial in glaucoma.

Flying. In Chapter 2.2.2, it was shown that the IOP measured by doctors – as defined from a physics point of view – is the difference between an absolute intraocular pressure and the current atmospheric pressure. A rapid decrease in the atmospheric pressure thus leads to a (relative) increase in the IOP. This normally poses no problem for a glaucoma patient on board a plane: there is an artificial atmospheric pressure inside the aircraft's cabin that compensates for most of the natural pressure drop experienced at high altitude. The eye adjusts relatively quickly to the new situation. A moderate decrease in atmospheric pressure will therefore not induce a significant rise in IOP.

Another aspect to consider is the quality of air inside the cabin with its somewhat lower concentration of oxygen at high altitude and, as a consequence, a lower availability of O_2. But here again, cabin ventilation provides the passengers with an almost normal level of oxygen. Nevertheless, glaucoma patients with advanced circulatory problems who fly frequently should discuss this with their ophthalmologist.

Music. Playing a wind instrument may lead to a transient increase in the intraocular pressure. Glaucoma patients who play these instruments should discuss this with their ophthalmologist.

8.3   Contact Lenses

The contact lens wearer can be reassured that these little optical devices do not affect the intraocular pressure. Indeed, IOP-reducing drugs can be given in even smaller doses to contact-wearing glaucoma patients. This is because a part of the drug is stored in or beneath the contact lens, forming a depot that continually releases the medication. However, keep in mind that some IOP-lowering drugs can render the corneal surface less sensitive. This increases the likelihood that an accidental injury occurring during lens insertion could go unnoticed.

After years of wearing contacts, certain changes occur in the patient's conjunctiva. This means there is a higher risk for the eventual obstruction of a fistula should a glaucoma operation become necessary. The introduction of mitomycin C has reduced this risk (cf. Chapter 7.4). Some glaucoma drugs can increase the symptoms generally known as "dry eyes," a condition that makes wearing contact lenses more difficult.

In short: Glaucoma patients can usually wear contact lenses, but should first consult their ophthalmologist.

8.4   Pregnancy and Nursing

On average, the IOP decreases during pregnancy. This (as well as the moderate increase after menopause) is an indication that sex hormones play a significant role in regulating the intraocular pressure. Since glaucoma is a chronic disease with a very slow progression, starting a therapy can often wait until after delivery. If there is already advanced glaucomatous damage or the IOP is extremely high, therapy during pregnancy is necessary and possible. The treating physician will know which IOP-lowering drugs are harmless for the mother and the fetus, and will choose the appropriate therapy.

Supplementary Chapters

This book describes the various diagnostic and therapeutic aspects of glaucoma. Even though it was the authors' goal that the text be straight-forward and easy to understand, nevertheless, to comprehend some aspects, a certain level of basic knowledge is required. Because not everyone has had the same opportunities to learn, or indeed, even the same desire to learn, about many of the topics covered, supplementary chapters have been written to provide detailed but basic information, for example, anatomy and physiology of the visual system.

Many of the methods used in diagnosing glaucoma are also used for other eye diseases. For those wishing more information on these procedures, the corresponding supplementary chapters will provide more detailed descriptions.

Because the glaucoma patient often has concomitant diseases, such as a cataract or macular degeneration, these diseases are also explained in more depth in the supplementary chapters.

It is not necessary to study these supplementary chapters in order to understand the main text. It is rather the authors' intention that the supplementary chapters be used as an opportunity to fill any gaps in knowledge and, depending on the reader's interest, to delve deeper into those topics he finds intriguing.

S 1 Anatomy and Physiology of the Visual System

In order to adequately comprehend those diseases that can affect an organ, a physician must thoroughly understand its anatomy and physiology [Gr. *anatemnein*: to cut open]. Structures of the human body have long only been studied by examining the dead, but with today's modern technology, e.g. magnetic resonance imaging (MRI), human anatomy can also be visualized in the living (cf. Fig. S 1.1).

Anatomy refers to the structures of the human body, while physiology is concerned with the functioning of a single organ or the entire organism [Gr. *physikos*: bodily/Gr. *logos*: word, study of]. The "visual system" refers to all structures that participate in vision [Lat. *visum*: that seen], from the eye to the brain (Fig. S 1.2). Vision basically refers to the perception of light, but first, an explanation of the nature of light is in order.

Light. In order to see the environment, a specific medium, i.e. light, is necessary. A star can only be seen because it emits light, light which eventually finds its way into the eye. An apple placed on a table is visible because it scatters and partially also reflects the light differently than the table.

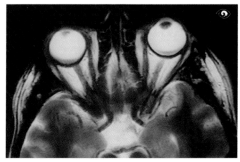

Fig. S 1.1: MRI showing the eyeballs, optic nerves and parts of the brain.

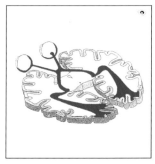

Fig. S 1.2: The visual pathway leads from the eye into the visual cortex

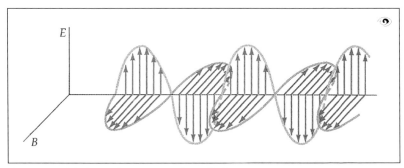

Fig. S 1.3: Light is an electromagnetic oscillation.

But what exactly is light? Even though light is something natural and commonplace, it is not an easy term to define or describe. From a physical point of view, light is a wave, specifically, a wave within an electromagnetic field (Fig. S 1.3). The electromagnetic field stretches across the universe and transports energy in the form of waves. The higher the wave's frequency, meaning the shorter the wavelength, then accordingly, the higher the energy that is transported. There is an infinitely wide range of frequencies within the electromagnetic field.

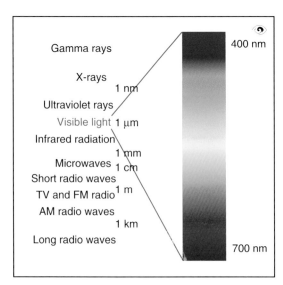

Fig. S 1.4: From among the broad spectrum of electromagnetic waves, only a small portion is perceived as light.

From among this broad spectrum, only a tiny section can be perceived by the human eye and identified by the brain as light (Fig. S 1.4). Within this extremely limited band, the human eye can distinguish between different wavelengths. These differences in wavelengths are perceived as different colors.

But light also has characteristics of corpuscular matter. It has a certain mass that is related to the energy it possesses. Therefore, it is drawn to, and deflected by, the planets or the earth, albeit only to a slight degree.

Light can pass through certain physical bodies: glass and water are classical examples. These bodies or substances are termed "transparent." A black object is black only because all colors are either partially or completely absorbed by the object. This is also the reason black objects in particular warm up when exposed to light: the absorbed energy is transformed into heat. Most matter does not absorb all wavelengths to the same degree. For example, a red apple absorbs all other wavelengths more than the wavelength for red light – this specific wavelength is scattered and thus makes the apple appear red (Fig. S 1.5). Light is reflected off surfaces. If such a reflecting surface is smooth or polished, it acts as a mirror.

Light travels with the "speed of light" in empty space. The progress of light slows down in a medium having some density. When light enters a denser material, such as glass, refraction occurs. Refraction is the basis for the optical effect of lenses.

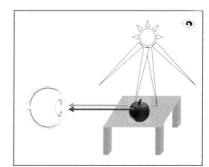

Fig. S 1.5: Objects appear to be colored because they absorb light of a certain wavelength.

What does "Vision" Imply? The visual system functions so automatically and perfectly that, in daily life, one is unaware of what a wondrous process is actually taking place. Before the individual aspects of vision are discussed, let's provide an example of how vision works: Imagine you are sitting around and talking with some friends. Someone brings out an old photo album. You browse through the pages, and suddenly, there is a picture of someone you knew in elementary school but have not seen in years. If one analyzes this situation, one could ask, "How did you recognize your former classmate?"

First of all, light must fall onto the picture. The photo scatters and reflects the light in different directions, and a very a small portion of that light enters the eye. The eye's optical system creates a second image on the retina. However, in order to get a clear image of the picture, and specifically of the section that shows the classmate, the eyes must move in such a way that the picture is located at your retina's area of highest resolution, the macula. Thus, a system for moving the eye must be present.

While still young and reading glasses are not yet needed, the image is automatically focused on the retina by the lens (which either increases or decreases in thickness to achieve a perfect focus). When the image is projected onto the macula, it must be transformed into neuronal impulses for the brain to be able to comprehend the visual information. When the same picture is observed with either sunlight or a light bulb shining on it, the light that reaches the eye is very different, both in brightness as well as in the color composition. Nevertheless, to the brain, both images are perceived as being quite similar because of a refined pre-processing of the incoming visual information by the retina. The information is transmitted from the eye to the primary, and later to the secondary, visual centers in the brain's visual cortex. Through a separate analysis of varying aspects of the different incoming information, such as direction, brightness, differences in light intensity, colors, movements, distances, etc., an "image" is created inside the brain; a process simply taken for granted.

You saw many people while browsing through the photo album, nevertheless, you recognized the classmate. The brain compared all the faces seen while browsing in the album with those faces kept in its "archives," i.e. the memory. Vision is thus something that can be fully utilized only when all visual impressions are compared with the memory.

This example demonstrates not only how complex, but also how amazing the visual function truly is. One is often surprised when something goes awry with this system, but what is even more astonishing is that this complex system works so well most of the time.

Some anatomical aspects of the visual system will be discussed before coming back to function.

The Eyeball. When talking about "the eye," one usually refers to that part which is visible from the outside, such as the eyelids and part of the eyeball (Fig. S 1.6). But most of the time, the eyeball or bulbus (bulbus oculi) is meant when speaking of the eye [Lat. *bulbus*: onion/Lat: *oculus*: eye].

If one looks straight into a person's eye, only a small portion of the eyeball is visible. The larger part is covered by the eyelids.

The eyeball is safely embedded within the eye socket (also called the orbit). If one looks at a cross-section of an eye, one notes that it is almost perfectly round (Fig. S 1.7).

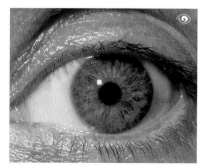

Fig. S 1.6: Usually only a small portion of the eyeball is seen.

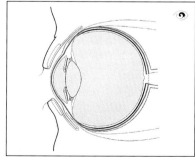

Fig. S 1.7: The eye is almost spherical and often compared to an apple.

This round shape permits a perfect focusing of the light and also facilitates movements in all directions.

In order to project an image from the environment onto the retina, the eye requires certain structures that aid in focusing light (refraction). At the same time, these structures have to be transparent which, in effect, also means that they should not contain blood vessels (Fig. S 1.8). The first refractive structure is the cornea [Lat. *cornu*: horn], and it focuses light. Figure S 1.9 shows a histological section through the cornea.

At the limbus, the cornea merges with the sclera [Gr. *skleros*: hard, tough]. Both the cornea and the sclera are relatively strong and solid, and form something akin to the eye's skeleton.

Behind the cornea is the space called the anterior chamber that is filled with aqueous humor (Fig. S 1.10).

The next anatomical structure is the iris [Gr. *iris*: rainbow], which functions as the eye's optical diaphragm (Fig. S 1.11).

The iris muscles determine the size of the opening where light enters, called the pupil [Lat. *pupa*: puppet, doll]. The latter term came into use because the observer sees himself reflected, tiny as a doll, when looking directly into the eyes of another person.

Behind the iris is the lens [Lat. *lens*: lens/Gr. *phakos*: lens] (Fig. S 1.12), which further focuses the light, a process started by the cornea. The lens is attached to the ciliary body by the fine, delicate zonular fibers. The ciliary body contains a circular muscle which, when it contracts, causes the zonular fibers to relax; the lens thus becomes more spherical. This further enhances the refraction of the incoming light, a process called accommodation [Lat. *accommodatio*: adjustment].

Accommodation specifically means the adjustment of vision to the changing distances of the objects being observed. The ability to accommodate gradually decreases with age and, usually between the ages of 40 to 45, most people require reading glasses. This age-related loss of accommodation is called presbyopia [Gr. *presbys*: old/ Gr. *opsein*: to see].

The small posterior chamber (Fig. S 1.10) and the much larger vitreous cavity (Fig. S 1.13) are located behind the iris and the lens.

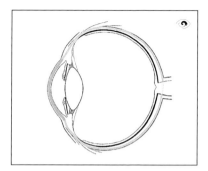

Fig. S 1.8: The cornea (blue) continues posteriorly as the sclera (gray).

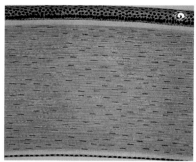

Fig. S 1.9: Histological section of the cornea: The multi-layer structure is easily recognizable.

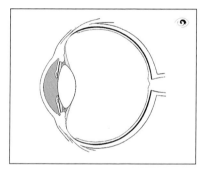

Fig. S 1.10: Anterior (dark blue) and posterior chamber (light blue), both filled with aqueous humor.

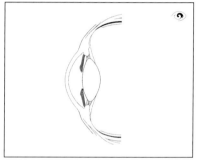

Fig. S 1.11: The iris (red).

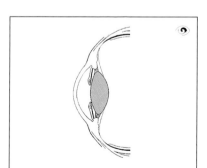

Fig. S 1.12: The lens (blue).

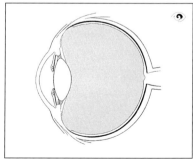

Fig. S 1.13: The vitreous chamber (gray).

The vitreous body consists of a highly viscous, transparent, gelatinous mass with a frame of supporting fibers. Throughout life, small opacities inside the vitreous body can develop, thereby casting shifting shadows onto the retina. If the patient is aware of these opacities, they are termed "mouches volantes" or flying mosquitoes. [Fr. *mouche*: mosquito/Fr. *volant*: flying]. During the normal aging process (particularly in myopic individuals), the vitreous body occasionally shrinks some and thus can become separated from the retina. This results in a normal posterior vitreous detachment. However, if the vitreous body adheres to parts of the retina during the detachment, holes can be torn in this sensitive structure. These holes and tears can lead to a retinal detachment.

The innermost structure of the eye's posterior segment is the retina [Lat. *rete*: net], which is highly sensitive to light (Fig. S 1.14) and consists of several different layers (Fig. S 1.15).

Behind the retina is the pigment epithelium that contains, as the name implies, much pigment, specifically, melanin [Lat. *pingere*: to paint/Gr. *melas*: black] (Fig. S 1.16). Melanin absorbs light and thus prevents any further dispersion. Figure S 1.17 shows a strongly magnified picture of pigment cells laden with melanin.

If these pigment cells lack melanin (a condition called albinism), the larger choroidal vessels can be directly observed (Fig. S 1.18).

Besides absorbing the light, the pigment layer serves several other important purposes with respect to the retina's nutrition. Behind the pigment epithelium is the choroid, which is primarily composed of blood vessels [Gr. *chorioidea*: similar to the chorion, chorion-like/Gr. *chorion*: placenta] (Figs. S 1.19 and S 1.20).

Together, the iris, ciliary body and choroid are also called the uvea [Lat. *uvea*: grape]. If the choroid is opened up, it indeed resembles the skin of a red grape. The intense degree of circulation that occurs inside the choroid (Fig. S 1.21) is essential for the retina's nutrition, and also provides a constant, stable temperature and regulates volume.

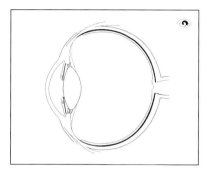

Fig. S 1.14: The retina (yellow).

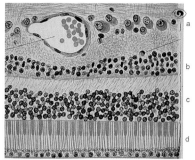

Fig. S 1.15: Histological section of the retina: a) ganglion cells, b) bipolar cells, c) nuclei of receptor cells, d) outer-segment of receptor cells.

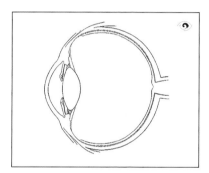

Fig. S 1.16: Pigment epithelium (brown).

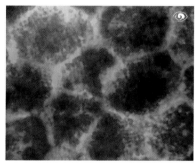

Fig. S 1.17: Pigment epithelium as seen under a microscope.

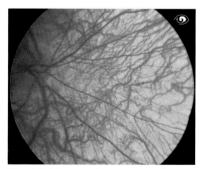

Fig. S 1.18: Posterior segment of a patient suffering from albinism. The large choroidal vessels are visible.

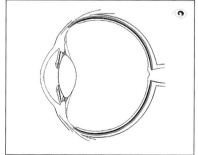

Fig. S 1.19: The choroid (red).

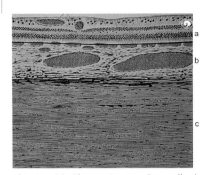

Fig. S 1.20: The eye's posterior wall: a) retina, b) choroid, c) sclera.

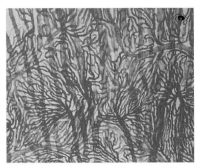

Fig. S 1.21: The choroid is primarily composed of blood vessels.

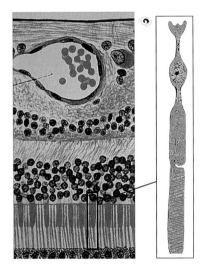

Fig. S 1.22: The external retinal layer contains the receptor cells; on the right, an enlarged sketch of a rod.

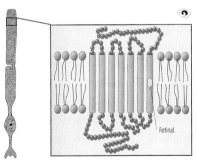

Fig. S 1.23: Rhodopsin, which contains retinal, can be found in the lamellae of the receptor cells.

Changing Light into Sight. The retina's sensory cells (Fig. S 1.22) contain a photosensitive substance called retinal (Fig. S 1.23). When retinal absorbs a photon (one unit of light), it undergoes a change in shape (Fig. S 1.24).

Other molecules recognize that this alteration has occurred, and a series of reactions is started which results in a closure of ion channels that lead into the cell [Gr. *ion*: walking]. This, in turn, alters the potential of the cell membrane and transforms the incoming information into a nerve impulse (Fig. S 1.25). The entire process of turning light into neural information is called phototransduction.

Fig. S 1.24: Retinal changes its configuration when it is exposed to light und thus starts the flow of information.
a = retinal before exposure to light;
b = retinal after exposure to light.

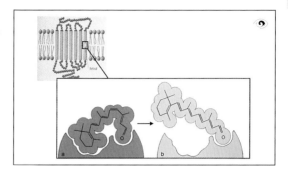

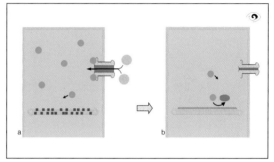

Fig. S 1.25: The messenger substance, cGMP (green), is broken down. Ion channels close and the cell membrane's potentials change.
a = before exposure to light;
b = after exposure to light.

There are two kinds of photoreceptors in the retina, the rods and the cones. The rods are very sensitive to intensity and function throughout a remarkably wide range of light, i.e. from brightness to almost total darkness; they thus enable vision even in dim light. The cones, on the other hand, require a more intense level of light to function, and provide greater resolution for details and the interpretation of colors. Both use the same light-sensitive molecule, retinal. Retinal is embedded within a large protein called opsin. Retinal and opsin together form rhodopsin [Gr. *rhodon*: rose, rose red].

There are different types of opsin: each type of opsin has a different amino acid sequence (i.e. the basic molecular sequence). Because rhodopsin is a combination of opsin and retinal, the various forms of opsin create diverse forms of rhodopsin – the primary difference being a slight spectral shift in the wavelength of the absorption maximum of the retinal component of rhodopsin. This enables

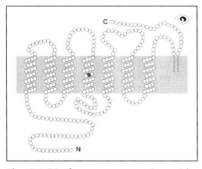

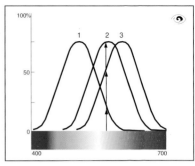

Fig. S 1.26: If one or more amino acids (red) are exchanged inside the opsin molecule, the spectral sensitivity of retinal is altered.

Fig. S 1.27: Spectral sensitivity of the three different kinds of cones: The impression of color is created by the relative contribution made by each of these three different cones (arrows).

cones containing different pigments to identify different colors (Fig. S 1.27).

Because the composition of opsin can also vary from one individual to another, not all humans share the same color perception. Sometimes one or two of the types of rhodopsin cannot be formed at all, and this results in a congenitally poor color perception.

From Vision to Recognition. The retina reduces the incoming information to the essentials, and the essentials are not absolute brightness or absolute colors, but rather contrast. If the green leaves of a tree are observed in the bright noontime sunlight and when the sun is setting, then the light that is scattered by these leaves and which reaches the eye has completely different physical characteristics. Nevertheless, the brain identifies "green leaves," and this phenomenon is known as color constancy. The same thing happens with different degrees of brightness: Even though the absolute brightness of the environment might change by a factor of several thousand, a very similar picture is still perceived. This is truly essential for vision and protects the brain from an overload of information while, at the same time, ensuring that the relevant information gets accurately transmitted.

Another example underscores this: Imagine someone sitting in a dimly lit room where a slide presentation is about to begin; the slides will be projected onto a screen. Before the presentation starts, the screen does not appear to be particularly bright, but it is still recognizable as a white surface. Then the presentation starts and a slide is projected that contains letters written in black on white; while there is no change in the room's illumination. Some spots on the canvas receive the additional illumination from the projector, while others, where the dark letters are written, do not receive additional light. It thus appears that something is written in "black on white." In reality, however, at those areas with the dark letters, the screen is still as white as it was before the projector was switched on. This means that the same information, emanating from the same spot on the screen, is first perceived as "white" and a moment later, in a different comparison, as "black."

This exemplifies the preselection capability of the retina: It does not absorb information indiscriminately, but rather starts a very sensitive process of selection and transformation. The brain assembles this information transmitted from the retina via the visual pathway to form a complete picture and constantly compares the content of this image with similar features stored in its "archives" – the memory.

Protecting the Eye. Because the eye is a delicate organ that can be easily injured but nevertheless must be able to move, it is safely embedded in the orbital cavity. The orbit's outer walls are bony structures; its internal surface is covered by cushioning fat (Fig. S 1.28). The lids (Fig. S 1.29) automatically close whenever danger appears, as well as during sleep (Figs. S 1.30 and S 1.31). An involuntary lid closure, i.e. a blink, occurs about every ten seconds or around 6000 times a day. This not only optimally distributes the tear layer across the ocular surface, but also wipes away any small foreign bodies.

A mucous membrane, called the conjunctiva [Lat. *konjugere*: to bandage], covers both the interior portion of the eyelid as well as part of the eyeball's surface. The conjunctiva's relatively loose struc-

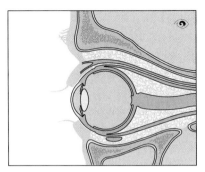

Fig. S 1.28: The eyeball is embedded in a fatty cushion within the orbit.

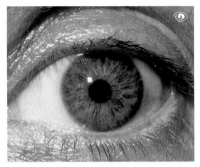

Fig. S 1.29: The eyelids protect the eyeball.

Fig. S 1.30: The lids contain cartilage (blue) and are covered by conjunctiva (red) on their backside.

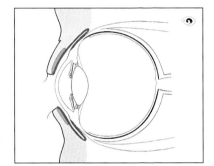

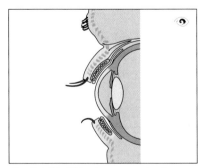

Fig. S 1.31: This picture emphasizes the fine muscle layer of the lids as well as the small oil-producing glands inside the cartilage.

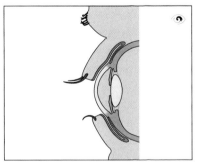

Fig. S 1.32: The good mobility of the eyeball is made possible by the loose conjunctiva of the eyeball and the lids (red).

ture contributes to the eyeball's mobility (Fig. S 1.32). In combination with the tear film, the conjunctiva also protects the eye from foreign bodies and infections. An inflammation of the conjunctiva – a quite common event called conjunctivitis – results in an increased blood flow. The conjunctiva becomes redder and redder, and the patient suffers from the proverbial "pink eye." But normally, the conjunctiva is transparent, and one sees through to the next – subconjunctival – layer, the sclera, which makes up the "whites of their eyes."

The surface of the cornea and conjunctiva is covered by the tear film. This part watery, part oily layer keeps the cornea smooth and also contributes to its superb ability to refract light. The tear film is produced by the lacrimal glands and is drained via the lacrimal duct into the nose and throat.

Moving the Eye. Imagine you see a fly walking across a desk and you observe its movements. What is actually happening with your eyes?

Both eyes move in such a way that the fly's image is constantly kept on your eye's macula [Lat. *macula*: spot]. The macula is a small spot on the retina that delivers the best visual acuity achievable (cf. S 9). When a certain object is closely observed, the eyes shift exactly to that one position which brings the object's image directly onto the macula. Back to the fly: the eyes steadily follow the fly. To do this, not only is a motor (muscular) apparatus required (Fig. S 1.33), but a center in the brain is also needed to coordinate the eye movements thereby ensuring that the image of the fly is constantly fixed on the maculae of both eyes. Another example: Imagine while you're taking a stroll, you see a hot-air balloon up in the sky. The balloon is first noticed when it enters your peripheral visual field, meaning the eyes are not yet fixated on the balloon. To achieve a better image of the balloon, your eyes turn, within milliseconds, in such a way that the balloon's image becomes focused on your maculae. These rapid eye movements are called saccade [Fr. *saccade*: jerk, jolt].

This rapid and not consciously-induced movement causes the image of the environment to quickly move across the retina. It

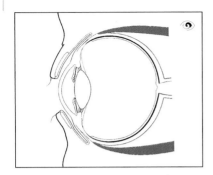

Fig. S 1.33: The outer eye muscles rotate and move the eye.

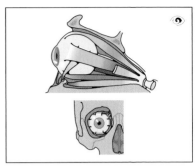

Fig. S 1.34: Six muscles ensure good eye mobility in every direction.

would be a most unpleasant experience if the surrounding world were perceived to be moving so rapidly. The brain has solved this problem in a unique fashion: The incoming image is suppressed for that short moment during which the eyes move so rapidly, a process called saccadic suppression [Lat. *suppressio*: suppression]. This process happens so quickly that one is not aware of the fact that, for a split-second, the eyes do not see anything at all. The size of the saccade can vary greatly and depends upon where the targeted object is located in the visual field, i.e. in a relatively more peripheral or central site. Furthermore, part of the necessary movement is not done by the eyes alone but also by a turning of the head. The brain precisely calculates the direction and the extent of the movement necessary before sending the impulse that triggers the movement. It divides the size of the movement into a larger portion for the eye and a smaller portion for the head. Once again, this is a very complex function of the brain that is simply not consciously recognized.

The subspecialty that deals with crossed eyes, i.e. strabismus [Gr. *strabos*: askance], eye movements and their disturbances is called orthoptics [Gr. *orthos*: straight/Gr. *opsein*: to see]. Figures S 1.33 and S 1.34 show the muscles that move the eyeball.

Structures Relevant for Glaucoma. In order to better understand the mechanisms of glaucoma, attention is now directed to certain components of the visual system. These include the ciliary body, which produces aqueous humor, the anterior and posterior chambers, through which the humor passes and, finally, the trabecular meshwork and Schlemm's canal where the aqueous humor leaves the eye. Alterations in any these structures can lead to a rise in intraocular pressure.

Glaucomatous damage occurs in the ganglion cells of the retina and the papilla, which is the reason why these structures at the posterior pole of the eye are also discussed.

The Ciliary Body. The ciliary body was defined above: it is a circular structure located in the anterior third of the eye (Fig. S 1.35).

Originating from the ciliary processes (Figs. S 1.36 and S 1.37), the zonular fibers [Lat. *zonula*: small belt] hold the lens in place. The ciliary body is covered by two layers of epithelium [Gr. *epi*: above/Gr. *thälä*: small wart].

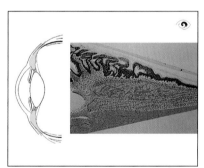

Fig. S 1.35: The ciliary body as seen: in a drawing (left) and in a histological cross-section (right).

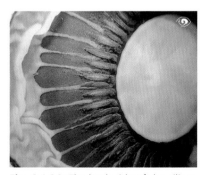

Fig. S 1.36: The back side of the ciliary body. (The picture was made from the eye of a cadaver.) The opaque lens is visible in the center.

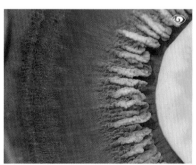

Fig. S 1.37: Ciliary body in high magnification.

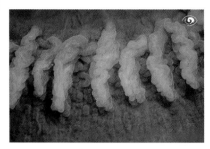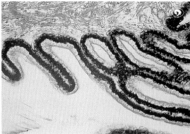

Fig. S 1.38: Ciliary body processes, in the eye of a cadaver (left), in a histological section (right).

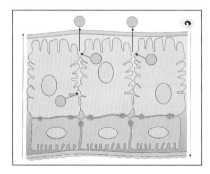

Fig. S 1.39: Aqueous humor is secreted via active transport by the bi-layer epithelium of the ciliary body.

The epithelium describes the outermost layer of the skin. Likewise, it is also used to refer to the outer layer of other structures, such as the cornea and the ciliary body.

The two ciliary epithelial layers are easily distinguished: The outer epithelial layer is pigmented and the inner epithelial layer is lacking in pigment (Fig. S 1. 38).

The aqueous humor is produced by these epithelial cells. Below the epithelium, there are fenestrated [Lat. *fenestra*: window] blood vessels, meaning there are small pores in the vessel's endothelial lining that permit ions and molecules of small or intermediate size to leave the capillaries. This creates a fluid-soaked layer directly between the blood vessels and the two epithelial layers.

From this fluid, the epithelium actively extracts various substances, transports them together with water into the posterior chamber, and thus forms aqueous humor (Fig. S 1.39).

This means that fluid is not simply squeezed out of the vessels. Quite the contrary: Certain ions and molecules have to be actively transported against a concentration gradient using specialized pumps within the cell wall, a process that induces water to follow the ion flow via osmotic forces.

Producing aqueous humor is essential for maintaining intraocular pressure and nourishing those segments of the cornea and lens that lack blood vessels. Aqueous humor carries oxygen, glucose and other nutrients; a high concentration of vitamin C is also found here. This vitamin protects the cornea and the lens from the damaging influence of free radicals.

To a large extent, the production of aqueous humor is independent of the IOP. Up to a certain level, when the intraocular pressure rises, humor production still continues. In extreme cases, such as in angle-closure glaucoma (cf. Chapter 3.5.1), the IOP can rise to a level of 60 mmHg or even higher. However, the IOP rises just until the ocular perfusion becomes cut off by the high pressure. This means an end to the blood supply with the result that the aqueous humor production slows down and finally stops. Because systolic blood pressure inside the eye rarely exceeds 60 or 70 mmHg, the IOP never significantly rises above this level.

The Anterior and Posterior Chambers. Aqueous humor flows from the posterior chamber, where it is produced by the ciliary body, through the pupil into the anterior chamber (Fig. S 1.40). The iris is normally in loose contact with the lens. There is thus no significant resistance that might hinder the humor's flow. In far-sighted individuals (hyperopes), the anterior chamber is comparatively shallow, leading to a stronger contact of the iris to the lens. Something similar happens in the eyes of a person with no refractive error as he ages: the lens gradually gets thicker and thus comes into a closer contact with the iris. As hyperopic individuals age, the two factors doubly increase the risk of developing a pupillary block (cf. Chapter 3.5.1).

Due to optical considerations, it is imperative that the aqueous humor be completely transparent. There are, however, patho-

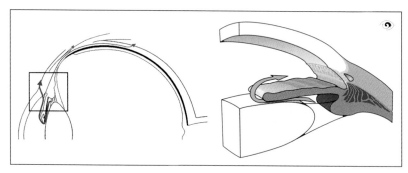

Fig. S 1.40: Aqueous humor flows from the posterior into the anterior chamber and then leaves the eye.

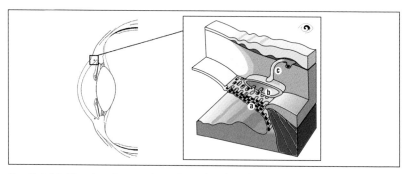

Fig. S 1.41: The chamber angle region: a) trabecular meshwork, b) Schlemm's canal, c) collecting channels.

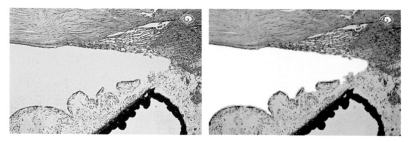

Fig. S 1.42: Histological section through a normal chamber angle region. In the picture on the right the chamber angle (normally filled with aqueous humor) is dyed yellow.

logical conditions where the aqueous humor is no longer transparent. For example, with an intraocular inflammation, white blood cells and fibrin might mix with the humor and cause an opacification (clouding). In the wake of an injury or operation, there might be bleeding into the anterior chamber. Red blood cells cause a particularly intense blurring of vision when present at this location.

The Aqueous Humor Drainage System. The aqueous humor flows from the anterior chamber through the trabecular meshwork into Schlemm's canal (Fig. S 1.41). The trabecular meshwork acts like a strainer (Fig. S 1.42), however, the spaces between the meshwork are not completely empty (Fig. S 1.43). These pores contain large molecules that provide some degree of resistance to the humor outflow.

Indeed, and quite important to the study of glaucoma, alterations in the meshwork structure are the cause of the IOP rise in primary open-angle glaucoma (cf. Chapter 3.4.1/Figs. 3.11 and 3.12).

From the trabecular meshwork, the humor drains through Schlemm's canal. Named after a German anatomist, this circular conduit is located below the area where the cornea merges into the sclera. From Schlemm's canal, the humor drains into small collecting channels (Fig. S 1.44) and then back into a system of tiny veins above the sclera where it becomes part of the bloodstream.

Some scleral veins can be viewed where the humor flows next to, and parallel with, the venous blood, and these are called aqueous veins (Fig. S 1.45).

A small portion of the fluid leaves the eye via the uveoscleral outflow (Fig. S 1.40).

This means that the humor flows between the cells of the peripheral iris and the ciliary body, and then enters the space between the uvea and sclera. From here, it is either taken up by the uvea's blood vessels or it drains through the sclera into the orbit. The uveoscleral outflow is believed to be particularly important at night during sleep, a time when the trabecular meshwork and Schlemm's canal regenerate. Uveoscleral outflow is enhanced by prostaglandins.

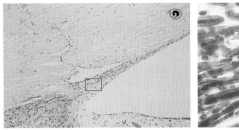
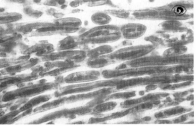

Fig. S 1.43: Aqueous humor trickles through the trabecular meshwork into Schlemm's canal (as seen in high magnification on the right).

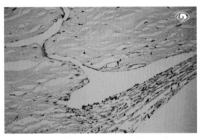
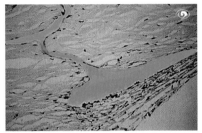

Fig. S 1.44: Histological section of the humor's outflow passages. In the picture on the right, the draining channels are dyed blue.

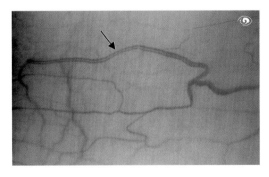

Fig. S 1.45: The white stripe inside the vein (→) is aqueous humor that has not yet completely mixed with blood.

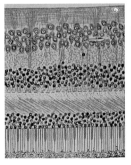
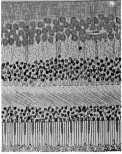

Fig. S 1.46: Histological section of the retina: in the picture on the right, the ganglion cells and the nerve fiber layer are dyed red.

Prostaglandins are locally effective, multifunctional hormones (cf. Chapter 7.2.5). With inflammation, there is an increased production of prostaglandins; this transiently enhances the uveoscleral outflow. This is one of the reasons why the IOP can be quite low during acute intraocular inflammation. This particular effect is exploited in glaucoma therapy (cf. Chapter 7.2.5).

This then completes a basic overview of the eye's structures that are essential for regulating intraocular pressure. Attention now turns to the parts of the eye that are damaged during glaucoma.

Retina, Disc and Optic Nerve. The retina transforms the light's information into neuronal impulses. The retina is composed of several layers (Fig. S 1.15), the most external of which contains light-sensitive receptors. These transmit the information to the next layer, consisting of bipolar cells. From here, the information is transmitted on towards the innermost retinal layer that is composed of ganglion cells (Fig. S 1.46).

Protrusions from these neural ganglion cells, called axons, leave the eye through the optic disc (also called the papilla or the optic nerve head) and lead directly into the brain (Figs. S 1.47 and 1.48).

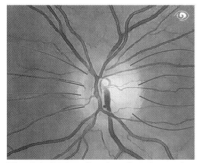

Fig. S 1.47: Fundus showing the optic disc, the red lines symbolize the course of the nerve fibers.

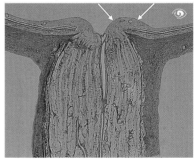

Fig. S 1.48: Histological section of a healthy optic disc and the anterior segment of the optic nerve. The cushion (→) of the nerve fibers is clearly visible.

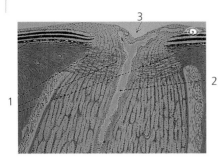

Fig. S 1.49: Histological section of a normal optic disc and the anterior segment of the optic nerve: Fig. 1. lamina cribrosa; Fig. 2. central retinal vein; Fig. 3. physiological excavation.

These axons form the optic nerve (Fig. S 1.49), which continues to the optic chiasm where half of the optic nerve fibers cross to the other side of the brain (Fig. S 1.2). From here, the nerve impulses are transmitted to the geniculate body [Lat. *geniculatus*: knee-like, knee-shaped] from where it is transferred, via synapses, to other nerve cells and then travels through the optic radiation into the visual cortex in the occipital portion of the brain [Lat. *caput*: head/Lat. *occiput*: back part of the head].

As noted earlier, the retina not only perceives and transports the information, but also preprocesses it. In order to achieve this, a complex connection between the cells is required.

In glaucoma, individual retinal nerve fibers or even entire nerve fiber bundles can be affected, the latter being called a nerve fiber bundle defect. Figure S 1.50 shows a longitudinal section, and Figure S 1.51, a cross section, of such a bundle of nerve fibers. The optic disc has a very special blood supply system. The superficial segments are supported by the retinal circulation, the deeper layers by the ciliary circulation that also supplies the choroid with blood (Fig. S 1.52). Even though the disc (and indeed the entire optic nerve) is actually part of the brain and thus has a blood-brain barrier, vasoactive substances from the optic disc's surroundings can find their way into this structure. This is one of the reasons why the optic disc is so vulnerable. In contrast to the optic nerve, the retinal nerve fibers do not have myelin [Gr. *myelos*: marrow], a special protective and insulating layer. If they did, they simply could not properly fulfill their function in the visual process because transparency is essen-

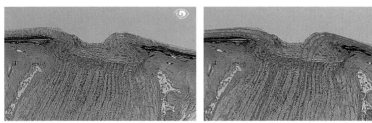

Fig. S 1.50: Histological section of the optic disc; in the picture on the right, some nerve fibers are shown in red.

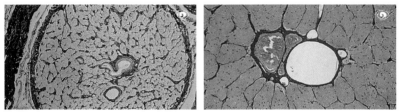

Fig. S 1.51: Cross-section of the optic nerve: an overview (left), highly magnified (right).

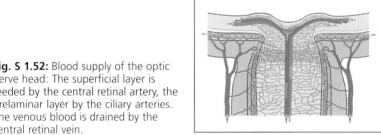

Fig. S 1.52: Blood supply of the optic nerve head: The superficial layer is feeded by the central retinal artery, the prelaminar layer by the ciliary arteries. The venous blood is drained by the central retinal vein.

tial: light has to find its way unchallenged through the fiber layer and reach the photoreceptors. The optic disc is devoid of any myelin as well – not because transparency is required here, but rather due to the lack of space at the lamina cribrosa where the nerve fiber bundles exit through the sclera.

The lamina cribrosa (Fig. S 1.49) is a slightly thinner continuation of the sclera that has tiny holes through which the nerve fibers leave the eye [Lat. *cribrum*: sieve/Lat. *lamina*: thin plate].

However, inside the optic nerve, the axons become myelinated as soon as they have passed through the lamina cribrosa. In demyelinating diseases, the optic nerve becomes damaged, but not that portion within the eye which is devoid of myelin. The most important and also most well known of these diseases is multiple sclerosis. When the optic nerve is afflicted with an acute inflammation (as, for example, with multiple sclerosis), the condition is termed "retrobulbar optic neuritis," i.e. located in the optic nerve somewhere behind the eyeball.

But back to the nerve fibers inside the eye: axons run from the retinal nerve layer towards the exit at the optic disc. This leads to an increasing thickness of the retinal nerve fiber layer as it approaches the optic disc.

The optic disc, the site where the nerve fibers exit the eye, contains a relatively constant number of fibers. But because the papilla is sometimes larger than the space that the nerve fibers require, it is usual that there is a variable open space right in the middle of the disc, referred to as an excavation [Lat. *cavum*: cave] or, more precisely, a physiological excavation. A healthy person can have a physiological excavation. However, the excavation that a glaucoma patient suffers is not termed physiological, but rather pathological. It is an acquired excavation that can become larger during the patient's lifetime if the glaucoma is left untreated.

The larger the optic disc, the larger the physiological excavation. In a healthy individual having an extremely small papilla, there

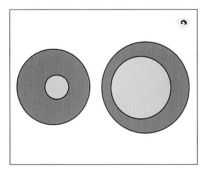

Fig. S 1.53: In healthy eyes, small optic discs have small excavations and large optic discs have large excavations. This is due to the fact that the area of the neuroretinal rim (red) has a fairly constant size.

is no excavation noted (Fig. S 1.53). This normal variation, from non-existent to noteworthy, is important to know when assessing a patient's optic disc, and thus a great deal of experience is required in the cup's evaluation, which is a decisive factor in diagnosing glaucoma (cf. Chapter 2.1.2).

A healthy eye has approximately 132 million receptor cells, approximately 1 million ganglion cells and, as a consequence, 1 million nerve fibers that run from the optic disc into the brain. During one's lifetime, even under normal conditions, there is a daily loss of ganglion cells and their axons. However, because of disease, a glaucoma patient suffers from a much more rapid demise of ganglion cells and nerve fibers (Fig. S 1.54). The accelerated death of nerve fibers leads to an enlargement of the excavation (Fig. S 1.55), which is then termed a pathological or glaucomatous excavation. Natu-

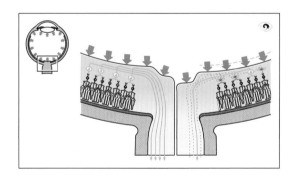

Fig. S 1.54: Loss of nerve fibers and progression of the excavation, possibly due to elevated IOP.

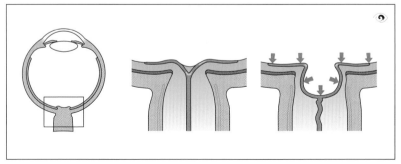

Fig. S 1.55: The loss of nerve fibers and glial cells results in glaucomatous excavation.

rally, there are corresponding alterations in the other tissues of the visual pathway down the line, such as the optic nerve and the geniculate body inside the brain. But because these structures are out of reach for daily diagnostic purposes, they are not discussed in detail here.

Table S 1: Ocular Anatomy – Some Average Numbers about the Eye

Diameter of eyeball		23 mm
Weight of eyeball		7.5 g
Thickness of cornea		0.6 mm
Thickness of sclera at the equator		0.3 mm
Thickness of sclera near the optic disc		1.3 mm
Thickness of choroid at the equator		0.12 mm
Thickness of choroid near the macula		0.26 mm
Thickness of retina at the equator		0.18 mm
Thickness of retina at the fovea centralis		0.10 mm
Thickness of retina next to the optic nerse		0.56 mm
Thickness of lens in a newborn		3.5 mm
Thickness of lens in a 20-year-old		4 mm
Thickness of lens in an 80-year-old		5 mm
Diameter of the optic nerve		4 mm
Daily tear production		1 ml
Daily aqueous humor production		3 ml
Number of photoreceptors		132,000,000
rods	125,000,000	
cones	7,000,000	
Number of retinal bipolar cells		2,000,000
Number of retinal ganglion cells		1,000,000

S 2   The Development of the Eye

When studying the anatomy and physiology of the eye (cf. S 1), the wondrous nature of this organ is most evident. Light that is scattered and reflected by the environment can be perceived in such a manner that objects can be identified. This process of identification works so perfectly that faces can be recognized or texts read without difficulty. As great a miracle as is the development of the eye, even more amazing yet is that of the organism as a whole.

Controlling Development. Ponder for a moment how the human body, starting from just one single fertilized egg cell, after undergoing cell division and multiplication, becomes a human being. Imagine that a fertilized egg cell has already divided and now consists of eight cells. How does each cell know in which direction it has to develop? Will this cell (or rather its offspring) finally contribute to the growth of the head or the creation of a foot? Until very recently, these questions still posed a great mystery to biologists. However, during the past few years, some insight has been gained into the regulation of embryonic development. Even the unfertilized egg cell inside the ovary contains information as to how certain parts must develop should fertilization occur. Using specific messenger substances, the surrounding cells inside the ovary provide the egg with this information. The concentration of these messenger substances varies in the different parts of the egg cell, depending on the side from which the messengers have entered the cell. The way in which the cell will develop is thus predetermined. After the first division, both cells contain different concentrations of these messenger substances and therefore both "know" that they have different tasks to fulfill. They thus grow to become different cells by expressing different genes (cf. S 3).

At a later developmental stage, the information that each cell receives from its neighboring cells becomes crucial: simply put, the cells "talk" to each other. An example to illustrate this: When blood vessels grow into the eye, small arteries originating from the same vessel may take a completely different path in their development.

This path depends on many factors, including their location and whether they form part of the retina or part of the choroid. The surrounding tissue informs the cells how they should develop. For example, choroidal capillaries form tiny pores; the information to develop these pores in their walls comes from adjacent pigment epithelium. On the other hand, blood vessels inside the retina have to be non-fenestrated since any uncontrolled outflow of fluid would have devastating consequences for vision. Here, the developing blood vessels receive the necessary information from retinal cells. If these blood vessels approach the pigment epithelium, which only occurs in the case of disease or malformation, then tiny fenestrations (pores) start to develop. Complex control loops in which the cells "converse" with, and influence, each other regulate the behavior of each of these cells.

The development of the eye begins relatively early, within the third to fourth week of pregnancy. But how is this process controlled and directed? Once again, research has arrived at fascinating conclusions. There are "regulatory genes" (cf. S 3) to which are relegated the task of regulating the expression of subordinate genes. If this regulatory "eye gene" expresses itself, eye development commences, driven by the expression of many subordinate genes carrying out this order to develop. These subordinate genes basically contain a blueprint for the eye. "Expression" means releasing the information stored inside a gene with the aim of synthesizing a certain protein (cf. S 3) [Lat. *expressio*: expression].

It has been possible to demonstrate the effect that such a gene has in regulating the eye's development by a most unique experiment. By artificially "switching on" such a gene at a specific time point on various body parts of flies, it has been possible to grow eyes on their legs and wings! Equally remarkable is the fact that this regulatory gene is practically identical in humans and in animals, even though numerous types of eyes exist in the animal kingdom. This means that the same gene controls the development of the many-faceted compound eye of the fly and the eye of a human being! The difference lies in the subsequent gene expression that makes each animal species develop its specific type of eye (Fig. S 2.1).

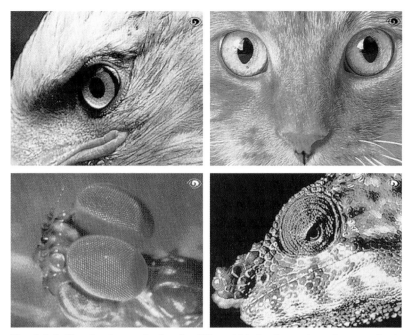

Fig. S 2.1: The development of quite different kinds of eyes in various species is ordered by the same regulatory gene.

The Genetic Blueprint of the Eye. Although many facts are known about the development of the eye and its regulatory genes, many questions still remain unanswered. Indeed, not all the genes that participate and direct the development of the eye and its function are known. Nevertheless, the genetic analysis of patients having various defects in ocular development has provided important clues. For example, those genes or rather gene products that play a role in phototransduction have been quite precisely identified (cf. S 1). A mutation at one of these genes can lead to a disease known as retinitis pigmentosa. Flaws in other genes can result in other specific diseases or developmental defects; many of these are discussed elsewhere (cf. A 3).

How Does the Eye Develop? A young embryo has three different primary germ layers: ectoderm, mesoderm and endoderm.

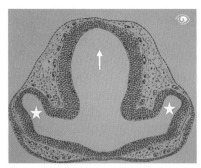

Fig. S 2.2: Cross-section through brain vesicle (→) and optic vesicle (*) in the third week of pregnancy.

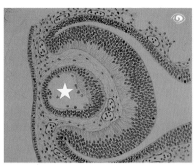

Fig. S 2.3: In the sixth week of pregnancy, the optic vesicle develops into the optic cup. The embryonic lens becomes visible (*).

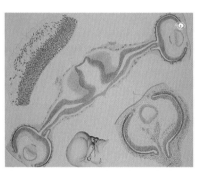

Fig. S 2.4: Cross-section through the brain vesicle and the embryonic eye (sixth week of pregnancy).

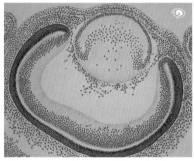

Fig. S 2.5: In the seventh week, the optic cup differentiates into the anteriorly located retina and the posteriorly located pigment epithelium (stained darker).

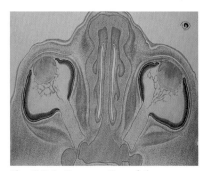

Fig. S 2.6: Cross-section of the embryo's head in the eight week of pregnancy. The eyes develop at the side of the nose.

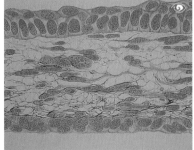

Fig. S 2.7: The embryo's cornea in the eighth week.

The ectoderm primarily develops into skin and the nervous system, mesoderm into muscles, connective and supportive tissues, and endoderm into the gastrointestinal tract, the liver and pancreas. Both mesoderm and ectoderm play a role in the formation of the eye. During the third gestational week, small optic cups form on both sides of the neural tube in what later becomes the forebrain region (Fig. S 2.2).

With increasing growth, the bulb-like optic vesicle invaginates in an anterior and downward direction, thus forming the optic cup (Figs. S 2.3 and 2.4).

The interior layer of the optic cup will become the retina and the exterior layer will develop into the pigment epithelium (Figs. S 2.5 and S 2.6).

The ectoderm forms a vesicle as well, which later separates from the dermal ectoderm and becomes the lens vehicle. This then provides the basis for future lens development (Figs. S 2.3 and S 2.6).

The dermal ectoderm will form the cornea (Fig. S 2.7) and, at a later embryonic stage, the eyelids (Fig. S 2.8). Choroid and sclera arise from mesoderm. In the embryonic stage, there are blood vessels that go to the lens, but these are normally completely resorbed by the eighth month of pregnancy (Fig. S 2.9).

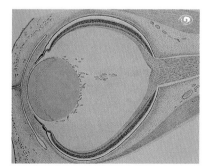
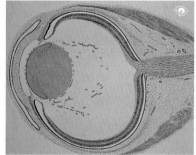

Fig. S 2.8: The eye in the third month of pregnancy: The anterior chamber is not yet formed, the lens is right behind the cornea.

Fig. S 2.9: Twelfth week: The anterior chamber exists as a small slit, the iris has barely been formed.

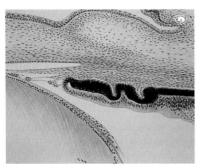

Fig. S 2.10: In the tenth week, the embryonic chamber angle is still closed.

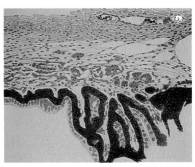

Fig. S 2.11: Sixth month: the ciliary body starts developing its processes.

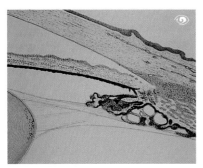

Fig. S 2.12: The chamber angle has developed by the eighth month.

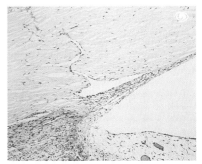

Fig. S 2.13: Normal, open chamber angle at the time of birth.

The maturation and differentiation of the various ocular tissues, particularly the retina, is quite complex and will not be described in detail here.

In the following, the focus is on the formation of the anterior chamber, the chamber angle and the optic nerve, all of which are relevant for glaucoma and, if malformed, for the pathogenesis of congenital glaucoma.

During the third gestational month, the lens is situated directly behind the cornea (Fig. S 2.8). The iris has only partially developed (Figs. S 2.9 and S 2.10), and the anterior chamber will gradually deepen during the weeks and months that follow.

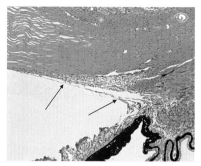

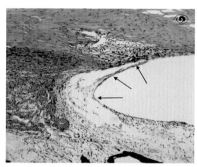

Fig. S 2.14: Incompletely matured chamber angle in congenital glaucoma. The trabecular meshwork is covered by a small membrane (→).

Fig. S 2.15: The chamber angle in congenital glaucoma: the arrows point to the tissue that blocks the humor outflow.

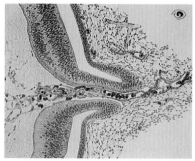

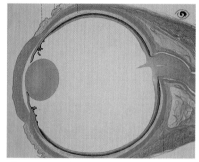

Fig. S 2.16: Second month of pregnancy: the first signs of the optic nerve appear.

Fig. S 2.17: The optic nerve is almost complete by the eighth month.

This leads to an increased distance between the lens and cornea. The ciliary body begins to form (Fig. S 2.11). The next step is the growth and maturation of the iris and the anterior chamber (Fig. S 2.12). Originally completely closed, it slowly opens up and becomes wider during the remaining months of embryonic development (Fig. S 2.13). If this process of differentiation is defective or incomplete (Figs. S 2.14 and S 2.15), the newborn's trabecular meshwork cannot properly drain the aqueous humor, thus resulting in an increase in intraocular pressure (cf. Chapter 3.1).

The retinal ganglion cells send their axons (cf. S 1) across the retina towards the optic disc (Fig. S 2.16). From here, they find their

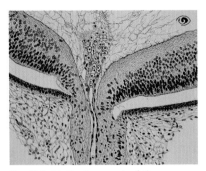

Fig. S 2.18: During most of the embryonic stage, there are blood vessels inside the vitreous body.

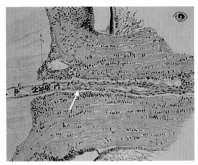

Fig. S 2.19: The central retinal artery (→) develops in the second month.

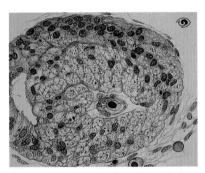

Fig. S 2.20: Cross-section through the embryonic optic nerve.

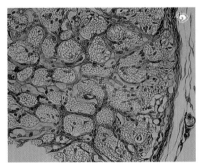

Fig. S 2.21: The nerve fibers are organized into bundles.

way through the disc and the optic nerve directly into the brain (Fig. S 2.17). An enormous number of fibers develop, but not all will find an acceptable contact inside the brain. Those cells that cannot establish contact degenerate and die.

In the center of the developing optic nerve are blood vessels (Figs. S 2.18 and S 2.19), and the nerve fibers become organized into bundles (Figs. S 2.20 and S 2.21).

This then basically completes our description of the development of the eye.

S 3   Genetics

Genetics is the science of heredity [Gr. *genesis*: origin]. Since early times, man has witnessed how children inherit characteristics from their parents. However, it wasn't until 1866 that the most important fundamental rules of genetic inheritance were recognized. The Augustinian monk, Gregor Mendel (1822–1884), made a series of breeding trials with plants and thus discovered (without realizing it) classical genetics. Taking what he learned with bean plants, he demonstrated that the form and color of the beans were determined by "factors," now known as genes. Mendel was completely correct in his assumption that these "factors" occur doubled, i.e. one from the mother and one from the father.

A gene is a genetic code for heredity, a heredity factor. The term "genome" is used to express the sum of all genes of an organism. There are genes that are the same for all healthy individuals within the same species, e.g. the gene that provides the code for the insulin hormone, thus explaining why all healthy humans have the same insulin.

There are also genes that can differ from person to person, e.g. the opsin gene. In Chapter S 1, it was explained that the light sensitive substance, retinal, is embedded within a large protein called opsin. Three different opsin molecules are responsible for the three color sensitivities of the cones. In addition, there are also inter-individual differences that can result in slight variations of the visual spectral sensitivity from person to person. This means that not all healthy people see colors in exactly the same way. One also speaks of "alleles." Alleles are genes that store the same basic characteristic (e.g. the opsin protein), but in slightly differing forms in various individuals. Alleles provide the basis for individual variations and are the source of our diversity.

Classical genetics systematically researches the laws of heredity. Since the middle of the 20th century, biologists have come up with new technologies to advance research: With developments in modern biochemistry and biophysics, biological processes can now be described at the molecular level and, as a result, it is now known how hereditary information is stored and transmitted. Important advances are being made in molecular biology and in molecular genetics and, using these and other technical advances, in molecular medicine as well.

Chromosomes. It is now known that genetic information is stored in the chromosomes of the cell nucleus. Relatively early in the history of genetics, it was noted that chromosomes stain with dyes, hence their name [Gr. *chroma*: color/Gr. *soma*: body]. Humans have 22 pairs of chromosomes, plus there are two X chromosomes in women, while men have an X and a Y chromosome (Fig. S 3.1).

A chromosome is nothing more than a very long molecular chain that is cleverly folded in such a manner that it fits within a tiny cell nucleus (Fig. S 3.2). Chemically, the chain is the DNA molecule (deoxyribonucleic acid).

The information along this chain is linearly arranged using four different bases (adenine, thymine, guanine and cytosine). In effect, the bases are the letters of the genetic alphabet (Fig. S 3.3).

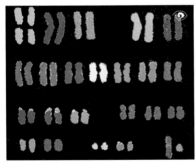

Fig. S 3.1: The 23 pairs of human chromosomes.

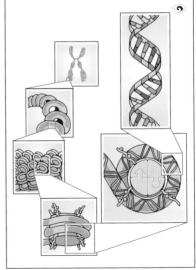

Fig. S 3.2: The very long DNA molecule is so tightly wound that it can even fit into a short chromosome.

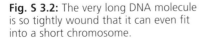

Fig. S 3.3: Double-stranded DNA with its three different base pairs.

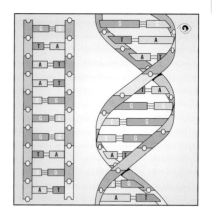

Three successive bases (called triplets) contain the information for one respective amino acid (cf. amino acid).

The information in the cell nucleus is stored in the form of a double chain. The chains are complementarily arranged [Lat. *complementare*: complete], i.e. there are fixed base pairings – certain bases are always positioned across from each other. Thus, thymine is always across from adenine and cytosine is always across from guanine, and vice versa. This permits a rapid doubling of the entire genetic information when a cell divides. When a double chain splits open, like a zipper, each chain is rapidly completed by the complementary chain. In humans, the entire genetic information is stored in the form of several billion base pairs that contain information for roughly 100,000 genes.

Such an enormous amount of information is difficult to imagine. If one could lay out the genetic information of a human being in a straight line and one base pair were placed every millimeter, then the entire length would stretch the distance between the east and west coast of America.

There are approximately one million cells in each cubic millimeter (1 mm³) of tissue. Every single cell has the entire genetic information stored twice: once from the father and once from the mother. This is an amazing concentration of information, information that allows a human being, with all of his physical, mental and emotional qualities, to grow and develop out of one fertilized egg!

Expression of the Genetic Information. Even the cells in an adult constantly rely on their genetic information in order to react correctly to all situations. Nevertheless, each cell knows that the genetic information stored in the nucleus is unique and must never be lost. Cells thus behave like a library that contains valuable books: they only lend out copies. The copy of the DNA information is called RNA (ribonucleic acid), and RNA's structure closely resembles that of DNA.

When a certain gene is "read" in a chromosome or copied onto the RNA, then one says that the gene has been "expressed." The copies, available singularly or in multiple form, leave the cell nucleus and are bound to the ribosomes during protein synthesis (Fig. S 3.4). A specific triplet (three base pairs) codes for a particular amino acid. In the end, a gene, independent of which properties it contains, always uses protein synthesis to develop its information. These proteins have many different functions. They can be active, as with enzymes, or built into the cellular structure, serve as ion channels, receptors for hormones, etc.

The proteins synthesized according to the RNA code are usually much longer in the beginning than the functional end product. Part of the protein serves as an "address." The newly synthesized protein has to "know" where it should go in order to commence its function. This can be compared to a telephone number: the first three digits determine the region, the next three digits the city, etc. The addressing of a protein functions in a similar manner: each wanders to its proper location. The information no longer needed (because the protein has arrived where it should be) is then split off. The information in the cell nucleus thus guides the structure and function of the cell in an extremely elegant fashion.

Cells can be totally different, both structurally and functionally, despite the fact that all carry the same genetic information. For example, a brain cell not only looks dissimilar but it also has other functions than a gastric mucosal cell. This is because not every cell expresses all the genes it possesses. Each takes out of its large library only those documents needed at that moment. Gene expression, that is, the decision as to what will be used, is guided by regulatory genes

Fig. S 3.4: The DNA becomes copied (transcribed) onto an RNA chain; the RNA controls protein synthesis.

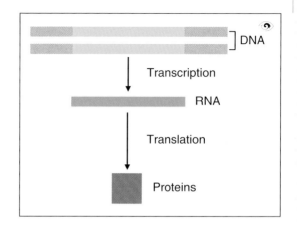

(cf. S 2). For differentiated cells, internal and external factors, such as hormones, contact with other cells, etc., also contribute to this process. It was noted earlier (cf. S 2) that cells communicate with each other. But even within a cell itself, there is a complex network of information that influences gene expression.

Medical Genetics. Medicine is primarily concerned with genetic errors. The large amount of information in the cell nucleus of every single cell, consisting of billions of base pairs, must double itself an innumerable number of times, namely, with each cell division. It is not surprising that errors occur. One refers to these as mutations [Lat. *mutare*: change]. A point mutation is when one single base becomes incorrectly replaced by another.

If the error or variation lies within a gamete (sperm or egg cell), it will be passed on from the parent to the child, and the error will be present in all of the child's cells. Errors can also be acquired during the course of a lifetime, e.g. through powerful radiation or chemical poisons. This type of error is not present in all cells. If a mutation occurs in the process of development, then all cells that are derived from the altered cell will have the same error. If the error arises only when the organism is fully developed, it is only present in one or a few cells; this is called a "somatic" mutation [Gr. *soma*: body]. An error in a single cell is usually not serious. However, if many significant errors accumulate in the same cells throughout a lifetime, this can lead to serious consequences. For example, a cell, regardless of contradicting information from its environment, can begin to divide and a tumor (unregulated growth) is created. A tumor is thus the result of errors in the cell's genetic information.

However, keep in mind that mutations are not always disadvantageous to an individual; certain mutations can indeed prove advantageous. Certain mutations in the heredity substance have proven useful in the ability to survive and therefore form a crucial basis for evolution.

What are the consequences of hereditary errors that can be transmitted from parents to children? When an error occurs in a gene and its corresponding protein, it is primarily manifested as an amino acid exchange, one amino acid exchange from among the hundreds of amino acids present in a particular protein. There are also errors in which a protein is not completely synthesized. A protein with an exchanged amino acid sometimes has slightly different physical and chemical characteristics. For example, the folding of the protein and its corresponding three-dimensional structure might change. Depending on the gene, this may or may not have a critical effect. When such damage occurs in a regulatory gene, severe disturbances in the embryonic development might ensue. As an example for the eye, the iris can be completely missing (called aniridia). When the defect is present in a gene that is activated at a later time, then only mild consequences could appear, e.g. possibly glaucoma later in life.

Many cells can function quite normally even with mutations because the mutated gene, embedded among such a large assembly of many other genes, is not definitively needed. However, when environmental damage is constantly brought into a cell during a person's lifetime and the repair mechanisms slowly fail, then the damaged gene can begin to make its presence felt. This is also the reason why some hereditary diseases become evident only in advanced age.

Different mutations in various genes can evoke very similar clinical pictures. For example, retinitis pigmentosa is an affliction in which part of the retina gradually dies. The disease manifests itself as night blindness and an increasing narrowing of the visual field. Phototransduction (cf. S 1) has been described; this is the chain of events in which a perception of light is transformed into a nerve impulse. A series of proteins are involved in phototransduction. Several different mutations of these proteins can thus lead to a very similar clinical picture, namely, that of retinitis pigmentosa.

Conversely, various mutations on one and the same gene can evoke varying symptoms. Additionally, a mutation that causes a disease in one person does not necessarily cause the same disease in another. In the manifestation of hereditary diseases, environmental factors also play an important role.

Currently, there are only a few genes known to be involved in the development of glaucoma. In most forms of glaucoma, the genetic form is still unclear, even though it is known to occur more frequently among certain families. Knowledge in this field is expected to grow rapidly within the next few years.

S 4 Optics of the Eye

The retina is the light-sensitive layer of the eye. Before impressions from the outer world can reach the brain as visual information, they must first be projected onto the retina. This can be compared to a photographic camera: the retina represents the film, and the refractive media of the eye, specifically, the lens and the cornea form the focusing (camera) objective.

The cornea plays a considerably more important role in light refraction (light focusing) than does the lens. But light refraction due to the cornea is constant, while the lens adjusts its focal power to the changing distance between the observer and that which is being observed.

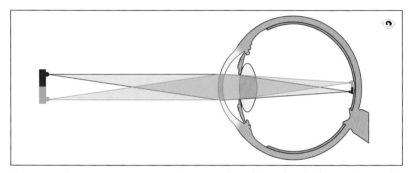

Fig. S 4.1: In emmetropic eyes, the external world is sharply focused onto the retina. (In theory, the observed object must be far away.)

Focusing Errors. In order for an image to be sharply in focus at the retina (and not at some distance in front of or behind it), the focal power of the optical system and the length of the eye from the cornea to the retina must match (Fig. S 4.1). This is guaranteed by a complex control system that develops while the eye is still growing. Only a seeing eye can guide growth in such a way that the imaging occurs at the right location. Unfortunately, the length of each eye does not always precisely match the focal powers of the cornea and lens' optical systems. If the eye is too short, a blurred image will

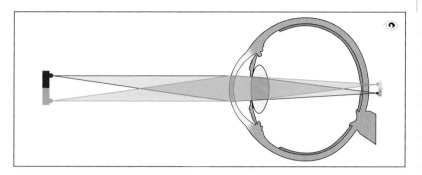

Fig. S 4.2: The hyperopic eye is too short and, theoretically, the image would be in sharp focus behind the retina. (Again, in theory, the observed object must be far away from the eye.)

appear at the retina (Fig. S 4.2). Theoretically, the picture would be sharply in focus behind the eye. Since the blurriness of an image decreases when the object is far away, one speaks of far-sightedness; i.e. these patients can see things (without glasses) better when they are at a distance than when they are up close.

If the length of the eye is too long in relation to the focal power, the retinal image is again fuzzy (Fig. S 4.3). In this case, the picture is sharply focused in front of the retina. When looking at an object up close, the blurriness is reduced. Here one speaks of near-sightedness because the patient sees (without glasses) near objects better than those farther away.

Emmetropia is the term for normal vision [Gr. *emmetros*: right amount/Gr. *opos*: sight]. Far-sightedness is called hyperopia or hypermetropia [Gr. *metron*: amount/Gr. *hypermetron*: excessive amount], while near-sightedness is called myopia [Gr. *myein*: to close the eyes]. The term myopia came into existence because near-sighted people see somewhat better when they squint and, before glasses, went around squinting with their eyes slightly closed.

Presbyopia. As mentioned above, the human lens can adjust its focal power to match various seeing distances, a process called accommodation.

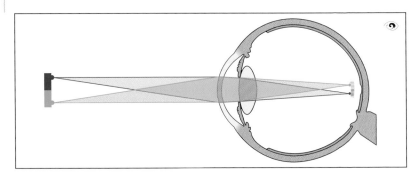

Fig. S 4.3: The myopic eye is too long and, theoretically, the image is in sharp focus in front of the retina.

In cameras, this regulation is achieved by adjusting the focusing distance of the lens. Certain animals can move the lenses in their eyes in a manner similar to a camera lens. But in the human eye, accommodation (focusing) takes place by a change in the lens shape. The lens has a natural elasticity and tends to take on a round shape. This is counteracted by a tight stretching of the zonular fibers, the eye's "support apparatus," which makes the lens elliptical. When the zonular fibers are relaxed, the lens becomes rounder and thus thicker. The degree of tension of the zonular fibers depends in turn on the ring-shaped ciliary muscle, to which they are also attached.

When an object is looked at from up close, the ciliary muscles contract (S 1), the zonular fibers relax and the lens becomes rounder, thereby increasing its focal power. As one gets older, the lens loses some of its elasticity and the ability to accommodate decreases; thus, age-related far-sightedness develops, medically referred to as presbyopia [Gr. *prespys*: old].

Astigmatism. Astigmatism [Gr. *stigma*: point] is a refractive error of the eye that causes the visual image in one plane to focus at a different distance from that of the plane at a right angle. This most often results from too great a curvature of the cornea in one of its meridians. When the refraction is ideal, a point-shaped object is projected as a point on the retina. If the eye has uneven refraction, e.g. due to a corneal deformation, a point becomes projected on the retina as a line, and there is astigmatism (not point-shaped).

Refraction. The focal power of the eye is also called refraction [Lat. *refringere*: break apart], and refractometry is the term used for its measurement. Units for the refractive power of a lens and thus also for the optical system of the eye are known as diopters. If a lens focuses parallel light at a point one meter (1 m) away, it has a focal power of 1 diopter. If it focuses parallel light at a point 50 cm away, it has a power of 2 diopters, 25 cm is 4 diopters, etc. A lens that does not focus light, but rather diverges it as if it were coming from a focus from behind, has a negative diopter value.

Correction Possibilities. Today there are numerous possibilities for correcting refractive errors of the eye. Well-known and proven are eyeglasses. Technology has made enormous progress here: thanks to new materials, today's eyeglasses are much lighter and thinner than ever before. Additional correction for near distances can be easily and usually invisibly included in the lens. Glasses additionally offer a mechanical protection against injuries and, in particular with special lenses, protection against ultraviolet light.

Contact lenses offer a second option for correction. Much progress has been made in this area as well, particularly in the materials employed that significantly improve their wearing comfort. Optically, contact lenses achieve excellent correction, and glaucoma patients can also wear them (cf. Chapter 8.3). Furthermore, a variety of surgical options are available. For example, an artificial lens can be implanted in the human eye, and astigmatism can be improved through tiny cuts made in the cornea itself. Nevertheless, both of these procedures are only practical in special situations.

A laser may also be used to thin the cornea, thereby either increasing or decreasing the focal power of the eye. Although the short-term results with laser treatment are usually quite good, cautious consideration and second opinions from neutral professionals are recommended before such interventions are undertaken. To date, long-term results from this procedure are still lacking, i.e. the condition of eyes thus treated in 20 or 30 years is still not known (S 13). Even when the initial success is excellent, complications down the road are quite possible. Laser correction is not recommended in glaucoma patients for several reasons, including the fact that after such an intervention, precise measurement of eye pressure is much more difficult.

S 5 Cataracts

The term, cataract, is used to describe a clouding, or opacification, of the eye lens [Gr. *kata*: down/Gr. *raegnymein*: to tear or break] (Fig. S 5.1).

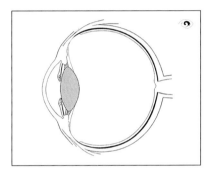

Fig. S 5.1: A cataract is a clouded lens (gray).

The term probably came into existence because the lens opacification was compared to a waterfall. A cataract is not the same as glaucoma, though sometimes both occur together, especially among the elderly.

On a worldwide basis, cataracts are still the most common cause of blindness. Approximately 20 million people are blind because of cataracts. In principle, cataracts can be "cured" with an operation where the clouded human lens is replaced by a clear artificial lens. In industrialized countries, it is rare that anyone goes blind or is severely visually impaired because of cataracts. However, in developing countries, cataract-based blindness is not so much a medical problem as it is a socio-economic problem (cf. A 5). There are not enough doctors or adequate funds to make this relatively straightforward operation available to the general population. Is it not a tragedy for mankind that millions of people are blind because of a lack of financial resources to pay for this basic operation?

The Role of the Lens. Since early history, learned people have been interested in the functioning of the lens. In antiquity, it was thought that this was where seeing occurred, a misconception that endured almost to modern times. Today, it is known that the lens has an optical function: it focuses the light and contributes to projecting images from the outside world onto the retina. Moreover, the lens can change its focal power and thus makes accommodation possible. Accommodation is the adaptation of vision to varying distances. In order for the light to be depicted accurately, the lens must be transparent. This is why the lens has no blood vessels. With cataracts, this transparency is reduced or may even be completely lost.

Lens Growth. The lens is a unique organ with regard to growth: the lens continually grows during one's lifetime. The outer layer contains cells that multiply and extend themselves in length, and these, in turn, form lens fibers that lay on top of the external fibers already present. The growth of the lens thus resembles that of a tree trunk – rings of growth are added year after year. To prevent the volume of the lens from getting too large, the internal portion becomes increasingly denser and hardened. This results in a loss of flexibility with age. A child can see an object sharply which is only few millimeters in front of his eyes, but a 50-year-old with normal vision has to hold the newspaper far away in order to read it without glasses.

The lens loses not only flexibility with age, but also transparency. Less light can enter unobstructed because more light is absorbed or scattered. The opacity lens meter (OLM) measures the scattering (and thereby the degree of lens clouding) (Fig. S 5.2). The transparency of the lens slowly diminishes throughout life (Fig. S 5.3). However, when this process appears relatively early and to a marked degree, it is known as a cataract. Figure S 5.4 shows a thin and still normally transparent lens of a 25-year-old woman; Figure S 5.5 shows the somewhat thicker and less transparent lens of a 70-year-old healthy woman.

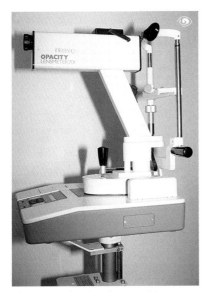

Fig. S 5.2: The Opacity Lens Meter: an instrument used for quantifying the degree of opacification (clouding) of the lens.

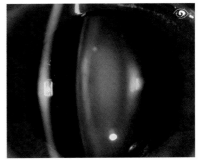

Fig. S 5.3: Opacification of the lens in healthy individuals. x-axis: age; y-axis: OLM value. With advancing age, the opacification of the lens increases and the transparency decreases, even in healthy eyes.

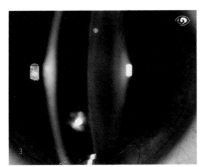

Fig. S 5.4: The lens of a 25-year-old woman; the lens is still relatively thin and quite transparent.

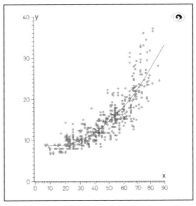

Fig. S 5.5: Transparency is somewhat decreased in the slightly thicker lens of a 70-year-old woman.

The Genesis of a Cataract. The lens contains proteins that are folded into a particular three-dimensional structure. These proteins are the chemical substrate of the crystallin of the lens. Throughout the course of one's lifetime, especially when damaging factors (see below) are present, the structure of these proteins becomes altered. Light can then no longer pass through the lens unimpeded, but rather it becomes scattered by these altered molecules. Clouding can affect the different parts of the lens with varying intensity. A few lenses become fogged mostly in the center (Fig. S 5.6 and Fig. S 5.7), while others are affected around the periphery (Fig. S 5.8) etc.

In these various cataract forms, the clouding progresses at different rates and patients experience varying degrees of subjective disturbance.

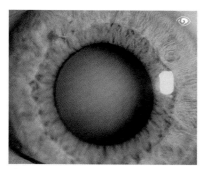

Fig. S 5.6: The eye of a 70-year-old male showing significant central lens opacification.

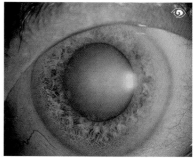

Fig. S 5.7: Advanced lens opacification with yellow-brown pigment deposits in a 75-year-old male.

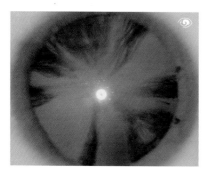

Fig. S 5.8: Spoke-like opacification in the lens periphery of a 65-year-old patient.

Cataract Symptoms. A cloudy lens both scatters the light and partly absorbs it, thereby making the image quality at the retina even poorer. What the cataract patient sees is blurred and fine print can no longer be read; additionally, he has the impression of being in a fog. Since various colors are scattered and absorbed to varying degrees in a cloudy lens, the world is no longer seen in exactly the same colors. Blue tones are especially weaker. But because these changes have occurred very gradually, the patient hardly notices them. When a cataract patient looks in the direction of a strong light, the light is perceived as blinding. Cataract patients perceive glare more frequently.

Even healthy people occasionally experience this phenomenon. When driving a car with a dirty windshield, light coming from oncoming cars is often blinding. This occurrence can be briefly explained by the following: Imagine an eye that is looking at a traffic sign. At the same time, the sun is shining and also sends light to the eye. If there is no clouding of the medium, the sunlight will fall on the outermost part of the retina (Fig. S 5.9) and the traffic sign can be read without difficulty, despite the sunlight. However, if there is clouding present, for example, in the lens, the light will be scattered at that point and part of the sunlight will fall onto the macula, the site of sharpest vision; in other words, on that site where the traffic sign is projected (Fig. S 5.10). The visual image of the traffic sign becomes mixed with that of the extra sunlight (Fig. S 5.11). This is annoying and perceived as blinding glare; it also explains why some cataract patients wear hats with broad brims. Glare can arise from other causes too, as described in Chapter 6.7.4.

Risk Factors. Even though not all aspects of cataract development are completely understood, increasingly more risk factors that contribute to its growth are becoming known. These factors are essentially the same as those that promote arteriosclerosis, specifically, smoking, increased blood pressure, diabetes mellitus, vitamin deficiency, etc. Furthermore, the type of light to which the eye is exposed also plays a role: UV light, for example, accelerates cataract development.

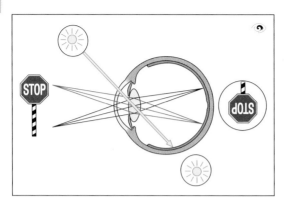

Fig. S 5.9: With a clear optical medium, sunlight blinds only slightly; the sunlight primarily falls on the peripheral retina.

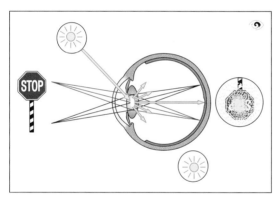

Fig. S 5.10: With opacification of the optical medium, sunlight is particularly blinding because light is projected not only to the peripheral retina but also partially scattered onto the macula.

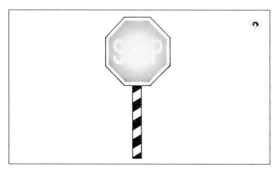

Fig. S 5.11: This is how a patient having severe opacification (e.g. with a cataract) perceives a traffic sign in bright sunlight.

Cataract Treatment. It has long been attempted to eliminate or even prevent lens clouding with medication but, to date, results have been less than satisfactory. The main difficulty has been in getting the medication to its site of action, specifically, the lens. Though this should eventually prove possible, for the time being, the only way to treat a cataract is to replace the cloudy lens with a clear artificial one.

Cataract Operations. Fortunately, today's operating techniques are so far advanced that only a short procedure is required to replace the natural cloudy lens with an artificial one. Indeed, this is often performed in a doctor's practice. Worldwide, cataract operations are the most frequently performed surgical procedures. In the USA, there are some 1.6 million cataract operations each year. The procedure basically consists of using ultrasound to make the lens material fluid so that it can be sucked out. A folded, flexible artificial lens is then inserted through a tiny opening into the eye and subsequently unfolds within the old lens capsule. Figures S 5.12 to S 5.16 show the main steps of a cataract operation.

After the operation, there is a rapid improvement in vision. Imaging is sharper, colors are more intense, and the world is again brighter. Since the deterioration in vision took place over years while the improvement after the operation is very dramatic, patients often have the feeling that they see better than ever. However, if other eye diseases are present, e.g. maculopathy (S 9), the improvement in vision is much less dramatic. If one compares the eye with a camera, one can say that even though the damaged objective lens was replaced, the picture is still unsatisfactory because of bad film (a damaged retina). Unfortunately, it is not yet possible to replace the retina as one replaces film in a camera.

Concurrent Incidence of Cataract and Glaucoma. Since both afflictions appear most frequently among the elderly, it is not uncommon that a patient has both a cataract and glaucoma. While a cataract operation can "cure" a cataract, a glaucoma operation cannot remove glaucomatous damage. It can only reduce the eye pres-

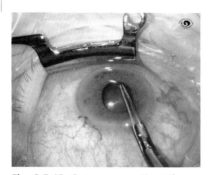

Fig. S 5.12: Cataract operation: The anterior lens capsule is first opened with forceps ...

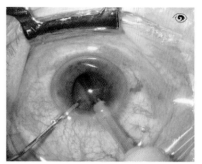

Fig. S 5.13: During phacoemulsification, the hard lens core is emulsified using ultra-sound and then suctioned out.

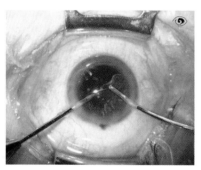

Fig. S 5.14: Here the softer lens rim is suctioned out.

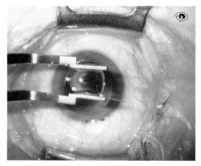

Fig. S 5.15: The plastic lens is folded ...

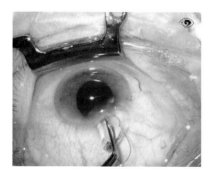

Fig. S 5.16: ... and inserted into the eye, where it then unfolds.

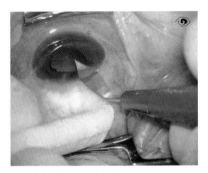

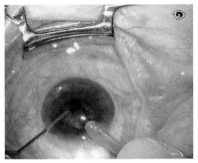

Fig. S 5.17: Opening the anterior chamber during a cataract operation in an eye that has previously been operated on for glaucoma. The bleb remains intact.

Fig. S 5.18: Phacoemulsification following an earlier glaucoma operation.

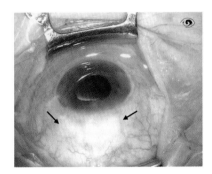

Fig. S 5.19: The artificial lens is inserted while ensuring that the bleb remains undisturbed.

sure and thereby improve the long-term prognosis for the patient's vision. While a cataract patient usually sees distinctly better after the cataract operation, after a glaucoma operation, the glaucoma patient does not enjoy improved vision. In fact, it is quite possible that vision is temporarily poorer.

Both diseases are not always equally severe. A patient might have an extensive cataract and only early glaucoma or vice versa, i.e. severe glaucomatous damage and an incipient cataract.

In principle, a cataract and glaucoma can be operated on in one session. The combined operation has both advantages and disadvantages, and each case must be individually considered (cf. Chapter 7.4.6).

It is important to be aware that glaucomatous damage, once it has appeared, cannot be reversed, while a foggy lens can be operated upon at any time and the visual handicap alleviated. For this reason, a glaucoma operation frequently has the higher priority. Likewise, a cataract operation following a glaucoma operation is possible at any time without endangering the success of the preceding glaucoma operation. A glaucoma operation will occasionally accelerate cataract development. Above are a few pictures of a cataract operation that followed a glaucoma operation (Figs. S 5.17–S 5.19). During the procedure, special efforts are made to ensure that the filtering fistula is not damaged.

Secondary Cataract (After-Cataract). During a cataract operation, in order for the artificial lens to be anchored in the correct position, part of the lens capsule is left in place as a support or holder. Months to years after the operation, these membranes can become cloudy. This is then termed a "secondary cataract" or "after-cataract" (because it appears after a cataract operation). Today, using a simple laser procedure (S 13), this secondary cataract can be eliminated so it no longer disturbs the patient. The cloudy posterior capsule is disrupted in the center and this procedure is known as a "sec-

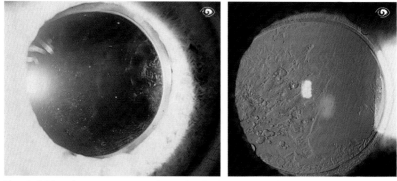

Fig. S 5.20: After-cataract. On the right, back-scattered from the fundus, and on the left, in focal illumination (back-scattered from the after-cataract).

ondary cataract dissection" [Lat. *diszisio*: splitting]. The dissection can be performed routinely in a few minutes on an out-patient basis and is completely painless.

Figure S 5.20 shows a secondary cataract preceding laser treatment and Figure S 5.21, a secondary cataract after laser treatment.

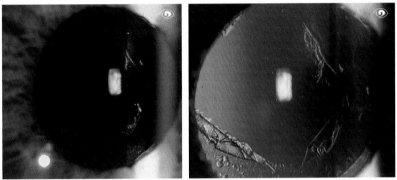

Fig. S 5.21: After laser treatment: The center of the posterior capsule is opened and the after-cataract has disappeared in the center.

S 6 Arteriosclerosis

The term arteriosclerosis is used to describe a thickening and hardening of the arterial wall [Gr. *skleros*: brittle, hard]. A few concepts should be explained at the beginning: Arteries are blood vessels that transport blood away from the heart; veins are blood vessels that transport blood back to the heart [Lat. *vena*: blood vessel]. At death, the arteries contract and squeeze out the remaining blood. Early anatomists therefore assumed that these vessels did not contain blood, but rather air, and thus named them "arteries" [Gr. *aaer*: air].

Figure S 6.1 shows a cross-section through a normal artery and a normal vein. The vessels depicted here are the central artery and vein of the retina, blood vessels that supply the retina.

Figure S 6.2 schematically depicts the structure of an arterial wall with its various layers. The innermost layer, the intima [Lat. *intimus*: innermost] is composed of endothelial cells. These cells form not only the barrier between the blood and tissue, they also regulate the vessel diameter and blood coagulation by releasing local messenger substances. The smooth muscle cells that lie beneath this layer can actively contract and relax, thereby regulating the blood vessel diameter. They receive their instructions from the above-

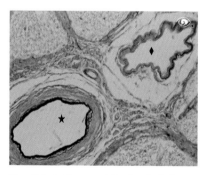

Fig. S 6.1: Shown at the level of the lamina cribrosa is a cross-section through the central retinal artery (on the left) and the central retinal vein (on the right).

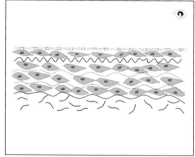

Fig. S 6.2: Arterial wall: yellow = endothelium, blue = smooth muscle cells.

mentioned endothelial cells and from fibers of the autonomic nervous system. Various forms of arteriosclerosis are known, the description being based on which cell layer is primarily affected.

Atherosclerosis. The most frequent form of arteriosclerosis is atherosclerosis, which starts with lipids being deposited under the intima. The resulting atheroma [Gr. *athera*: porridge] can be limited to a local area, and then it is called an intimal pad. This occurs most frequently at arterial bifurcations. The spot-shaped changes are also known as "plaques" [Fr. *plaques*: plate, spot].

Not only are lipid deposits associated with atheromatosis, but there are also chronic structural changes that take place within the vessel wall. Oxidized lipids that have been deposited between the vascular layers are phagocytized (eaten) by inflammatory cells, and muscle cells from the vascular wall divide and then migrate into the intimal pad. Atheromatosis is thus a type of inflammation but it is not yet clear what role chronic infection plays in its development. Changes in the vascular wall precipitate its hardening, which is referred to as sclerosis [Gr. *skleros*: brittle, hard]. Figure S 6.3 shows a cross-section through a blood vessel that has undergone atheromatous changes, while Figure S 6.4 shows a schematic representation of the altered cell wall.

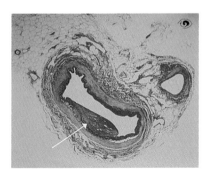

Fig. S 6.3: A histological section showing arteriosclerotic wall thickening (at the arrow) of the ophthalmic artery.

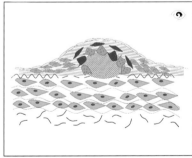

Fig. S 6.4: Vessel wall showing atheromatous changes of the vessel wall with increased cell numbers from migrated muscle cells (blue). The necrotic core (orange), macrophages (green) and foam cells (red) are easily seen.

Thrombosis. Because there are atheroma that pad the lumen, i.e. the inner blood vessel diameter, it becomes progressively smaller [Lat. *lumen*: light, width]. If the vessel narrowing is severe, blood flow can be impeded. The intimal paddings are especially dangerous when they break off, as shown in Figure S 6.5. With this ulceration [Lat. *ulcus*: abscess], blood comes into contact with the tissue, as occurs in an injury, which then leads to a local coagulation. With injury, blood clot formation is useful: bleeding is checked and the vascular wall can undergo repair processes. However, with atheromatosis, such clots can lead to dangerous complications. This type of clot is called a thrombus [Gr. *thrombos*: congealed mass of blood] and the disease caused by a thrombus is known as thrombosis.

The thrombus that forms where the atheromatous plaque has been broken off disrupts the blood flow. Through the subsequent release of local hormones, vascular contraction occurs which, in the worst case, causes a complete occlusion of the blood vessel. Tissues past this occlusion receive little or no blood and they become ischemic [Gr. *ischein*: hold back/Gr. *haima*: blood].

Ischemia that lasts for a prolonged period leads to an infarct, i.e. tissue death [Lat. *infarcire*: to cram or pack in] in the corresponding area that had been supplied by this vessel.

Emboli. A thrombus growing into the lumen of an artery can also be torn off by flowing blood which then carries it away and transports it to a peripheral site. Since the blood vessels become smaller at every bifurcation, the broken-off thrombus eventually

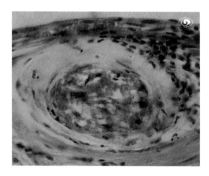

Fig. S 6.5: A blood vessel occluded by a thrombus.

gets stuck, often at such a site. The term embolus describes the floating mass, and when the embolus becomes lodged and causes obstruction, it is then termed an embolism [Gr. *ballein*: throw/Gr. *emballein*: throw into].

Emboli generated in the arteries are differentiated from those originating in veins. The latter are often transported to the pulmonary circulation leading to a pulmonary embolism.

Atheromatosis is a frequent cause of death and severe disease. Classical examples are heart attacks and brain infarctions (also known as strokes).

In the blood vessels leading to the eye, atheromatosis is observed relatively frequently and early in the disease course. This may cause an infarction in the eye. As an example, Figure S 6.6 shows a retinal infarct; in Figure S 6.7, an embolus is visible in a retinal artery.

Arteriolosclerosis. Atheromatosis primarily affects large and medium-sized blood vessels. However, within the eye itself, the blood vessels are relatively small, and thus do not undergo much atheromatous change. However, arteriolosclerosis can occur in the eye. An arteriole is a small artery. In arteriolosclerosis, there is tissue thickening that primarily occurs in the middle layer of the vascular walls. Figure S 6.8 shows a normal retinal arteriole; Figure S 6.9 a sclerotically-altered arteriole.

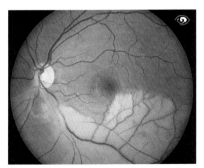

Fig. S 6.6: Retinal infarct (light area) due to occlusion of a branch artery.

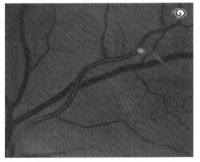

Fig. S 6.7: An embolus (bright spot) has become wedged at a bifurcation, thereby partially occluding an arterial branch.

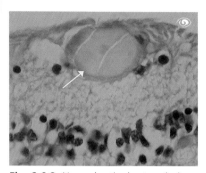

Fig. S 6.8: Normal retinal artery (→).

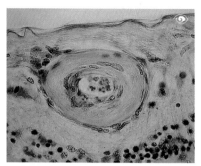

Fig. S 6.9: Arteriolosclerosis of a retinal artery.

The precise mechanisms of development for the various forms of arteriosclerosis are complex and not yet fully understood. However, the risk factors that promote the appearance of arteriosclerotic changes are relatively well researched and include smoking, high lipid blood levels, elevated blood pressure, a sedentary lifestyle, diabetes mellitus (S 7), and even perhaps chronic infections.

Interesting to note is that, in addition to an elevated risk for infarction, patients having arteriosclerosis also have an increased risk for developing early cataracts (S 5) or maculopathy (S 9). Neither of these diseases is probably the result of a disturbance in the blood flow, but rather, both have mechanisms of development similar to arteriosclerosis. This thus explains why these eye diseases occur more frequently in patients suffering from arteriosclerosis.

Patients with arteriosclerosis also have a slightly increased risk for an elevated intraocular pressure, though arteriosclerosis on its own is hardly a risk factor for glaucomatous damage. It was known for decades that patients having glaucomatous damage exhibited decreased blood circulation in their eyes, but a correlation between arteriosclerosis and its risk factors on one, and glaucoma on the other side could not be firmly established. Finally, in the 1980's, after we realized that the blood flow disturbances in glaucoma were less related to arteriosclerosis than to dysregulation of the blood vessels (S 8), did it become possible to solve this apparent contradiction.

S 7   Diabetes Mellitus

There are various forms of diabetes, but diabetes mellitus [Lat. *mellitus*: sweet], or "sugar diabetes" is the most prevalent and well known. In this disease, the glucose (a type of sugar) concentration in the blood and in the urine is elevated. When the glucose concentration exceeds a certain level, urine production increases. In untreated diabetes, there is excessive urine production [Gr. *diabainein*: to pass through]. This is caused by the osmotic effect of sugar (cf. Chapter 7.2.6); urine that contains glucose smells sweet.

Blood glucose is an important source of energy: the brain and the retina are completely dependent on glucose because they cannot use other substances for energy. When the glucose falls below a critical level in the blood, the patient experiences certain typical symptoms; however, when the glucose level is too high, there are other serious problems, as shall be discussed below.

After a meal that contains carbohydrates, there is an immediate increase in the blood glucose level, even in healthy people. To counteract this increase, specialized cells in the pancreas [Gr. *pan*: whole/Gr. *kreas*: flesh] that are grouped together into little islands become activated to secrete the hormone insulin [Lat. *insula*: island]. Insulin promotes sugar (glucose) absorption into the cells, especially in the liver. This lowers the blood sugar concentration back to its original level.

With diabetes mellitus, the level of glucose in the blood is too high, especially after a meal. There are two possible causes for this: In type 1 diabetes, the insulin production is severely reduced or even halted because the insulin-producing cells in the pancreas have been destroyed by a chronic inflammatory process. This form of diabetes is most often seen among young adults and even in children. In type 2 diabetes, the pancreas continues to produce insulin; the insulin concentration in the blood may even be elevated. But in this case, the number of the insulin receptors is reduced – the insulin cannot find an attachment site on the cells. One speaks of an increased insulin resistance [Lat. *resistere*: set back]. If one compares insulin to a key and the receptors to a keyhole, then there would be many keys, but too few keyholes on the cell doors. The glucose cannot enter the cell in sufficient quantities and so it remains in the bloodstream. This second type of diabetes mellitus is seen especially among overweight patients in the second half of life.

In 1921, the Canadian physician, Sir Frederick Banting, first isolated insulin from animal pancreases. Before this, diabetes – especially type I – was a fatal disease. However, with the isolation procedure, it became possible to treat patients with animal insulin. Animal insulin is no longer widely used because human insulin can now be manufactured with genetic technology. Since insulin is a protein, it must be injected; if it were given orally [Lat. *os, oris*: mouth], the protein molecule would be broken down in the gastrointestinal tract and would no longer be functional.

In diabetes mellitus, there is a distinction made between acute complications, such as hyperglycemia (too much blood glucose) or hypoglycemia (too little blood glucose) [Gr. *hyper*: above/Gr. *hypo*: below] and late (or chronic) complications. If treatment is inadequate, the disease eventually leads to damage in various organs, especially the kidneys, nerves and eyes.

Consequences for the Eyes: Diabetic Retinopathy. Diabetes can lead to various alterations in the eye, e.g. to an accelerated cataract development or to optic nerve disease. From a clinical point of view, diabetic retinopathy, that is, the changes that occur in the retina, are most relevant.

Diabetics are afflicted more frequently, and at an earlier age, with arteriosclerosis; specifically, with atheromatosis (S 6). In addition, the small blood vessels (arterioles) are subject to diabetes-specific changes: the glucose binds itself to various molecules, especially to protein molecules, a process called glycosylation. In turn, glycosylation causes changes in the characteristics of the tissues. The small blood vessels are especially affected and can even become completely occluded. In the eye, this has special consequences: due to the closed vessels in the retina, there are areas that are poorly perfused with blood. Furthermore, the glucose-damaged vessels start to leak – fluids escape from the retinal blood vessels and leave fatty deposits behind. Small hemorrhages may also arise in the retina. All these events lead to the clinical picture that is known as non-proliferative diabetic retinopathy [Lat. *rete*: net/Gr. *pathein*: to suffer].

Figure S 7.1 shows non-proliferative diabetic retinopathy with mild changes. Several small blood vessels are dilated and spot-like hemorrhages are visible. The yellow spots correspond to fatty deposits.

Figure S 7.2 shows a more advanced stage of the disease. The few white, fuzzy spots scattered throughout correspond to nerve fibers that have swollen as a result of perfusion disturbances, and are thus no longer transparent. They are often called "cotton-wool" spots because they look like small balls of cotton. The sharply-delineated spots are hard exudates and correspond to fatty deposits [Lat. *exsudare*: sweat out].

The poorly-perfused retinal areas produce substances that stimulate local blood vessels in the retina and vitreous body to new growth (neovascularization), as shown in Figure S 7.3. This form of retinopathy is no longer termed non-proliferative diabetic retinopathy, but rather proliferative retinopathy [Lat. *proliferatio*: rampant growth, excrescence].

There may be hemorrhages in the retina as well as in the vitreous body from these newly formed blood vessels, as shown in Figure S 7.4.

The newly formed tissue can also shrink. This may cause a detached retina in which the retina becomes separated from the pigment epithelium.

Less frequently, but especially when the lens is missing, new vessels can also form on the iris. If the vessels reach the chamber angle, a sharp rise in intraocular pressure may occur (cf. Chapter 3.6.2). Figure S 7.5 shows vessel proliferation on the iris.

Because the iris appears red due to the newly formed blood-filled vessels, one speaks of a rubeosis iridis [Lat. *ruber*: red]. Since these newly formed vessels often bleed, the resulting glaucoma is termed hemorrhagic glaucoma [Gr. *haem*: blood/Gr. *raegnymein*: tear/Gr. *haimorragia*: blood flow, blood drop].

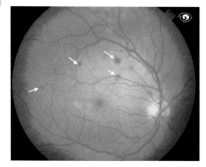

Fig. S 7.1: Diabetic retinopathy: isolated hemorrhages (→).

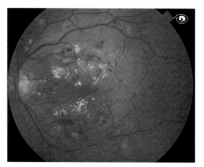

Fig. S 7.2: Diabetic retinopathy: lipid deposits.

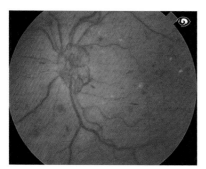

Fig. S 7.3: Proliferative diabetic retinopathy: newly formed vessels (neovascularization) at the papilla.

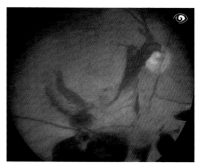

Fig. S 7.4: Proliferative diabetic retinopathy: hemorrhaging into the vitreous body.

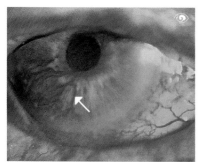

Fig. S 7.5: Rubeosis iridis: newly formed blood vessels visible on the iris (→).

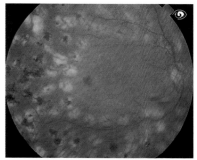

Fig. S 7.6: Condition following a photo-coagulation: partly pigmented and partly non-pigmented laser scars are visible.

Treatment. The late complications of diabetes mellitus can be prevented or at least greatly slowed by optimal treatment and active patient cooperation. Not only must the blood glucose be well controlled, but also blood pressure and blood lipids should be regularly checked and treated, if necessary. Some patients might have to lose weight. Severe complications in the eye can often be prevented, or at least slowed, using laser treatment. Those areas of the retina that have insufficient perfusion are scarred with a laser so that they can no longer produce vascular growth promoting substances. A diabetic should be checked regularly by his ophthalmologist so the ideal moment for the laser procedure is not missed. Figure S 7.6 shows diabetic retinal changes following laser coagulation therapy. The spotted, partly dark colored points are laser scars (also termed laser foci) (S 13).

Diabetes and Glaucoma. Just like anyone else, a patient with diabetes mellitus can also develop glaucoma. Diabetics have a slightly increased risk for developing an elevated intraocular pressure. Fortunately, severe pressure increases resulting from rubeosis iridis, described above, are rare because of the optimal treatment and preventive measures that are now available.

In contrast to what is written in most textbooks, patients with diabetes mellitus rarely have an increased sensitivity to high intraocular pressure. This means that therapy for a diabetic patient with glaucoma is basically the same as for a non-diabetic.

However, when the eye pressure in a diabetic is reduced too much, there is a risk that any developing diabetic retinopathy could be accelerated. Each individual case must be carefully weighed as to which risk poses the greater threat: that from glaucomatous damage or that from diabetic retinopathy. Frequently, eye drops containing beta-blockers (cf. Chapter 7.2.3) are administered to reduce intraocular pressure. A diabetic must know, however, that beta-blockers may mask the symptoms of hypoglycemia.

S 8   Vascular Regulation and Dysregulation

A failure to properly regulate the body's blood flow is called vascular dysregulation [Gr. *dys*: faulty]. Before turning to the various types of dysregulation, a description of how normal circulation is regulated will first be presented.

S 8.1 Regulation of Blood Flow

Blood Flow is Crucial for the Survival of the Body's Organs. There is a constant flow of blood through almost all parts of the body. Blood transports nutrients, hormones and other essential substances into the tissue and carries away waste products. Many tissues can build up a small deposit of certain nutrients, such as fat or glucose. However, there is no way to store oxygen, an element essential for life. The first effect of an interruption in the blood flow is a lack of oxygen. Everyone is aware of the strange feeling when, during blood pressure measurement, the cuff has been pumped up to the point where perfusion in the arm stops; a numb hand results. If this interruption in the blood flow persists for a few minutes, the arm and hand start to hurt. Should this cessation of the circulation continue, the hand would virtually die within a few hours. The same thing happens, albeit more slowly, in heavy smokers who are often afflicted with gangrene of the feet. They experience a slow but progressive cut-off of the circulation and thus of oxygen [Gr. *gangrein*: festering ulcer]. The brain is even more sensitive to a lack of oxygen. If blood flow to the head is interrupted, morbidly exemplified by strangling, consciousness is lost within a few seconds and death ensues within minutes. Blood flow is vital to all organs; interrupting the perfusion will lead to tissue death in that part of the body within minutes or hours.

Blood Flow also Assists in Keeping the Temperature Stable. Blood not only transports important molecules and cells, but also heat. Whether one experiences the cold from a winter day or suffers from the summer heat, the temperature inside the body stays astonishingly stable, even despite the different levels of energy production by the various organs. This thermoregulation [Gr. *thermos*: warm] not only functions via evaporation of perspiration, but also by adjusting the amount of body heat otherwise released from the skin. If there is an increase in blood flow to the skin, the skin gets warmer and thus gives off more heat to the environment. Keeping a constant temperature is crucial for most organs to function properly. Consider the eye, an organ very exposed to the environment. When one is skiing in the cold and an icy breeze blows onto the face, one could expect that the eyes would cool down considerably; perhaps the aqueous humor might even freeze under extreme climatic conditions. Fortunately, this is not the case and the eye temperature stays more or less constant, even in extreme conditions. The choroid, with its high rate of blood flow, functions like central heating. Experiments have shown that choroidal perfusion increases immediately after a stream of cold air hits the face. In short, the regulation of the blood flow not only has to ensure an adequate supply of nutrients and oxygen to the different tissues but, at the same time, also has to keep the temperature stable in vital organs, such as the brain, the eyes and the liver. If, for example, in a cold winter we would go out from a warm room, our eyes would cool down very quickly if blood flow in our eyes would remain constant. To avoid this situation the circulation in the eye is increased within seconds. This is in part due to the coldness-sensitive temperature sensors in the sclera. If you put a drop of local anesthetics in one eye, the increase of circulation in that eye is diminished.

Blood Flow and Sleep Behaviour. The regulation of circulation and temperature is related to a number of other biological functions such as sleep. Before we fall asleep a mandatory redistribution of temperature takes place. The temperature of the trunk decreases and the temperature of the feet increases. If this redistribution of temperature takes longer for some reasons, it takes longer to fall asleep.

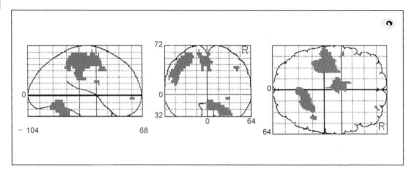

Fig. S 8.1: A PET makes it clear which areas of the brain are active (red). This scan illustrates someone moving the fingers of his right hand (seen from the side, from the back and from above).

The Heart as the Driving Force. The blood circulation requires a motor to adequately perform its complex task, and this function is fulfilled by the heart. Similar to a pump, it forces the blood into the major arteries and thereby builds up the blood pressure. The pressure gradient that stretches from the arteries into the capillaries and on to the veins is the driving force that moves the blood through the vessels. The heart adjusts its pumping power to what the situation demands. A good example is the increased heartbeat that is experienced after rapidly climbing stairs.

Blood Distribution to the Various Organs is not Constant. As described, the skin's perfusion rises when heat production increases. This is also the case with ocular blood flow in a cold environment. There are many more examples that show how the tissue perfusion adjusts to changing circumstances and the actual requirements. Blood flow in the brain, for instance, increases precisely in those centers that are active at the moment. This can be demonstrated with P̲ositron E̲mission T̲omography (PET). Figure S 8.1 shows which brain areas experience an increase in blood flow when the fingers of the right hand are moved. The impulse – or the "order" – to move the fingers, comes precisely from those cerebral regions with the higher perfusion rate. With this technology, one can therefore determine which areas of the brain are responsible for a certain function; in this example, areas controlling finger movements are shown. When a person watches TV, the blood flow increases in the visual cortex.

When hiking, perfusion to the legs increases; after dinner, the same thing happens in the stomach and intestines. Organs or body parts receive more blood than usual when demands are temporarily above average. The blood flow must react almost immediately to the changing requirements. When lying flat on a bed, with head and legs at the same level, blood pressure at both sites is almost identical. After suddenly rising, within seconds, blood pressure in the legs is considerably higher than in the head. However, it is essential that the brain receive its constant blood supply too. There must thus be a rapid adjustment to the new situation, and this process is called autoregulation [Gr. *autos*: self]. Under normal circumstances, a constant blood supply to the brain is guaranteed through local regulatory mechanisms as this is paramount to survival; this occurs in spite of fluctuations in the blood pressure. The same applies to the retina.

How is the Blood Flow through the Organs Regulated? In Switzerland, the first author's native country, there is a traditional irrigation system used by farmers in the Valais, where the Swiss Alps are located. Using long pipes, water is directed downhill into the valley communities. From this lower location, there is an intricate system of smaller pipes and streams that leads to each farm, letting the farmer drain water, according to his needs, onto his fields by opening or closing the sluice-gates. Quite the same thing happens in the body: The blood vessels, large and small alike, dilate or constrict, respectively, to direct more blood to an organ which has a higher temporary demand and less to other body parts currently not in particular need of nutrients and oxygen.

Even Blood Vessels have their own Muscles. Blood vessels are not rigid pipes with fixed calibers. When pressure is applied to an artery at the wrist, the vessel can be closed or opened. The veins at the back of the hand are even easier to compress. The innermost layer of the blood vessels is covered by the thin endothelium. It is a very delicate skin made up of just one cell layer; more attention will be directed to the endothelium below. Next, in the vessel wall, is a variably thick layer of smooth muscle cells. Smooth muscle cells – in contrast to skeletal muscles – do not show any transverse striations under the microscope. When the smooth muscle fibers contract, the vessel's lumen becomes narrower; when the muscle fibers relax, the blood vessel dilates. The muscle force that opposes the blood pressure determines the diameter of the vessel and thereby the amount of blood that will actually flow through a defined area. But how do these muscle cells know whether they should contract or relax?

Regulating the Vascular Tone. A number of factors participate in regulating the tone of the blood vessels; some have already been presented. There are both general as well as local interests that contribute to the dilation or the constriction of a blood vessel. During physical activity, the locomotor system requires an increased blood supply. Such a marked increase cannot be satisfied by just redistributing the available resources, since other vital organs (e.g. liver and kidneys) still have their requirements in spite of the physical activity going on. Therefore, it is not just a redistribution that takes place; the heart increases its output. The number of beats per minute (heart rate) and the pressure with which it pushes the blood through the arteries is increased. While at rest, after dinner for instance, there is not only an increase of blood flow to the gastrointestinal tract, but also a decrease in the heart rate due to a reduced overall demand. Correspondingly, this leads to a slight drop in the blood pressure. Organizing an adequate supply on a global level is mainly the task of the autonomic nervous system. It is called autonomic because it works independently of one's consciousness. The term "vegetative nervous system" is sometimes used as well. The autonomic nervous system contains a sympathetic portion, which is mainly activated by stress (fight or flight), and a parasympathetic portion, which is active when the organism is at rest (rest and digest). There are also some local and specific interests of the body's organs that the autonomic system can satisfy to only a limited extent. This explains why a local regulation of the distribution process must also be present; in this respect, the endothelial cells play a decisive role.

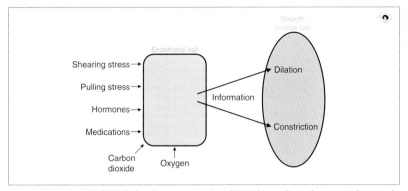

Fig. S 8.2: The endothelial cells process signals and regulate the smooth muscle cells of the blood vessels.

Endothelial Cells as the Circulation's Policemen. As explained above, endothelial cells form the delicate, innermost layer of the blood vessels. They are in a strategically important position at the border between the blood and the other tissues. Endothelial cells regulate the exchange of molecules and cells from the blood into the tissue and vice versa. They also provide instructions for the smooth muscle cells by telling them when to contract and when to relax, thus regulating the vessel's lumen. Endothelial cells are highly sensitive to the information they receive from their immediate surroundings and to the demands of the neighboring tissues. Among other things, they chronicle the friction that the blood streaming along exerts upon the vessel's walls, and the tension which is created by the blood pressure inside these walls. They also have "a feeling" for whether the oxygen supply is sufficient and whether too much waste material has accumulated. Endothelial cells collect these bits of information and process them into signals that are then transmitted to the smooth muscle cells. Within the past few years, the "language" that is used by the endothelial cells has been largely decoded. A simplified overview of this is provided in Figure S 8.2. For more information on how these cells work, please refer to the literature reference mentioned in the bibliography, A 3, "Basic Research."

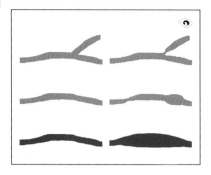

Fig. S 8.3: A drawing showing vascular dysregulations (arteries are red, veins are blue).
Left: normal; right: dysregulation.

In summary: The circulation is constantly under the influence of control and regulatory mechanisms that have to consider many varied interests. It should come as no surprise that occasional dysregulations arise in such a complex system.

Causes of Circulatory Problems. As can happen to any body part, blood vessels can also be afflicted with disease or dysfunction. Inflammation or arteriosclerosis may compromise efficiency (cf. S 6). Blood flow can be hampered or even blocked by thrombosis or embolism, but even anatomically healthy blood vessels can be misguided if given incorrect information from e.g. the vegetative nervous system or from the endothelial cells. This is called vascular dysregulation.

S 8.2 Vascular Dysregulation

Many people suddenly get red or white spots on their faces or throats when placed under emotional stress. This is a harmless, though plainly visible dys-regulation. It is indeed a dysregulation because the increase or decrease of perfusion (in this case: perfusion of the skin of the face) is not at all related to the actual demand of the body or one of its parts.

Figure S 8.3 schematically shows how blood vessels behave during such dysregulation.

Vascular dysregulation denotes an inappropriate local regula-

> Vascular dysregulation implies an inadequate constriction or an insufficient dilation of an artery, an arteriole or a capillary, sometimes in association with a simultaneous dilation in other sections of the circulatory system, particularly in the veins.

tion of arteries, veins, or capillaries. As a consequence local blood supply does not correspond to the local demand. This can imply over- or underperfusion. Sometimes a simultaneous overperfusion occurs in one part of the organ, while other parts are underperfused.

While overperfusion of a tissue rarely leads to damage, an underperfusion can lead to symptoms and in extreme situations even to infarctions. This is the reason why more emphasis is given to underperfusion. This local reduction of blood flow is either due to an insufficient vasodilatation if needed or to an inappropriate vasoconstriction. The latter is also called vasospasm. If vasospasm tend to occur in different organs and at different times it is called a vasospastic syndrome. In this context we will use the term "vascular dysregulation", keeping in mind that it is more or less synonymous to the "vasospastic syndrome".

We differentiate a primary vascular dysregulation from a secondary vascular dysregulation. While the primary vascular dysregulation (PVD) is an inborn predisposition to respond different to various stimuli, a secondary vascular dysregulation (SVD) is a local or systemic dysregulation as a consequence of an underlying disease.

S 8.2.1 The Primary Vascular Dysregulation (PVD)

What is a PVD? PVD is an inborn propensity to respond different to stimuli. Most of the subjects with PVD are healthy people. Under balanced conditions there is little distinction compared to other persons. When challenged, however, they respond differently to a number of stimuli or so called trigger factors.

PVD and Temperature. Very classical is the response to coldness. Subjects with PVD have strikingly cold hands even when there is only a moderate decrease in the outside temperature. Some of them even complain of being cold at all times whereas others get cold hands under psychological stress. Again others suffer rather from cold feet.

PVD and the Eyes. While all these symptoms on hands and feet are quite harmless, a parallel reduction of blood flow occurs often in the eyes and sometimes also in other organs. This explains why people with PVD, although mostly healthy, have a higher probability to acquire some eye diseases as e.g. glaucomatous damage (cf 5.3 Reperfusion Damage).

PVD and Sleep Behaviour. As discussed before it is necessary that our feet warm up before we can fall asleep. This is the reason why people with PVD have a longer sleep onset time. Sleep onset time is reduced if such patients take a warm bath before they go to bed or if they warm their feet with socks.

PVD and Psychological Stress. Coldness is not the only trigger, that induces symptoms in patients with PVD. We already mentioned psychological stress. Everybody experiences from time to time psychological stress. But the way our body responses to this stress is individually different. People with PVD often respond by reducing their blood flow, both in the extremities like the hands and in the eyes. In very rare, extreme situations this can even lead to an infarction, e.g. to an infarction of the optic nerve head. We observed such infarctions e.g. in stock market trader when share values dropped dramatically; or in a student who failed an exam. While such extreme reduction of blood flow in PVD patients is exeedingly rare, a mild reduction, leading to a repeated mild reperfusion stress is very frequent. This explains why this type of circulation problems can contribute to a disease process that develops over years or decades as e.g. the glaucomatous damage.

PVD and Mechanical Stress. Some of the PVD subjects also have high sensitivity to mechanical stress. When working e.g. with a compressor they get cold hands or even sometimes white fingers. When PVD patients sustain a whiplash trauma they suffer more and longer from corresponding symptoms like headache or visual disturbance.

PVD and Drug Sensitivity. When drugs are prescribed to patients with PVD they often respond stronger, sometimes even violently to some classes of drugs, but less than the average to a few other classes. When treated e.g. systemically with calcium channel blockers, betablockers, and others they sometimes feel sick and have more side-effects than expected. If however, the same drugs are given to a much lower dose the desired effect can still be observed but without or with much less side-effects. On the other hand, when suffering pain they often need painkillers at higher doses or more frequent than others. This difference in sensitivity to drugs can be explained by a different expression of the so called ABC-transport proteins in subjects with PVD. These are proteins that are, among other things, involved in the transmembranal transport of drugs.

PVD and Thirst. Patients with PVD are often less thirsty than others. Normally they drink enough, but rather because they are aware of the necessity to drink, than driven by thirst. This symptom like many others can be explained by a slight increase of the hormone Endothelin in the circulating blood. Endothelin is a peptide produced by the endothelial cells. It is secreted abluminally to regulate local vascular tone. A small part of it is secreted intraluminally. As a consequence it induces some systemic effects. One of these effects is a slight suppression of the center of thirst in the brain (via an upregulation of another hormone, namely prostaglandin E_2 (PGE_2)).

PVD and Sensitivity. On the average, people with PVD have a higher sensitivity, not only to drugs, but also often on a psychological level and also in terms of sensory perception. They can smell things that others cannot or to a much lesser extent. But unfortunately they also have a higher sensation of pain. This is also explained by the increased level of Endothelin. Endothelin influences the threshold of pain sensation. In extreme situations PVD patients may suffer from so called fibromyalgia. Other types of pain also occur more often in these patients, e.g. headache. In addition, when they suffer from migraine, they tend to have more accompanying symptoms like visual disturbance or cold hands. Although PVD patients suffer more often from migraine, migraine and PVD are not identical. Unfortunately, these two entities are often confounded.

PVD and Blood Pressure. On the average, patients with PVD tend to have a low blood pressure, specially at night and particularly when they are young. Some of them suffer from orthostatic hypotension. The major cause for this systemic hypotension is a reduced salt reabsorption in the proximal tubuli of the kidneys. This is also due to an increased level of Endothelin. These people therefore loose more salt and need to eat more salt to keep their blood pressure at a normal level.

PVD and Social Behaviour. Fortunately PVD is not only associated with downsides. People with PVD also have advantages. On the average they are more successful in professional life. They tend to be very exact and diligent. These are the types of people one can rely on.

What is the Underlying Mechanism of PVD? Patients with PVD are characterized by a number of other attributes. While they are weak in producing temperature when they are at rest, they are physically strong. Not infrequently they are very good runners. This can be explained by the fact, that they have an unimpaired production of ATP (Adenosintriphosphat) in their mitochondrias. ATP is the most important energy transporter in our body.

While we use ATP we also automatically produce heat. Under conditions, however, in which we do not use much ATP (e.g. when we are at rest), mitochondrias are able to produce heat by an

Table S 8.1: Frequency of Primary Vasospastic Syndrome

Women suffer more frequently than men
Younger people suffer more frequently than senior citizens
White collar workers suffer more frequently than blue collar workers
Japanese suffer more frequently than Europeans
Europeans suffer more frequently than South Americans
Thin people suffer more frequently than heavier people
Non-diabetics suffer more frequently than diabetics
Ambitious perfectionists suffer more frequently than those who are tranquil and calm

alternative pathway. It is this alternative pathway that seems to work insufficiently in PVD patients. This also explains why the symptoms (e.g. cold hands) are boosted when patients reduce their food intake.

On the average, subjects with PVD have a lower BMI (body mass index), in other words, they are on the average slimmer and the symptoms are mitigated when they gain weight. Already the intake of some gram of sugar leads to some warming up of the hands and interestingly also increases the blood flow in the eyes. In old days it was (correctly!) recommended to people with sleep disorders to drink some water with sugar or honey.

Although there is a number of indications, that the main cause of PVD is a dysregulation of mitochondrial function, the exact underlying causes and mechanisms are not yet known.

Risk Factors for PVD. Although patients with PVD are born with this propensity, the symptoms mostly begin during puberty and decline with age, particularly after the menopause. It occurs more often in females than in males. Estrogens obviously play a role. This also explains why the symptoms often aggravate or return in the postmenopausal phase if these women take estrogens.

PVD occurs more often in some populations like e.g. in Japanese and Koreans. This may partly be explained by genetic differ-

Table S 8.2: Organs that Frequently Experience Vasospasm

Hands	+++
Eyes	++
Heart	++
Ears	+
Feet	++
Brain	(+)

ences, but also by the way of life including the differences in nutrition. This also explains why Japanese people suffer less often from high-tension but more often from normal-tension glaucoma (Table S 8.1).

Which Organs are Involved in PVD? PVD can involve many different organs (Table S 8.2), although there is a clear predilection for hands and eyes. The coronary arteries and probably the auricular vessels are also involved to some extend whereas the brain vessels seem to be less dysregulated in such cases.

Correspondingly this can lead to a number of additional symptoms (Table S 8.3) , such as tinnitus, sudden hearing loss, or in extreme and fortunately rare situations it may lead to myocardial infarction. A mild myocardial ischemia without pain (so called silent myocardial ischemia) is very often observed.

Dysregulation of Barrier Function. The brain and retinal tissue is separated from the blood by a so called blood-brain- (or blood-retinal-) barrier. Certain molecules in the blood would otherwise disturb proper brain function. A dysregulation of the diameter of the vessels is often paralleled by a dysregulation of the barrier function. This might be due to the fact, that the regulation of the diameter of the vessels is influenced to some extend by the same molecules as the regulation of the barrier.

This explains, why patients with PVD (with or without glaucoma) often show small splinter hemorrhages at the border of the

Table S 8.3: Frequency of Symptoms in Primary Vasospastic Syndrome

Cold hands	+++
Diffuse visual field defects	+++
Reduced thirst	++
Low blood pressure	++
Increased response to certain drugs	++
Cold feet	+
Migraines	+
Tinnitus (ringing in the ears)	+
Hearing problems	(+)
Reduced visual acuity	((+))

optic nerve head (Fig. 2.8). The barrier dysfunction is mainly in the peripapillar area (Fig S 11.15). This is explained by the fact, that regulating hormones like Endothelin or MMPs can diffuse from the choroid into that area of the retina.

The barrier dysfunction also explains, why the so called central serous chorioretinopathy (CSC) occurs much more often in patients with PVD. In this disease a reversible breakdown barrier of the pigment epithelial cell layer separating choroid from the retina leads to a liquid accumulation between retina and pigmentepithelium. In contrast to glaucoma it occurs however more often in young males, specially when they are under professional stress. The testosterone hormone obviously plays a role. We observed an older lady with serous chorioretinopathy. We were puzzled by the fact that she was older and female. However, she had a classical patient history of PVD. After questionning, she indicated that she was taking testosterone tablets to improve professional performance. This observation underlies a role of PVD and testosterone in the occurrence of CSC.

S 8.2.2 The Secondary Vascular Dysregulation (SVD)

A number of diseases can lead secondary to local or systemic vascular dysregulation (Table S 8.4). An increase of oxidated low-density lipoproteins (oxidized LDL) can lead to vasoconstriction both in the eye and in the periphery and most probably also in other organs. From the point of ophthalmologists all diseases leading to an increased level of circulating Endothelin are of special interest, as this hormone nearly always tends to reduce ocular blood flow. In the brain, however, increased level of Endothelin reduces blood flow only if a local damage of the blood-brain-barrier occurs. The difference between the eye and the brain is due to the fact, that we have fenestrated blood vessels in choroid of the eye and the blood-brain-barrier in the optic nerve head is not fully developed.

The level of Endothelin in the circulating blood is increased in a number of diseases like multiple sclerosis, giant cell arteritis, chronic polyarthritis, fibromyalgia, and in untreated HIV infections. This explains why in these diseases patients often demonstrate pale optic nerve heads and often show (mostly unrecognized) visual field defects.

While PVD interferes with the autoregulation and therefore contributes to glaucomatous damage, SVD reduces blood flow under basal condition, but seems to interfere less with autoregulation and therefore contributes less to the glaucomatous damage.

S 8.2.3 Additional Aspects of Vascular Dysregulation

Mechanism of Disease. In his 1892 thesis, Raynaud described an illness involving local ischemia of the hands. This led to the term "Raynaud's disease." The term, "Raynaud's *syndrome*," was later coined to describe a similar, but clearly weaker entity. With respect to the hands, the symptoms of Raynaud's syndrome are about the same as the symptoms of patients with vasospastic syndrome. As early as 1895, reduced perfusion in the hands was first attributed to local vasoconstrictions. Today this is taken for granted, however, the mechanisms that lead to a dysregulation are not yet completely understood. It is known that there is a genetic predispo-

Table S 8.4: Possible Causes for Secondary Vascular Dysregulation

Autoimmune Diseases	Multiple Sclerosis
	Giant Cell Arteritis
	Lupus Erythematosus
	Antiphospholipid Syndrome
	Rheumatoid Arthritis
	Preeclampsia
Infectious Diseases	Some bacterial infections
	e.g. bacterial meningitis
	Some viral diseases
	e.g. viral liver cirrhosis
	AIDS
Other Possible Causes	Cerebral Hemorrhage
	Head Injury
	Anorexia Nervosa
	Mitochondriopathies
	Some tumors, e.g. prostate cancer
	Ulcerative Colitis
	and Crohn's Disease
Drugs (in patients having a predisposition)	Adrenaline
	Alpha II Interferon
	Sumatriptane
	etc.

sition for acquiring primary vasospastic syndrome. These patients typically tell us that their parents, especially mothers, suffered from cold hands and low blood pressure as well. Additional studies have demonstrated that there is an increased endothelin blood level in both primary and secondary dysregulations. Endothelin is a protein with a strong vasoconstrictive effect, which is primarily produced by the blood vessel's endothelial cells. Vasospastic patients have a permanently increased endothelin level, even when no vasospastic activity is actually going on. This means that an endothelin increase alone cannot be solely responsible for vasospasms. Rather it seems to heighten the sensitivity of the blood vessels to other triggering factors. A hyperactivity of the sympathetic nervous system also seems to participate in this process. The patient's decreased sense of thirst is due, at least in part, to an endothelin-induced inhibition of the thirst center in the brain. The low blood pressure also seems to be a result of an increased loss of salt in the kidneys.

It is not yet known why these spasms occur in such a localized pattern. Certain local factors seem to play a role as well. As mentioned above, hands and feet are frequently afflicted, a more or less harmless event. There are relatively frequent vasospasms in the coronary arteries, which are obviously not that harmless. On the other hand, the brain is less susceptible to the primary vasospastic syndrome due to its special and very sophisticated system of blood flow regulation. Nevertheless, vasospasms can occur due to migraine headaches, cerebral hemorrhages and head injuries. To date, only little is known about vasospasms in the ear, but tinnitus and temporary hearing loss are not rarely seen in vasospastic patients.

Primary vascular dysregulation has its origins primarily in a malfunction of endothelial cells. Decoding these malfunctions has become our primary scientific focus.

Triggering Factors. Primary vascular dysregulations usually occur when predisposed individuals encounter certain triggering stimuli.

Once again, traffic story can serve as a good example: No policeman can be adequately equipped to handle all unexpected situations. If the problem presented is too large for one policeman alone, traffic is unsatisfactorily controlled which, in the worst case, results in a traffic jam and chaos. Under normal circumstances, endothelial cells of these patients behave appropriately most of the time. If they are confronted with an additional stress, then symptoms of malfunctioning may start to appear. Not all individuals with primary vasospastic dysregulations react to the same triggering factors. Common

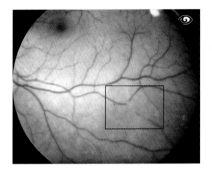

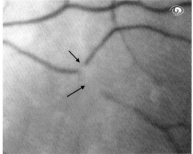

Fig. S 8.4: Fundus of a patient experiencing a migraine attack.

Fig. S 8.5: An enlarged section from Fig. S 8.4. showing local vasospasms (→).

triggers include cold, drugs, migraine attacks, hunger, mechanical stress and, based on the authors' experiences, emotional stress, which plays an important role (cf. A 3).

Migraine headaches and primary vasospastic syndrome are not identical. Yet patients with primary vasospasms suffer more often from migraine headaches which, in turn, can also act as triggers. As has been seen, perfusion to the visual cortex increases when TV is watched. In some migraine patients, this local adaptation of the cerebral perfusion is lacking during an attack. This renders these patients extremely sensitive to light and makes them prefer to temporarily stay in a darkened room.

The Consequences of Vascular Dysregulation at the Eye. In 1910, Blessig, an ophthalmologist, identified a retinal vasospasm in a patient who was experiencing a migraine attack at that very moment. Figure S 8.4 shows the fundus of a patient actually suffering an attack associated with unilateral visual problems. Figure S 8.5 shows an enlarged section of Figure S 8.4; note the local vasoconstrictions with the interrupted blood flow, a condition called "retinal migraine." These temporary reductions of retinal blood flow are quite rare but they can impressively demonstrate vasospasms during an acute phase of dysregulation. More frequent, yet invisible to medical science, are dysregulations in the underlying choroid. In 1939, Lisch, another ophthalmologist, published his hypothesis linking dysregulations in ocular blood vessels to those in the capillaries of the fingertips. Unfortunately, his observations were long forgotten.

With regard to glaucoma, it had long been assumed that perfusion played a role in the origin of tissue damage. But because most scientists were unaware of functional vascular dysregulations, no research was performed in this area. Attempts to establish a link between arteriosclerosis or its risk factors and glaucoma proved futile. Since the correlation between arteriosclerosis and glaucomatous damage is weak or even non-existent, reduced ocular blood flow was widely regarded as a consequence, not a cause, of glaucoma. As already discussed (cf. Chapter 4.2.7), a decline in perfusion is less the result but rather the origin of glaucomatous damage.

In the early 1980s, a young lady suffering from normal-tension glaucoma was examined in the authors' clinic. Her hands were strikingly cold. Examining her nailfolds with capillary microscopy demonstrated clear vasospasms. The question was posed: Does this patient, by chance, suffer from two separate diseases, normal-tension glaucoma and vasospastic syndrome, or is there a relationship between these illnesses? In other words: Can glaucomatous damage be interpreted as a manifestation of vasospastic syndrome? To obtain more clues, the patient was treated with calcium antagonists, a type of drug which, when taken in low dosages, exerts a beneficial effect on vascular dysregulation. Within just a few days, the patient's visual field significantly improved. Next, other patients were examined who had vasospastic syndrome but no glaucoma. Frequently discovered were visual field defects – of which the patients themselves were unaware. Usually these defects were relatively diffuse, changing from day to day, deteriorating when the patient was exposed to cold and improving when they were treated with drugs that enhanced their ocular blood flow (calcium antagonists for example). As a result of these observations, we postulated the potential participation of the eye in the vasospastic syndrome, and the term "ocular vasospastic syndrome" was introduced.

The Ocular Vasospastic Syndrome. Today, it is well known that the eye is an organ frequently involved in a primary vasospastic syndrome; fortunately, this is harmless in most cases. For example, even children experiencing stress at school can develop significant, but reversible, visual field defects of which they are not aware. When the initial observations were made by the authors' group with the young lady mentioned above, it was not yet possible to measure ocular perfusion on a quantitative basis. Several years later, when new technologies became available, such as color duplex sonography, measurements confirmed that ocular blood flow in these patients was indeed reduced (albeit transiently in most cases).

The proof was also provided that reduced ocular perfusion, as part of the vasospastic syndrome, constitutes a relative risk factor for certain other eye diseases, such as venous stasis (congestion) syndrome, retinal and optic nerve ischemia in young patients, and central-serous chorioretinopathy (Table S 8.5). An analysis of glaucoma patients revealed that the majority of the normal tension glaucoma patients, and many high tension glaucoma patients having only moderately increased IOP, suffered from primary vasospastic syndrome. More recent studies carried out by the authors have been able to detect evidence of vascular dysregulations increasing the eye's sensitivity to blood pressure drops and IOP peaks. This explains why some people tolerate a low blood pressure or a high IOP without developing damage while others do not. Of course, other factors also play a role, as discussed in Chapter 4.2.

Table S 8.5: Patients with Ocular Vasospasms frequently Suffer from

Visual field defects (diffuse, mostly reversible, generally unnoticed)	++++
A pale or occasionally excavated optic disc	+++
Retinal vein occlusions	++
Central-serous chorioretinopathy	+
Retinal ischemia and infarction	+
Optic disc ischemia and infarction	+

Table S 8.6: Indications of a Primary Vasospastic Syndrome

What the patient relates (symptoms)	Cold hands (occasionally cold feet)
	Low blood pressure
	Reduced feeling of thirst
	High sensitivity to certain drugs
What the ophthalmologist sees (signs)	Altered conjunctival capillaries
	Shiny spots on the retina
	Dilated veins or constricted arteries in the retina
	Pale optic disc
	etc.
Diagnostic examinations	Extended flow interruption in capillary microscopy (cf. S 11)
	Increased flow resistance in duplex sonography (cf. S 11), especially with low blood pressure
Lab findings	Increased blood concentration of endothelin-1
Special examinations	Increased sensivity to endothelin when blood pressure is low
	Measuring response of the choroidal circulation to an isometric exercise

How is a Vasospastic Syndrome Diagnosed? Diagnosis of primary vasospastic syndrome is based on several signs and symptoms, as listed in Table S 8.6. In secondary vasospastic syndrome, the symptoms are similar though not identical. They appear only in connection with the underlying disease and may affect the eye. Usually, the blood concentration of endothelin is even more significantly increased. Important for further diagnosis and therapy is the primary disease that has evoked the secondary vasospastic syndrome. Naturally, there are patients who have both congenital primary vasospastic syndrome and an acquired secondary vasospastic syndrome.

Treatment. Although many people suffer from a vasospastic syndrome that can, though rarely, result in serious illness, to date, there exists only scant scientific data available on this syndrome (cf. A 3). As a result, therapy is still in an early stage of development. Recommendations for treatment are only in part based on controlled studies; most suggestions arise from the authors' clinical experiences. Whenever possible, measures that enhance the body's overall circulation should be pursued. These include proper physical exercise, healthy nutrition, regular sleep and avoiding major stress situations. Vasospastic patients should refrain from certain activities that could be beneficial to other individuals, such as a prolonged fasting. In contrast to patients with high blood pressure, these patients should have sufficient salt intake and drink enough water, particularly in the evening. Patients who suffer marked BP dips when rising should wear supporting stockings. The intake of magnesium is also beneficial. Some patients respond well to acupuncture, and others to the Kneipp Water Cure, etc. Other recommendations can be found in Chapters 7.5 and 7.6. If serious symptoms occur, the physician will try to enhance blood flow with medication (cf. Chapter 7.5).

In this specific context, there is still no answer to the question as to whether estrogen replacement therapy for women after menopause is beneficial. Without doubt, estrogens (female hormones) have some positive effects. Nevertheless, in individual vasospastic patients, symptom exacerbation has been observed with estrogen therapy. Therefore, the recommendation for post-menopausal female patients having vascular dysregulation is to measure (ocular) blood flow before initiating estrogen replacement therapy and again three months after its introduction. If blood flow stays the same or even improves, the ophthalmologist will not object to long-term estrogen replacement.

S 9   Age-related Macular Degeneration (AMD)

Age-related macular degeneration (AMD) is a disease of the central retina associated with advancing age; it leads to a reduction in central vision.

It is the retina's task (cf. S 1) to absorb and transform light into neural signals. Both structure and function differ in the various areas of the retina.

If one looks at a distant object, such as the moon, the eyes are brought into a position which ensures that the moon's image is projected directly onto the center of the retina by the optic system. This center, which appears slightly yellow due to the pigment xanthophyll, is called the macula lutea, or the "yellow spot" [Lat. *macula*: spot/Lat. *lutea*: yellow]. Figure S 9.1 is a picture of the posterior segment of the eye (fundus) showing the optic disc, macula, and peripheral retina. While the latter is specialized in the perception of movements (mainly of larger objects), the center is designated for spatial resolution. This means that, at the retinal center, even tiny objects can be seen, and two points extremely close together can be identified as being separate and distinct. The capability of the resolution power can be expressed as the "visual acuity." A healthy person (with corrective lenses, if necessary) has a visual acuity of 100% or, in the vernacular of ophthalmologists, 1.0, or 20/20. The high capacity for resolution arises from the fact that photoreceptors are much more densely packed in the macula than in any other area of

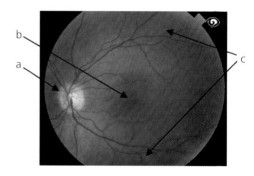

Fig. S 9.1: Ocular fundus:
a) optic disc, b) macula,
c) peripheral retina.

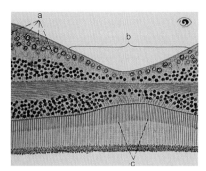

Fig. S 9.2: Macula: a) ganglion cell, b) foveola, c) receptor cells.

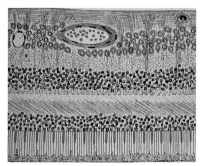

Fig. S 9.3: Cross-section through the retinal periphery.

the retina. Furthermore, at this site, the ratio between cone cells and ganglion cells is almost to 1:1; the macula's receptors are therefore connected via downstream retinal nerve cells directly to the brain.

Figure S 9.2 shows a histological section through the macula; and for comparison, Figure S 9.3 is a section through the peripheral retina. If the quality of the image on the retina is less than perfect, such as when a myopic person is not wearing glasses, visual acuity will be less than 100%. A 50% visual acuity (i.e. 0.5) means that in order to distinguish two points as being separate, they must be twice as far apart from each other as two points that would normally be seen as distinct in 1.0 vision. This distance is four times as large with 25% visual acuity, etc. With test charts, a patient having 0.5 vision will identify only letters or numbers twice as large as those that a person with 1.0 vision can see. If a myopic individual is tested with adequate glasses (or contact lenses), the results are again normal. However, if the retina itself is altered by, say, a loss of receptor cells or their misalignment, visual acuity will be decreased without the possibility of correction with glasses. This is particularly problematic for the macula.

The Aging Macula. As is the case with all organs, the retina also undergoes an aging process throughout life. Receptor cells and nerve cells slowly decrease in number, even in a healthy individual.

The pigment epithelium, located directly behind the retina and which has to continuously absorb and digest parts of receptor cells, gradually shows signs of waste material (indigestible) deposits. The perfusion of the next layer, the choroid, also decreases with age. The choroid's ability to transport warmth and adjust the blood volume according to demand likewise diminishes with age. At the same time, the choroid can no longer totally fulfill its role of nourishing the retina as efficiently. The deposits of undigested, mostly fatty material furthermore hinder transport from the retina to the choroid, and vice versa.

Even a healthy macula receives relatively little oxygen from the retinal vessels; instead, it is primarily supplied by the underlying choroid. This is the reason why the macula particularly suffers from age-related diffusion problems caused by these deposits. Another factor that plays a role is that the macula is much more exposed to light and its deleterious effects than other retinal areas.

There is no absolute and sharp division between normal aging and certain pathological processes. Many elderly people develop pronounced changes of the macula that can lead to severe impairment of vision. A precursor of such defects is the visibly increasing number of retinal deposits, called drusen (Fig. S 9.4). Drusen are small, clot-like formations primarily composed of fat and located between the pigment epithelium and choroid. In an eye examination, they can be identified as small yellowish spots beneath the retina (Fig. S 9.5).

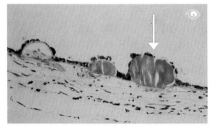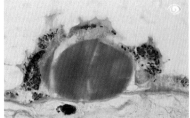

Fig. S 9.4: Drusen (→) shown in a histological section

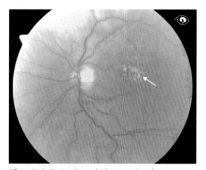

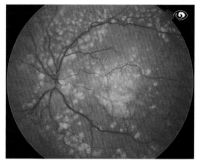

Fig. S 9.5: Isolated drusen in the macula. (→)

Fig. S 9.6: Large and partially confluent drusen.

Pathological Aging. If the aforementioned drusen are relatively large, without clearly defined boundaries and display a tendency to merge together (become confluent) (cf. Fig. S 9.6), then the risk of developing macular degeneration increases [Lat. *degeneratio*: degeneration]. Degeneration is defined as the restructuring of a tissue from a more complex into a simpler form, as well as from a well-functioning level to an impaired level. The first stage of AMD is an irregularity in the pigment epithelium visible in an eye examination (Fig. S 9.7).

Examination reveals that there is no longer a uniform fundus reflex showing red with a touch of black, but rather there are darker and brighter areas. A patient with these alterations will not see 100% but, depending upon the severity of these changes, anywhere between 20% and 80%.

The lowest visual acuity that is just "adequate" to read a newspaper (perhaps using reading glasses) is about 30%. AMD can either stop at this first stage (changes in the pigment epithelium) and develop no further. Otherwise, it can deteriorate into an atrophic form or can even progress to a "wet" form of the disease [Gr. *atrophein*: without nutrition]. Atrophic degeneration may be associated with a danger of advanced tissue loss and consequently impairment of visual function. This is seen in Figure S 9.8. These macular alterations just described are also called "dry" AMD.

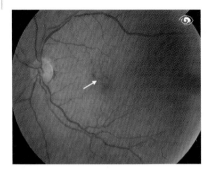

Fig. S 9.7: Pigment changes in the macula.

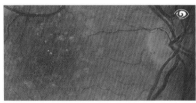
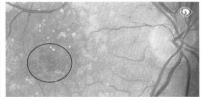

Fig. S 9.8: Atrophic AMD. In the color picture on the left, the atrophy is barely visible; it can be better seen in the picture on the right, where it is circled in red.

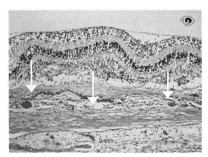
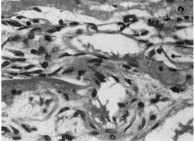

Fig. S 9.9: Wet AMD: Fibrovascular tissue has grown beneath the retina (→); this is shown under higher magnification on the right.

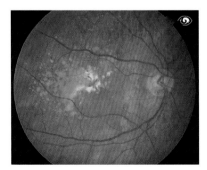

Fig. S 9.10: A fundus showing the pathological changes of wet AMD.

Dry AMD can progress into "wet" AMD. Nature strives to repair defects in the body whenever possible. Therefore, blood vessels may grow from the choroid into the degeneratively transformed macula and under the pigment epithelium. They can even break through the pigment epithelium and continue to grow between this layer and the retina (Fig. S 9.9). Under these circumstances, the efforts by Mother Nature to repair matters actually do more harm than good. In contrast to healthy capillaries, the newly created blood vessels are not "water-tight." Fluid, occasionally even blood, may leak and flow beneath and into the retina, thus giving rise to wet AMD (Fig. S 9.10).

These blood vessels and the exuded fluid lead to local detachments and dislocations of retinal receptor cells. As a consequence, the rods and cones are not where they are supposed to be, while at the same time, nourishment to the retina becomes ever more inefficient. If an image is projected onto the partly detached retina, the brain receives information that is topographically (spatially) incorrect. This is the reason why a patient suffering from wet AMD might not see a doorframe as a rectangle, but rather as a bowed or a wave-like structure. This phenomenon, called metamorphopsia [Gr. *metamorphopsein*: to see something bowed, tilted], is pathognomonic (strongly indicative) of macular disease.

Symptoms of AMD. To reiterate the most important symptoms of AMD: In dry AMD, there is a variably pronounced reduction in visual acuity; in wet AMD, there is a major reduction in vision associated with metamorphopsia.

The loss of vision is a heavy burden for the elderly. Comforting, however, is the fact that a patient will not go blind because of AMD. He may have serious problems reading or trying to identify faces, but will be spared complete blindness if there are no additional eye diseases (such as glaucoma) because other areas of the retina remain intact.

A patient suffering from AMD has a relatively good orientation ability and can freely move around because the peripheral retina is not affected by the disease.

How Frequent is AMD? There are some very rare, inherited forms of macular degeneration which can occur in childhood or when the patient is a young adult. These macular degenerations should not be confused with AMD which, specifically, is an affliction of the elderly. In middle age, AMD is quite rare, but the probability of developing AMD strongly increases with age. About 1.5% of people aged 52–64 suffer from AMD, while the rate is 10–20% among those 65–75 years of age, and approximately 35% among those between 75 and 84-years-old. One could almost even go so far as to say that anyone who lives long enough will almost certainly develop AMD. Since the average life expectancy continues to rise, one anticipates a corresponding increase in the number of AMD patients in the future.

Pathogenesis and Prevention of AMD. The pathogenesis of AMD is not well understood. This is the reason why attempts to treat it are still in the earliest stages.

Without a doubt, there is a certain genetic predisposition (cf. S 3) for this disease; children of parents suffering from AMD face a higher risk of later developing the disease. Individuals with fair skin who tend to be very sensitive to bright lights also suffer from the disease more frequently. It occurs more often in females than in males.

As with most age-related disorders, oxidative stress has been implied in the pathogenesis of AMD. What exactly does the term oxidative stress mean? If you have ever seen a brown apple or a rusted iron fence, then you have seen the results of oxidation. In strictly chemical terms, oxidation stands for removal of electrons from an atom or molecule. Due to the fact that oxygen can be very eager to receive additional electrons from other atoms and molecules, oxidation refers often to the binding of a molecule with oxygen. Oxygen is present everywhere, but it is fortunately in an inert state. This is the reason why flamable material like wood does not burn spontaneously. We first need to add some energy, e.g. with matches, to start the process of burning. If however, oxygen has gained an addition electron or if oxygen has received additional energy (so called singlet oxygen) then this oxygen is escharotic and will attack other molecules. Such a situation is called oxidative stress. Oxidative stress is a general term describing the level of oxidative damage taking place in a cell, tissue, or organ.

Our body constantly interacts with oxygen as part of the energy producing processes in the cells. Ironically, oxygen is not only the molecule which we cannot live without, but it is also the molecule that can harm us the most. The metabolism of oxygen can lead to the production of active, damaging forms of oxygen, known as reactive oxygen species (ROS). ROS can interact with other molecules within the cell, causing oxidative damage to proteins, membranes and genes. Under normal circumstances, cells have multiple protective mechanisms in the form of antioxidants and repair enzymes which succeed in protecting the cell from oxidative damage caused by ROS. Although oxidative stress occurs throughout life, it worsens as we age. It is hypothesized that as we become older normal defense mechanisms preventing oxidation decline, making it more difficult to fight off age related deterioration in physical and mental function. Our retina is particularly susceptible to oxidative stress as its need for oxygen is large, it is exposed to high levels of light (can induce the formation of ROS), and its membranes are rich in readily oxidized polyunsaturated fatty acids.

The other risk factors of AMD are similar to those causing arteriosclerosis: AMD is more frequently seen in association with smoking and increased lipid blood levels. There are also indications that a lack of vitamins, especially of vitamins E and C, but also vitamin A, seems to hasten AMD development. The general rules that have been established for preventing arteriosclerosis can also be regarded as preventive measures for AMD: refrain from smoking, a diet rich in vitamins and low in fat, plenty of physical exercise, etc. Since light most probably plays a role in the pathogenesis of AMD, wearing high-quality sunglasses that specifically absorb UV-light is recommended, particularly when at sea and near the water, in the snow, and in the mountains.

Treatment of AMD. There is no specific therapy for dry AMD. A diet rich in vitamins is usually recommended, as is occasionally a gingko preparation supplement.

In wet AMD, destruction of the new abnormal blood vessels (neovascularization) is attempted with a laser (S 13). These vessels indeed recede after laser treatment. It should not be overlooked, however, that: a) as in all laser treatment, healthy tissue is also destroyed; and b) the underlying cause of AMD is not influenced at all.

Recently, laser therapy has been improved by "photodynamic therapy." To carry out this therapeutic approach, a light-sensitive chemical is intravenously injected. This substance adheres primarily to the walls of the new and abnormal blood vessels and, to a lesser degree, to the walls of healthy blood vessels. Activating this substance by a non-thermal laser leads to a biochemical reaction that results in a closure and finally in the destruction of the "marked" newly formed blood vessels. Frequent and quite extensive follow-up examinations and repeated treatment are necessary in most cases because the causes of the disease are not eliminated. Photodynamic therapy has raised high hopes but it remains to be seen how substantial the long-term benefits of this treatment actually are.

In other therapeutic approaches, the newly formed blood vessels are surgically removed or the entire retina is detached, rotated and fixed in a position which brings the macula into contact with a section of still healthy pigment epithelium. However, such treatment is possible in only a very few cases, and the final outcome is still unclear.

Researchers who study wet AMD have found that a certain chemical in our body is critical in causing abnormal blood vessels to grow under the retina. That chemical is called vascular endothelial growth factor, or VEGF. Recently, scientists have developed several new drugs that can block VEGF (anti-VEGF). Blocking VEGF reduces the growth of abnormal blood vessels, slows their leakage, and helps to slow vision loss. It is therefore particularly useful in treating the wet or exudative form of AMD. Anti-VEGF treatment is a step forward in the treatment of wet AMD because it targets the underlying cause of abnormal blood vessel growth. Ranibizumab, Pegaptanib, and Anecortave are examples of anti VEGF drugs that may have potential in the treatment of wet AMD. Ranibizumab and Pegaptanib exert their anti VEGF effect by blocking specific VEGF receptors and thereby preventing VEGF from acting at its specific site. Anecortave is a steroid which exerts its anti VEGF effect by inhibiting the activity of enzymes that break down proteins.

Another drug which is often used by ophthalmologists in the form of an intravitreal injection is triamcinolone. Triamcinolone is also a corticosteroid and its potential as a treatment option for the wet form of AMD is due to its antiinflammatory and antiproliferative effects. Ophthalmologists often use this corticosteroid injection in conjunction with photodynamic therapy to reduce the persistence or growth of abnormal blood vessels. One main side effect of steroid injections is the possibility of an intraocular pressure rise. We therefore advice patients to have their intraocular pressure checked and monitored by their ophthalmologist when treated with steroid injections.

The anti-VEGF drugs must be injected into the eye with a very fine needle. The ophthalmologist cleans the eye to prevent infection and will administer an anesthetic to the eye to avoid pain. Usually, patients receive multiple anti-VEGF injections over the course of many months. As with any medical procedure, there is a small risk of complications following anti-VEGF treatment. Most complications that might occur, result from the injection itself, which in very rare circumstances can injure the eye or lead to an infection.

For many AMD patients, the hardest challenge is adapting to life with impaired vision. However, by training remaining peripheral vision, modifying the patient's environment and using available low vision devices and aids, AMD patients can continue to maintain their lifestyle and independence. It is important that patients seek assistance from low vision specialists and vision rehabilitation experts. These experts can help patients use their remaining sight to its full and teach new ways to accomplish everyday tasks. There are magnifying devices that can restore some ability to read, thus occasionally enabling patients with advanced AMD to read at least some documents and texts.

Low vision rehabilitation is a team effort often involving the low vision specialist (an optometrist or ophthalmologist skilled in the examination, treatment and management of patients with visual impairments), rehabilitation teachers, mobility and orientation specialists, occupational therapists, technicians, and other professions as needed.

AMD and Glaucoma. AMD does not occur more frequently among glaucoma patients than among the general population, but if it does occur in these patients, it is particularly disturbing. Characteristic for glaucomatous damage is that peripheral visual defects develop, while central vision remains normal almost to the very end. If a patient suffers simultaneously from glaucomatous visual field defects and an AMD-related loss in visual acuity, his vision is doubly impaired. This, once again, stresses the importance of treating glaucoma even if no subjective disturbances are noted. A glaucoma patient has to be aware of the possibility of developing AMD in later life, thus making preservation of the visual fields all the more important.

S 10 Visual Field Examination / Perimetry

The term, perimetry, is used to describe the scanning and measuring of the visual field [Gr. *peri*: around/Gr. *metron*: the measure/Gr. *metrein*: to measure].

The Visual Field. The visual field is the space or area that is seen by a fixed (non-moving) eye. An example to illustrate this concept: With his arm outstretched, a person is instructed to look at the tip of his thumb. Still staring at the tip of his thumb, keeping it in sharp focus and without moving the eye, the person notes that surrounding objects are still perceived, even though these are seen in less detail. The surrounding space that is perceived (plus the thumb) is called the "visual field." If the eye moves, the area observed becomes even broader, and this enlarged space is called the field of vision.

While concentrating on the tip of the thumb, other visual functions are perceived in the surrounding area, and these include not only brightness, but also colors, forms and even movements. This underscores how many different visual functions are included in the visual field; the sensitivity of these various functions can be measured and quantified.

The simplest function is light perception: Imagine a person sitting in a totally dark room fixating on a tiny point of light. Additional points of light could then be created in the visual field. The absolute light sensitivity threshold can be determined by how bright these other lights must be in order to be perceived. Though interesting, there is no practical purpose in measuring the light sensitivity threshold because it is not useful in disease diagnosis.

Perimetry. The next function, just a bit more complex, is the differential light sensitivity (DLS). Here the patient no longer sits in a completely dark room but rather in a room that is uniformly illuminated. There is thus a background light intensity, i.e. a brightness that exists throughout the entire visual field. Next a particular light, brighter than the background light intensity, is added at a local spot.

As soon as the second light can be discerned, the difference in intensity between the second light and the background light is recorded. This is termed the differential light sensitivity. The measurement of the differential light sensitivity, or perhaps more accurately, the threshold of the differential light sensitivity, is quite useful diagnostically and forms the basis of modern perimetry. Performing the measurement in a cupola (cf. Fig. S 10.1) provides results that are quite reliable. A defined background light intensity is created within this cupola and then additional light spots (stimulus lights) are introduced.

For most visual functions, the highest sensitivity is located in the center of where the eye is fixated. Sensitivity decreases markedly towards the periphery. This is most noticeable for visual acuity but clearly less pronounced with motion perception. Specifically, this means that the visual acuity is good in the center but decreases rapidly towards the periphery. In the peripheral visual field, for example, only large numbers or letters are recognized. Movements, on the other hand, are perceived in the periphery almost as well as in the center.

Differential light sensitivity decreases slowly from the center to the periphery. The decrease is not as abrupt as it is with visual acuity. One could figuratively describe this as a "hill of vision." The height of the hill represents the differential light sensitivity (Fig.

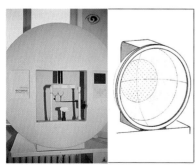

Fig. S 10.1: Cupola of a perimeter instrument in which a background light and stimulus lights are presented.

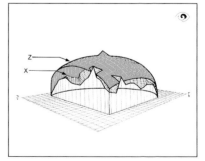

Fig. S 10.2: The "hill of vision" Z (green): age-corrected normal values; X (yellow): one patient's results.

S 10.2): it is highest in the center and decreases slowly as the periphery is approached.

Measurement Strategy. There are two possibilities to determine the shape of this sensitivity hill: a light too dim to be perceived is slowly moved from the periphery towards the center until it is noted (Fig. S 10.3). This light is called a stimulus [Lat. *stimulus*: goad, spur, incentive].

The location where this light is perceived is recorded as a point on a visual field map. The procedure is then repeated with the same light, but this time, the light comes from a different direction. After this has been done for a number of directions, the points marked on the "map" can be joined together with lines, called isopters [Gr. *isos*: same/Gr. *opsein*: to see] (Fig. S 10.4).

Next one uses a dimmer stimulus light that is seen only closer to the center. Again, the points that have been marked for this stimulus from a number of directions are connected, and a second isopter can be drawn that corresponds to the next higher level of sensitivity (Fig. S 10.5). The isopters can be compared to the contour lines of a topological map. The procedure described here in which the stimulus is moved is called kinetic perimetry [Gr. *kinein*: to move].

The other possibility for quantifying (measuring) the thresholds of the various light sensitivities consists of leaving the stimulus light at the same location, but gradually changing its brightness, step by step, until it is perceived (Fig. S 10.6). Conversely, one could also start with a bright light and gradually dim it until it is no longer seen. This procedure is called static perimetry, static because the stimulus light is not moved.

Both methods have proven useful in their own way. Kinetic perimetry is tested, for example, to identify certain brain diseases and static perimetry is used in diagnosing glaucoma. For this reason, the focus here is on static perimetry.

With static perimetry, there are also two methods that can be used and these are: threshold perimetry and suprathreshold or semi-quantitative perimetry. In threshold perimetry, the threshold itself is measured and then correspondingly printed out. In suprathreshold

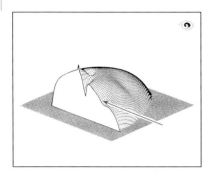

Fig. S 10.3: The principle of kinetic perimetry: A defined stimulus is moved towards the center of the visual field (red arrow) until it is perceived.

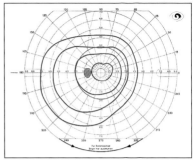

Fig. S 10.4: Connecting the visual field locations of the same sensitivity yields the isopters (red).

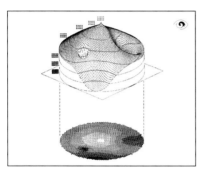

Fig. S 10.5: The gray scale representation (below) of the hill of sensitivity provides the same information as that shown above in three dimensions or as isopters.

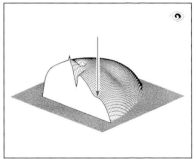

Fig. S 10.6: The principle of static perimetry: The brightness of a stimulus light is increased until it is perceived (red arrow).

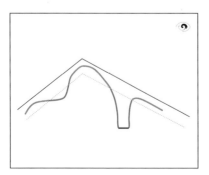

Fig. S 10.7: Semi-quantitative perimetry simply examines whether the threshold is normal (green), relatively destroyed (red) or totally destroyed (blue).

perimetry, the task is simpler. The precise threshold value is no longer investigated, but rather simply whether the observed threshold is at least at a certain level (Fig. S 10.7).

Concretely, this means that lights having a brightness somewhat greater than the expected threshold are presented. If the patient sees these light points, then the sensitivity at this test location is perceived as "normal" and if not, then the results are "abnormal." This suprathreshold perimetry saves time and is quite useful in diagnosing certain diseases. However, with glaucoma, it is important to know the precise threshold so that any changes occurring later, even though they might be slight in nature, can be established. Glaucoma therefore requires the more sophisticated threshold perimetry.

The Test Location Grid. Theoretically, one would like to measure the differential light sensitivity threshold at each point in the visual field. However, this would be extremely time-consuming and therefore not feasible. Instead, one performs a sort of sampling procedure: the threshold is simply measured at a certain number of locations in the visual field (usually between 50 and 100). In so doing, one must accept the possibility that very small visual field defects may go unnoticed on the test location grid and simply not be discovered. The test location grid can be adapted to specifically test for the disease one suspects. For example, we developed location grids for the Octopus automated perimeter programs, G1 and G2, as shown in Figure S 10.8, specifically for glaucoma diagnosis.

Bracketing the Differential Light Sensitivity (DLS). How is the threshold concretely measured? As mentioned above, one starts with a weak stimulus light and gradually increases its brightness until it is perceived by the patient, or conversely, one makes a bright light dimmer until it is no longer seen. However, these methods in which the threshold is approached from only one side have not proven useful in practice. This is due to the fact that when the patient doesn't concentrate fully, there is an apparent shift of the threshold. This problem has been solved by an ingenious method, the bracketing procedure (Fig. S 10.9).

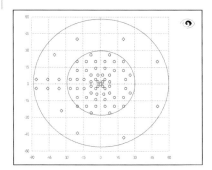

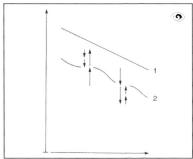

Fig. S 10.8: Test grids of the Octopus G1 and G2 glaucoma programs.

Fig. S 10.9: Principle of the bracketing procedure: 1 = normal value, 2 = sensitivity threshold of the patient.

To carry out this test, one starts with fairly large intervals that then become smaller as it crosses the actual threshold value. The threshold is approached from above and below the expected value. In other words, the light is increased or decreased in a step-wise fashion. When a patient sees the stimulus light, it is then again dimmed until it is no longer identified. Conversely, if light is decreased in a step-wise fashion until it is no longer distinguished, it is then gradually made brighter until it is again perceived. To express whether he has seen the light, the patient pushes a button. If no light is seen, he does not push the button. This is done at random for each test location in the test location grid. It is important that the patient not become distracted or frustrated when he realizes that the he does not perceive a stimulus light that is presented. This is part of the measurement strategy, and even someone with a normal, intact visual field will only be able to see about half of the stimuli.

The results obtained with this method are surprisingly independent of the "patient" factor. This means that the measurement outcome hardly depend on the patient's disposition. Patients occasionally complain that they are sure their visual field is poorer on a certain day because they just cannot concentrate as they should. Nevertheless, the examination findings agree with those from previous examinations. Simply stated, this method is more informative than the patient's subjective impression of it.

Fig. S 10.10: Principle of automated perimetry: The perimeter (A) displays stimulus lights and records the patient's responses. The perimetrist programs the computer (B).

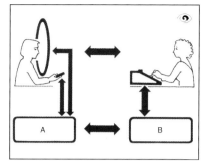

As complex as the examination may appear, there are only two possible responses that the patient can provide, either "seen" or "not seen." This is confirmed by the patient pressing a hand-held button when the light stimulus is seen, and not pressing it when it isn't seen. This poses a challenge for the examiner: he must make the stimulus light appear at various test locations with varying degrees of brightness. As the test evolved, this task became transferred to a computer, and is now called "automatic perimetry" or "computer perimetry"; however, it does not fundamentally differ from "manual perimetry." The computer presents the stimulus lights in varying degrees of brightness at different sites on the test location grid, registers and processes the patient's responses and from these, calculates the location and brightness of the next stimulus presentation (Fig. S 10.10).

Displaying the Results from the Measurement. With kinetic perimetry, the results are depicted as isopters. In computerized static perimetry, various possibilities are available for displaying the findings. One simple form is the gray scale (Fig. S 10.11).

Here the computer represents those areas having a higher sensitivity with a lighter symbol and uses a darker symbol for less sensitive areas. Many variations are possible: for example, instead of displaying the sensitivity directly, one could depict the difference between the measured value and the expected value as a gray scale, or the visual field as a colored map, etc.

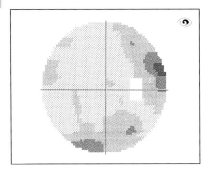

Fig. S 10.11: The examination results are shown using the gray scale. The region of the blind spot is intentionally left out.

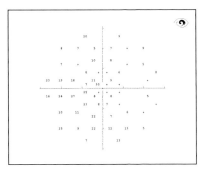

Fig. S 10.12: The examination results are shown using a comparison printout: The numbers correspond to the difference between the actual values measured and the expected normal values.

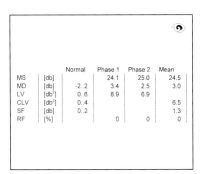

		Normal	Phase 1	Phase 2	Mean
MS	[db]		24.1	25.0	24.5
MD	[db]	-2..2	3.4	2.5	3.0
LV	[db²]	0..6	8.9	6.9	
CLV	[db²]	0..4			6.5
SF	[db]	0..2			1.3
RF	[%]		0	0	0

Fig. S 10.13: The examination results are shown using visual field indices.

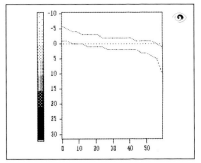

Fig. S 10.14: Normal range for the Bebie curve. The values on the left are better than expected while those on the right are poorer. Such deviations are completely normal, even for healthy persons.

The results can also be shown in numerical form. This has proven useful when showing the difference between the expected values and the actual threshold values measured (Fig. S 10.12).

When there are large quantities of numbers that have to be processed, as occurs in a census, mathematical procedures can be used to summarize them. For example, mean values and standard deviations can be calculated. We introduced such statistical procedures in perimetry and termed the outcomes "visual field indices" (Fig. S 10.13).

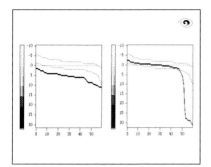

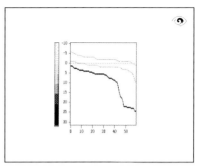

Fig. S 10.15: The visual fields are represented using Bebie curves. On the left, diffuse damage can be noted, while on the right, local visual field damage is indicated.

Fig. S 10.16: The visual field is represented using Bebie curve: combined diffuse and local damage.

The Bebie curve has proven useful in the investigation of diffuse components of visual field defects. The deviations between the measured and expected thresholds are calculated. These values are then ranked graphically so that the test locations with the largest positive deviation from the expected values are shown on the left, and those with the largest negative deviation are depicted on the right. For this cumulative defect curve, we introduced the term, "Bebie curve," in honor of Hans Bebie, a professor from the University of Bern, Switzerland, and a brilliant physicist who significantly contributed to the development of perimetry.

By measuring a large number of normal individuals, we have established standard values for Bebie curves. Even among healthy individuals, the values spread over a certain range (Fig. S 10.14).

When a given patient has a normal visual field, then his Bebie curve lies within the normal range. However, if the patient has a local defect somewhere in the visual field, the curve will fall steeply down on the right. With diffuse damage, the Bebie curve is shifted parallel to the normal curve (Fig. S 10.15).

Frequently, combinations of both forms of damage are present (Fig. S 10.16).

The Bebie curve is especially helpful (naturally in combination with other visual field representations) because certain forms of glaucoma cause diffuse visual field loss, with or without scotomata [Gr. *skotoma*: site of reduced vision]. It is particularly important to identify these diffuse visual field losses in patients having a vasospastic syndrome (S 8).

As with all technical instruments, there are many different products available from various companies. The first automated static perimeter that appeared on the market was the "Octopus," developed by Prof. Franz Fankhauser in Bern and manufactured by Interzeag in Schlieren, Switzerland. Professor Fankhauser also made other pioneering achievements in ophthalmology (cf. S 13). Similar instruments followed the Octopus, including the "Humphrey Perimeter" and the "Tübinger Perimeter," just to name two others.

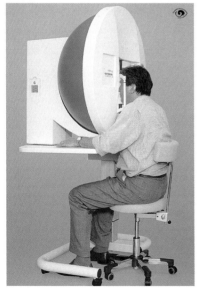

Fig. S 10.17: Patient undergoing an automated perimetry examination.

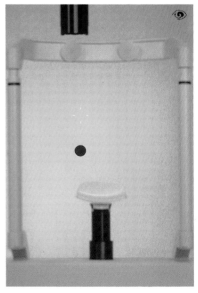

Fig. S 10.18: Chin rest and forehead bar on the perimeter. The background light in the cupola is visible.

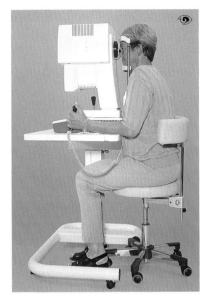

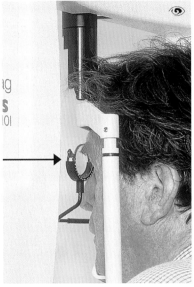

Fig. S 10.19: Patient undergoing an automated perimetry examination (Octopus 123); both the background light and the stimulus lights are projected directly onto the retina.

Fig. S 10.20: A corrective lens (→) is often required so the patient sees the stimulus in sharp focus.

How is an Examination Performed? The measuring procedure is first explained to the patient, who then sits down at the instrument (often fitted with a cupola) and which is equipped with a button that the patient pushes with his hand (Fig. S 10.17).

The patient fixes his gaze on a light or mark in the center of the cupola (Fig. S 10.18).

The computer then randomly presents light stimuli that have various levels of brightness at different test locations within the cupola. When the patient detects the stimulus, he confirms this by pressing the button. There are modern perimeters that no longer require a cupola because they project the background light as well as the stimuli directly onto the retina in the eye. This type of instrument is shown in Figure S 10.19.

The patient determines how fast the examination takes place. When the button is quickly pressed after the stimulus presentation, the computer rapidly presents the next light stimulus. If the patient prefers a slower pace, then this is likewise noted. The perimeter operator can also set the speed to comply with the patient's wishes. Should the patient close his eyes or blink during Octopus perimetry, he need not worry that a stimulus has been missed. The computer system registers the lid closure using an attached camera. When the lid closure occurs simultaneously with the presentation of a light stimulus, then the computer just repeats the very same stimulus at a later time. If the patient becomes fatigued during the examination and wishes to take a little break, he can just close his eyes or hold down the button. The computer waits until the patient is again ready to proceed before the next light stimulus is presented.

If a corrective lens is needed for the examination, as when a patient wears glasses, it is simply placed in the lens holder in front of the eye being examined. This ensures that the displayed stimuli are seen in focus at the appropriate distance. Contact lens wearers can keep on their lenses during the examination (Fig. S 10.20).

It is important that the patient does not feel intimidated by the instrument. The examination is actually quite straightforward and usually provides the physician with the needed information, even when the patient feels he wasn't cooperating as much as desired. Because of the prolonged viewing of the white background surface, the patient often subjectively perceives strange light formations. He might suddenly have the feeling that everything has gotten darker or that colors change. However, the patient should be reassured that these sensations are quite normal and arise from the eye's ability to adapt itself to a constant light level.

It was mentioned above that several different instruments from various companies are currently on the market. The examination procedure just described is based on Octopus perimetry, but basically, the investigation is similar with all the instruments.

Special Forms of Perimetry. Thus far, we have concentrated on measuring the differential light sensitivity that is carried out with white light, also called white light perimetry. Colored light and colored stimuli can also be used. For example, with glaucoma, perimetry is sometimes performed using blue stimuli against a yellow background. This has the advantage that glaucoma loss can be recognized relatively early, but also the disadvantage that the results are more affected by intraocular lens clouding. Therefore, we employ these only in special cases and not on a routine basis.

The stimuli can also be presented in a flickering rather than a constant manner. For example, the technique presently in evaluation, the frequency doubling technology makes use of an effect created by a stripe pattern undergoing rapid counterphase flicker (pattern reversal), thereby producing the appearance of twice as many light and dark bars than are physically present. Frequency doubling technology determines the contrast sensitivity for detecting the frequency doubling stimulus.

S 11 Measuring Perfusion

Diagnosing disturbances in blood perfusion has assumed increasing importance in medicine. When a specific organ does not have an adequate blood supply, it becomes damaged, and in extreme cases, the organ may die. The central motor of the circulatory system is the heart, which rhythmically pumps the blood throughout the entire body. A prolonged cessation of the heartbeat leads to death. Frequently though, it is only a small part of the organism that is not – or only poorly – perfused, and this can result in a variety of diseases. Thus physicians from almost all fields of medicine are interested in measuring blood perfusion. This delivers important information about the condition of the various organ systems and also serves as a means of checking the efficacy of a specific treatment. Many methods are currently available for measuring and graphically displaying perfusion.

Procedures with Image Display. Various methods of x-ray diagnostic procedures can show perfusion and perfusion disturbances. When a contrast dye is injected into the bloodstream, the blood column can be seen on the x-ray. Figure S 11.1 shows an angiogram [Gr. *aggeion*: vessel/Gr. *graphein*: to write] of leg arteries in the pelvic region. On the left is the native picture where the arteries have been filled with a contrast medium, in the middle, the image is shown after "digital subtraction" which exposes the differences between the images with and without the dye; on the right is a view from a patient having an occluded vessel.

In Figure S 11.2, the same recording technique has been applied to the leg arteries of a healthy person and one afflicted with an arterial occlusion.

The left and middle pictures of Figure S 11.3 show the occlusion of an artery in the head; on the right, the corresponding improvement in perfusion following lysis [Gr. *lysis*: loosening], i.e. after dissolving the thrombus with medication.

Figure S 11.4 shows the angiographic picture of the ophthalmic artery (arteria ophthalmica) which supplies the eye and its

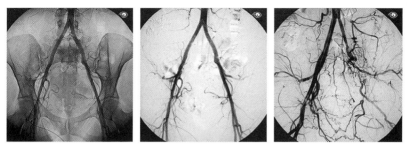

Fig. S 11.1: Angiogram of pelvic arteries.

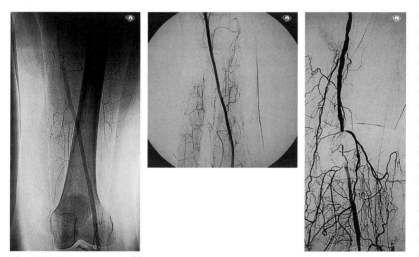

Fig. S 11.2: Angiogram of leg arteries.

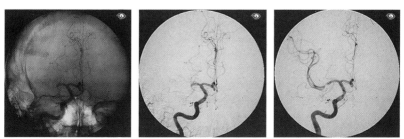

Fig. S 11.3: Angiogram of cranial arteries.

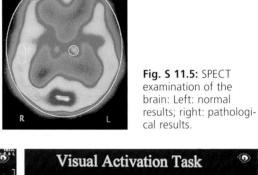

Fig. S 11.4: Those arteries that supply the eye are shown.

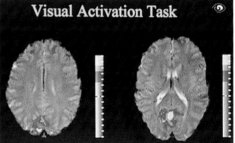

Fig. S 11.5: SPECT examination of the brain: Left: normal results; right: pathological results.

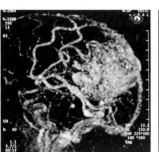

Fig. S 11.6: Brain perfusion shown with magnetic resonance imaging. The two pictures on the right show increased perfusion of the visual cortex during visual activity.

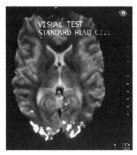

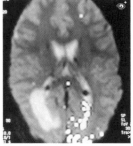

Fig. S 11.7: These images obtained using magnetic resonance tomography show normal activation of the visual cortex on the left and, on the right, abnormal activation due to multiple sclerosis.

surroundings. The left picture is the normal view and that on the right is after digital subtraction.

It is also possible to depict not the blood column but rather to show how much blood is actually flowing. An example of this is the "SPECT examination" which registers the quantity of blood flowing through the brain.

Figure S 11.5 shows brain perfusion as measured with the SPECT (Single Photon Emission Computed Tomography): The picture on the left is from a healthy individual while that on the right is a picture showing the pathology of a patient with a blood vessel inflammation.

Modern magnetic resonance procedures can also reveal perfusion, e.g. in the head. The picture on the left in Figure S 11.6 shows the blood flow in the brain; those in the middle and the right illustrate the increase in brain perfusion (located on the occipital, i.e. posterior, pole at the back of the brain) that occurs with visual activation.

Figure S 11.7 the responses to a visual stimulation: The image on the left is from a healthy individual while that on the right is from someone who has multiple sclerosis. Due to the disease, one half of the brain does not respond to the visual stimulation.

Evaluating the Ocular Blood Vessels. The ophthalmologist is particularly interested in perfusion, on the one hand because the eyes, as is the case with all body organs, are dependent on the blood flow, and on the other, because blood vessels within the eye can be directly observed. From this direct observation of the ocular perfusion, certain conclusions can be drawn about the general blood circulation. Moreover, as explained above, blood flow disturbances are crucially involved in the formation of glaucomatous damage.

Normally, there is such little blood that flows through the conjunctiva of a healthy eye that the underlying white sclera is visible. When the eye becomes irritated (e.g. during a viral infection or even simply while cutting onions), it appears red (Fig. S 11.8).

Looking at an irritated eye through a microscope on a slit-lamp, one has the impression that there are many reddened blood

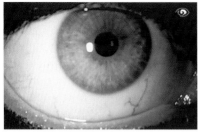
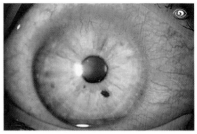

Fig. S 11.8: Left: The conjunctiva is barely visible in healthy persons. Right: due to blood vessel enlargement, the conjunctiva appears red.

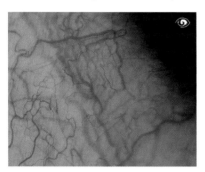
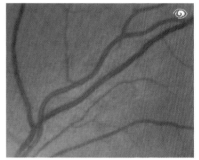

Fig. S 11.9: Reddened (hyperemic) conjunctiva with marked vessel enlargement.

Fig. S 11.10: The blood columns are visible on this fundus picture, but not the vessel walls.

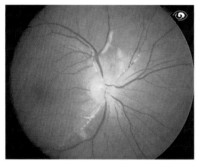
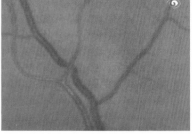

Fig. S 11.11: Altered blood vessel walls due to inflammation.

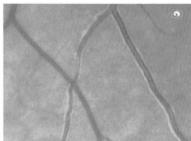

Fig. S 11.12: Arterial hypertension has caused changes in the blood vessels.

vessels. In reality, these are not blood vessels but rather the blood itself. The vascular walls are normally rather transparent so that one actually sees through them to the blood column (Fig. S 11.9).

The same applies to the retina where the blood columns can be directly observed, as with a contact glass (cf. Chapter 6.3) (Fig. S 11.10).

The blood vessels in Figure S 11.10 are healthy, i.e. they are transparent and the caliber of the arteries and veins is normal throughout. Figure S 11.11 shows vascular inflammation in which the vessels are no longer completely transparent.

In Figure S 11.12, severely constricted arteries can be recognized. For the physician, this is a sure sign that something is amiss in the circulatory system. In this particular example, the patient has severely elevated blood pressure.

With the slit-lamp, only the form of the blood column can be seen; one cannot determine how much blood actually flows through the vessel. Observing the blood vessels provides only an indication of the health status of the blood vessel, but does not provide information about the blood circulation. Below, methods are described with which the perfusion can be made more evident.

Fluorescein Angiography. In fluorescein angiography [Gr. *aggeion*: the vessel/Gr. *graphein*: to write], retinal blood vessels, or rather, the blood column, is made visible with a fluorescing dye, fluorescein sodium. After excitation by light of shorter wavelengths, fluorescing substances emit light of longer wavelengths; these wavelengths are characteristic for the specific fluorescing compound. Fluorescein angiography takes advantage of this phenomenon: The (non-toxic) fluorescein is injected into the patient's arm vein and, after passage through the heart, spreads out into almost all parts of the body, including blood vessels in the eye. When blue light is then shone onto the back of the eye, the fluorescein is stimulated to emit green-yellow light. The subsequent image of the retinal vessels (or more specifically, their contents) can be made visible with recording methods, for example, a photographic or video camera (Fig. S 11.13). To differentiate the fluorescent light form the stimulation light in the

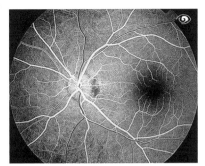

Fig. S 11.13: Fluorescein angiography: In the arteriovenous phase, the arteries are completely filled with dye while the veins are only partly filled.

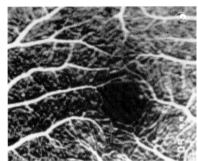

Fig. S 11.14: Even the fine capillaries around the macula (→) can be made visible using fluorescein angiography.

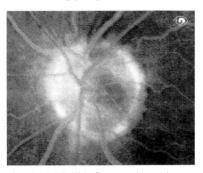

Fig. S 11.15: This fluorescein angiography shows a diffuse staining of the papilla in a glaucoma patient. This indicates that the blood vessels are "leaky."

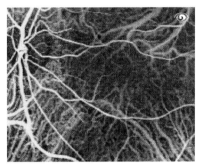

Fig. S 11.16: Deeper blood vessels of the choroid can be displayed using indocyanine angiography.

recording, a blocking filter is placed in front of a photodetector that only permits passage of green-yellow light, but not blue light. This increases the image contrast.

This method has the advantage that one can: a) picture the blood columns even in the capillaries (Fig. S 11.14); b) identify leaky places in the blood vessels since the dye flows out from these sites (Fig. S 11.15); and c) draw conclusions about the general perfusion situation: the more rapidly the fluorescein travels from the arm vein into the eye, the faster the blood flow.

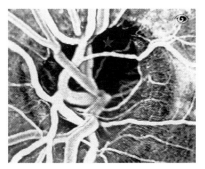

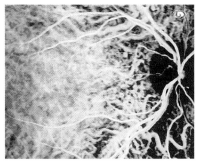

Fig. S 11.17: Fluorescein angiography of a glaucomatous papilla. Parts of the papilla remain black, i.e. they are not perfused (*).

Fig. S 11.18: Delayed filling of the choroid vessels near the papilla in a glaucoma patient. These are made visible using indocyanine green videoangiography.

With modern recording instruments and picture processing computers, blood flow velocity can be easily measured or calculated in the various parts of the retina.

There are disadvantages to these methods and they are: a) expensive instruments are required; b) in rare cases, the dye injected causes allergic reactions; and c) although information about retinal perfusion is gathered, not much is learned about the perfusion of the choroid or papilla.

A different dye, indocyanine green, is used for demonstrating perfusion of the choroid. The light absorbed by indocyanine green has a longer wavelength than that absorbed by fluorescein sodium; longer wavelength light can better penetrate into deeper sites. In addition, indocyanine green binds more strongly to certain proteins in the blood and thus does not leave the circulation as readily as fluorescein sodium, even in the fenestrated choroidal blood vessels. For these reasons, indocyanine green is better suited for examining the choroid than fluorescein (Fig. S 11.16).

In diagnosing glaucoma, angiography is employed more for research purposes than in routine clinical practice. Fluorescein angiography reveals e.g. poorly perfused areas in the optic nerve head of glaucoma patients (Fig. S 11.17).

In indocyanine angiography, delayed perfusion can be observed in the region around the optic nerve (Fig. S 11.18), especially in patients with vascular dysregulation (S 8).

Temperature Measurement. The average body temperature is 37°C (98.6 °F). Most people live in areas that are distinctly cooler than this and thus their bodies release heat to the environment. Because surface areas cool, hands are usually colder than livers, just to mention one example. A body part on or near the surface that has poor perfusion is provided with less warmth from the body, but still releases heat. This is why a poorly perfused foot feels cooler. The physician also notices this when he places his hand on a patient's leg: If one leg is colder than the other or than is expected, he knows that, in all probability, a perfusion disturbance is present. The physician thus welcomes "objective" and accurate instrumental temperature measurements that provide pertinent information about the perfusion situation.

How can temperature be measured? When a hand is placed on a cool table, the hand releases heat to the environment. A portion of the heat is delivered directly to the table. This process is termed heat conduction [Lat. *conducere*: conduct]. Another portion of the heat is released to the surrounding air, i.e. heat is conducted to the air. However, because the air in the immediate vicinity of the hand is made warmer, conduction here is quite weak. If, however, the wind blows, then the envelop of warm air around the hand is quickly replaced by cold air. This additional transport of heat is called convection [Lat. *vehere*: to carry]. Because the skin is always a bit moist, there is also a continuous slight water evaporation [Lat. *evaporatio*: evaporation]. Heat loss due to evaporation escalates during increased sweating.

Additionally, the hand gives off heat in the form of infrared radiation. Indeed, all objects do this. This means that the hand not only sends out radiation, but also receives it, e.g. from a wall.

There are instruments that measure this infrared radiation. Based on the spectral composition of the radiation, one can deduce the temperature of the object that emits it, in this case, the hand. A thermographic instrument [Gr. *thermä*: heat/Gr. *graphein*: to write] calculates the temperature of a body based on the radiated heat and displays it as an image. The newer ear thermometers also use this principle. In Figure S 11.19, a relatively warm and a relatively cold hand are depicted using a thermographic instrument. The temperatures calculated by the instrument are displayed in color.

The infrared radiation of a face and, in particular, the eye, can also be measured. Figure S 11.20 shows the facial temperature of a healthy subject under normal conditions while Figure S 11.21 shows that of a patient with a unilateral (one-sided) occlusion of the carotid artery in the neck. The eye and its surroundings are less well perfused on the side with the occlusion and are thus cooler than the other side.

A method has been developed that simply and quickly evaluates eye perfusion by employing corneal temperature measurements. In Figure S 11.22, temperature changes of the cornea are shown before, during and after a stream of air has been applied. One notes that the cornea cools very rapidly and then only slowly warms

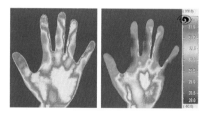

Fig. S 11.19: Thermogram of the hand: on the left is a warm hand; on the right is a cold hand.

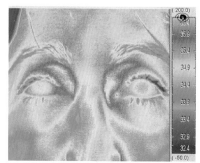

Fig. S 11.20: Thermogram of a face of a healthy individual.

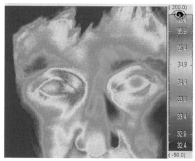

Fig. S 11.21: With the occlusion of the left carotid artery, the left side of the face is cooler than the right.

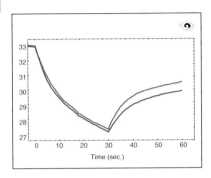

Fig. S 11.22: The change in corneal temperature before, during and after exposure to a stream of air. Healthy individual (green); patient with disturbed ocular perfusion (red).

back up. In patients having perfusion disturbances in the eye, the restoration of normal temperature is slower with the same stream of air.

This method is simple and convenient for the patient as well as for the doctor. The disadvantage is that there is not yet any long-term experience with this instrument. Further validation is necessary.

Color Doppler Imaging. With color Doppler imaging (abbreviated CDI), the location, the direction and the velocity of blood flow in an organ are examined using ultrasound. The flow direction is encoded in the display and this information is derived from sound frequency changes due to Doppler effect. The flow direction is encoded in color, thereby giving the method the name, "color Doppler imaging."

Ultrasound waves have such a high frequency that humans cannot hear them [Lat. *ultra*: beyond]. A probe is used to conduct sound waves into the tissue. When the waves encounter tissues having differing densities, some of these waves become reflected. The instrument that transmits the ultrasound also serves as a receiver for the echo that comes back. If the echo returns quickly, then it arises from a structure near the surface; if it arrives later, then it comes from a deeper site. The ultrasound instrument is thus able to construct a picture based on the varying echo information (Fig. S 11.23).

Many organs can be examined with the ultrasound instrument. For example, using this method in the eye, one can ascertain

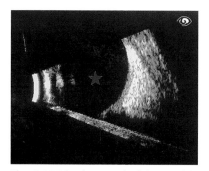

Fig. S 11.23: Ultrasound of the eye (*) and surroundings.

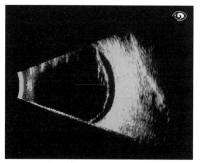

Fig. S 11.24: Ultrasound of an eye with retinal detachment (→).

whether behind the hemorrhage there is an underlying retinal detachment or tumor (Fig. S 11.24).

When the ultrasound is reflected by a stationary layer, the echo has the same frequency as the sound that was transmitted. However, if the echo arises from a moving object, the frequency of the echo is no longer the same. If the reflecting object (e.g. a blood cell) moves towards the probe, the frequency of the reflected signal is higher; if it moves away, it is lower. This is called the Doppler shift. Christian Doppler [1803–1853] was an Austrian mathematician and physicist who was the first to explain why light from stars moving towards the earth is bluer than that from receding stars which, in turn, is redder than that from stars having little or no movement towards or away from the earth. This phenomenon, which is encountered in acoustics and optics, is known as the Doppler effect or Doppler shift.

If the change of the sound frequency (Doppler shift) is displayed in color, one immediately sees whether, and in which direction, the object is moving (the object is normally blood) (Fig. S 11.25). Usually the blood that is moving towards the ultrasound probe is displayed as red while that which moves away is blue.

A third dimension can be introduced in color Doppler imaging: If the examiner has been able to display the blood vessel with ultrasound, he can determine the blood velocity in a field of interest by additionally applying a pulsed ultrasound (Fig. S 11.26). The in-

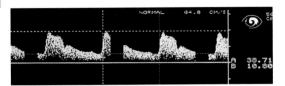

Fig. S 11.26: Display of the blood flow velocity in a blood vessel behind the eye using CDI.

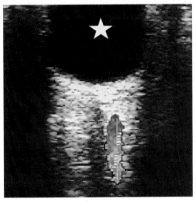

Fig. S 11.25: Ultrasound of the eye (*) and its surroundings. The colors indicate the presence and direction of blood flow (color duplex sonography).

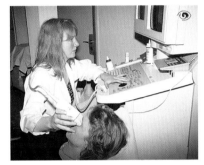

Fig. S 11.27: Patient being examined by a medical technician using CDI.

strument sends out a series of rapid surges – or pulses – from the probe.

Because blood in the arteries does not flow with constant velocity, but rather it pulsates, variations in the flow velocity arise. The blood flow velocity and, in particular, the ratio of highest to lowest velocity provides important information. It enables the ophthalmologist to measure the perfusion of the vessels behind the eye, specifically, those that supply the eye. Figure S 11.27 shows an examination being performed using color Doppler imaging.

Color Doppler imaging has proven useful as a valuable tool in the evaluation of glaucoma patients. It can assist in determining whether or not a glaucoma patient suffers from reduced perfusion in the eye. The advantages of this method lie in the many years of experience using it; normal values for healthy individuals are known (thus helping to better define abnormal values) and the examination is not uncomfortable to the patient. The disadvantages of the method are that the instrument is expensive and one must be trained in the measuring technique. Finally, though this method yields information about the blood flow velocity, it does not contribute direct information about the amount of blood actually flowing.

Capillary Microscopy. The capillaries are the body's smallest, "fine as hair" blood vessels [Lat. *kapillum*: hair]. Using a magnifying glass or microscope, the surface capillaries can be observed directly, especially in those places where the tissue is relatively transparent (e.g. on the lips) (Fig. S 11.28).

In clinical practice though, the examination of the capillaries in the nailfold has proven constructive and convenient because these capillaries all lie in the same layer and have the same direction (Fig. S 11.29). Additionally, the tissue can be made largely transparent with a drop of oil. If one observes the nailfold under a microscope, one sees individual blood cells as they wander through the capillaries. The velocity of the blood cells can be measured and also influenced: If the finger is somewhat cooled using a stream of cold air, the flow velocity is reduced, possibly even to total cessation for a short while (Fig. S 11.30).

For a patient with vascular dysregulation, this cessation in blood flow induced by the cold provocation lasts clearly longer than in a healthy person (cf. S 8).

If the perfusion before, during and after the cold provocation is recorded on a video, important variables for diagnosis can be cal-

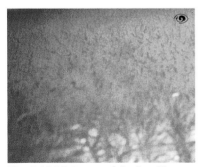

Fig. S 11.28: Image of the lips: The capillaries are barely recognizable.

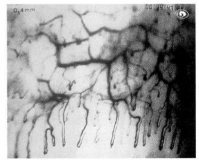

Fig. S 11.29: Blood vessels of a nailfold in the finger.

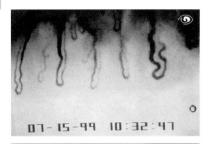

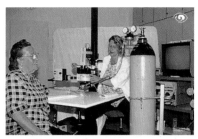

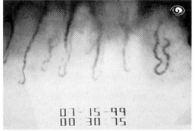

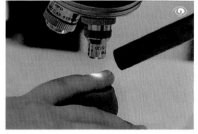

Fig. S 11.30: Nailfold capillaries: above: a normal flow; below: flow cessation after cold provocation.

Fig. S 11.31: Above: examination conditions for capillary microscopy. Below: The finger is placed under a microscope; for the provocation test, cold air is introduced from the tube.

culated or measured (e.g. the duration of the flow cessation). This is then termed video capillaroscopy (Fig. S 11.31).

For about the past 20 years, we have widely used capillary microscopy in perfusion diagnostics. It affords a simple method for determining vascular dysregulation without bothering the patient. But it does have some disadvantages: a) that although a proven dysregulation in a finger raises suspicion of the same problem in the eye, it does not prove it; b) dysregulation due to cold provocation can be measured, but that due to other stimulations (e.g. emotional stress) are more difficult; and c) this measurement only represents what is happening at a single point in time. A patient with unremarkable examination results can nevertheless have vascular dysregulation, it was just not provoked during the examination.

Up to this point, the measuring methods described have yielded indirect indications about the perfusion situation of the eye. To date, measuring the perfusion in the eye itself has long been only partially possible despite modern technology. Described below are the methods that have been developed for this purpose.

Blue Field Entoptics. Entoptic phenomena are optical perceptions that are generated by the body itself. When looking into a diffuse blue light (e.g. towards the blue sky), moving structures can be seen. These structures correspond to slight opacities (cloudings) in the vitreous body. White point-like objects that move are also noted. These points are the white blood cells that move in the retina. The normal blood columns of the retinal vessels are not noted because the retina has accustomed itself to the associated shadows. However, when there is a small transparent gap in the blood column (e.g. a white blood cell), a slight brightening is noted at these sites. The number and speed of these shining points provide information about the perfusion of the central retina. For the patient to be able to describe the amount and velocity of the moving points, comparison pictures are simulated for him on a computer monitor (Fig. S 11.32).

The simulation can be adjusted until it matches the entoptic impression perceived by the patient. The evidence provided by this method is limited because: a) the results depend on the concentration of the patient; b) there is a large inter-individual distribution; and c) only information about the perfusion of the central retinal capillaries is obtained.

Laser Doppler Velocimetry. When a stationary object is illuminated by light of a specified wavelength, the light is reflected or scattered back with the wavelength remaining unchanged. If the re-

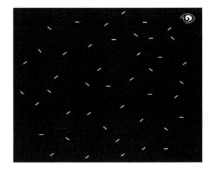

Fig. S 11.32: Computer simulation of the entoptically perceived moving light points.

flecting or scattering object moves, the wavelength changes. Once again, a Doppler shift is involved, similar to what was encountered with ultrasound (above). The frequency shift can be exploited to measure the blood flow velocity and thus the term, velocimetry [Gr. *velos*: fast/Gr. *metrein*: to measure]. Laser light (S 13) is focused onto a blood vessel and the blood flow velocity can then be calculated from the Doppler shift of the light that is reflected or scattered back towards the light source. While this method measures the velocity in a given blood vessel, it provides no information about the perfusion throughout the entire eye.

Laser Doppler Flowmetry. In contrast to laser Doppler velocimetry, with laser Doppler flowmetry (LDF), the laser light is not directed at a large vessel but rather at an area between large vessels. These regions normally contain numerous capillaries. The Doppler shift is again employed here, but this time to calculate the blood flow in this area. For example, this method can be used to measure the perfusion in the region of the optic nerve head (Fig. S 11.33). The disadvantage though is that the perfusion can only be measured in selected, relatively small regions and that, due to the limited penetration of laser light into the tissue, the perfusion is only measured to a relatively shallow depth. For these reasons, the method is suited primarily for studies in which two situations are compared (e.g. the perfusion before and after a certain therapy). This approach plays a minimal role for evaluating glaucoma patients.

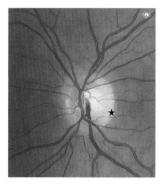

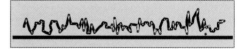

Fig. S 11.33: Using the LDF, perfusion is measured at a site on the papilla (*). The curve above shows typical blood flow variations.

Scanning Laser Doppler Flowmetry. With this procedure, a laser ray scans a certain area (e.g. the papillary region). Using rapid, automatic repetitions of the scanning process, it is possible to calculate the Doppler shift for each location scanned. The calculated velocities or the blood flow can then be graphically displayed (Fig. S 11.34).

The examination is relatively simple for both the patient as well as for the examiner, and the results are easily displayed. The disadvantages are that very high and very low velocities cannot be measured and that not only the Doppler shift but also other causes for temporal variations of the brightness enter into the calculations and influence the measurement results.

Measuring the Pulsations. Blood in arteries does not flow at a constant rate, but rather in pulsates. Correspondingly, blood in the eye does not flow in a constant manner. Since the eye sheath can stretch only slightly, pressure inside the eye varies in a pulsating fashion. The size of these pressure fluctuations permit one to derive the extent of perfusion. In the ocular blood flow (OBF) system, the pulsations are recorded (Fig. S 11.35) and, from these, the blood flow can be calculated.

The method is simple but has the disadvantage that the perfusion information provided by the pulsations is relatively vague and only the pulsatile portion of the perfusion can be registered.

It is also possible to measure the blood pressure in the eye by applying pressure to the eye. When the eye pressure exceeds the di-

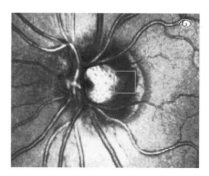

Fig. S 11.34: The blood flow is displayed (with artificial colors) using the Heidelberg Retina Flowmeter. Green: measurement window in which the perfusion can be quantified.

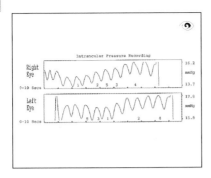

Fig. S 11.35: Measurement of the pulsations in the eye as an indirect measure for ocular perfusion (Langham's OBF instrument).

astolic blood pressure, the arteries begin to pulsate. When the pressure exceeds the systolic pressure, the arteries collapse. There are various methods to demonstrate this effect (e.g. the "SmartLens®").

Measuring the Diameters of Retinal Vessels. Using an instrument called the Retinal Vessel Analyzer (RVA), the blood column of the retinal blood vessels can be directly observed. These vessels, involved in the regulation of retinal blood flow, are neither rigid nor inflexible. Indeed, to continuously satisfy the ever-changing metabolic requirements of the retina they must constantly adapt to the perfusion needs.

The RVA can monitor, record and analyze the diameter of the retinal vessels and its fluctuations (cf. Fig. S 11.36). For this analysis, the boundaries of the blood column of a particular vessel are determined, and from these, the computer calculates the vessel diameter. The built-in algorithms not only allow automatic identification of the vessels located within a pre-determined window, but also minimize the impact of possible eye movements.

Results from such a measurement are shown in Fig. S 11.37, which displays the various diameters of a vascular section. The left side of the picture shows the eye fundus with a measuring window above the venous section examined. The diagram indicates both changes occurring at different points along one blood vessel (z-axis), and changes in the diameter over time (x-axis), as provided by the frequent measurements made within a short time period. In other

Fig. S 11.36: The Retinal Vessel Analyzer. On the right side is the fundus camera, on the left is the measuring unit. The fundus is shown on the right monitor, then the measuring window is adjusted, and the measuring values are continuously displayed on the left monitor.

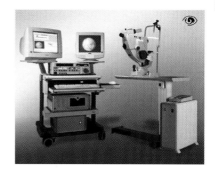

Fig. S 11.37: Representation of the retinal vessel diameters of a fixed vascular section using the RVA. Constriction resulted after provocation, i.e. the patient breathed 100% O_2.

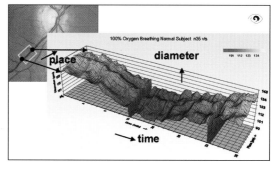

words, the RVA measures a particular blood vessel's diameter as a function of both location and time. Because this measuring procedure is still relatively new, not much is known about the behavior of the retinal vessel diameter or of the functional or clinical significance. Nevertheless, it is of interest to know how retinal vessels react to a particular treatment, just to provide one example of its application.

Blood Pressure Measurement. Blood pressure is an important factor for perfusion and thus its measurement is discussed here.

The heart moves the blood: it is pumped into the arteries by the rhythmic contractions of the heart chambers. The pressure produced in the arteries is known as the blood pressure. Since the heart does not pump continuously, but rather rhythmically, the pressure varies in the arteries and thus the blood pressure pulsates. These pulsations can be felt in the large arteries. The highest (top) value of this pulsation is called the systolic blood pressure and the lowest (bottom) value is the diastolic blood pressure. The systolic blood pressure, also known as the peak blood pressure, occurs at the moment when the heart chambers contract, the diastolic blood pressure occurs when the heart chambers relax [Gr. *systellein*: contract/Gr. *diastellein*: expand].

Blood pressure pulsations are used for measuring the blood pressure. When a blood pressure cuff is inflated on the upper arm, the pressure of the cuff is transmitted to upper arm. When the pressure exceeds the systolic blood pressure, the blood can no longer flow towards the hand. When the cuff pressure is below the diastolic pressure, the blood can flow through the arteries without impedance. When the cuff pressure lies between the systolic and diastolic pressure, the blood flows for a short time with each heartbeat and then stops again. The sound this makes in the arteries can be heard with a stethoscope [Gr. *stethos*: breast/Gr. *skopein*: to observe].

Some of the other instruments that measure the blood pressure function without a stethoscope. The blood pressure can additionally be measured at other sites, such as the wrist.

Since the establishment of high blood pressure as an important risk factor for cardiovascular diseases, much medical attention has been focused on blood pressure measurements. Included among the cardiovascular diseases are heart attacks, brain infarctions (strokes), arterial occlusions in the legs, etc.

However, it has only recently been learned that blood pressure which is too low can also be a risk factor, less so for cardiovascular disease but certainly for some eye diseases, such as glaucoma.

The blood pressure undergoes extreme variations throughout the day. A single blood pressure measurement provides a certain indication about someone's blood pressure, but little about its course throughout the day. If the blood pressure is somewhat elevated at the doctor's office, for example, it is quite well possible that it is normal for the rest of the day. On the other hand, significant drops in the nighttime blood pressure cannot be excluded just because a normal pressure was measured at the doctor's office. For this reason, a

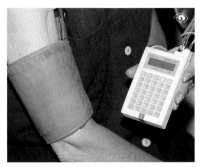

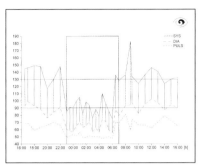

Fig. S 11.38: Portable blood pressure measuring instrument for registering the blood pressure during a 24-hour period.

Fig. S 11.39: Original printout of a 24-hour blood pressure measurement. The dashed line indicates the pulse.

method for measuring the 24-hour blood pressure has been developed (Fig. S 11.38).

This helps in identifying both blood pressure peaks in patients with hypertension (high blood pressure) as well as blood pressure dips in those with hypotension (low blood pressure). In glaucoma patients, it is particularly important to establish the presence of these blood pressure dips that occur primarily during the night.

The patient is thus given an instrument that measures and registers the blood pressure in pre-determined (e.g. hourly) intervals. When the patient returns the instrument to the doctor's office, a print-out of the blood pressure values can be made and analyzed (Fig. S 11.39).

Measuring perfusion after provocation. As much as it is important to obtain the information about the perfusion at baseline steady-state, sometimes it is even more important to impose a challenge on circulation and to observe the response. Thus, one can estimate the level of functional circulatory reserve in a given organ. As mentioned before, ocular blood flow is determined by the difference between the blood pressure and the IOP on one side, and by the vascular resistance on the other. All of these equation components can get modified. For example, blood pressure can be increased by means of physical exercise. Or, IOP can shortly be artifically increased by means of suction cup. This is s small plastic cup placed on the sclera with a negative suction pressure, thus causing the scleral / eyeball deformation and an increase in IOP. The vascular resistance can be manipulated in many ways. For example, shortly breathing pure oxygen or carbon-dioxide leads in general to the vasoconstriction and vasodilation, respectively. This response is different in various ocular tissues. Exposing retina to the flickering light, usually at frequences between 5 and 65 Hz, causes a widening of the retinal vessels, a phenomenon called neurovascular coupling. The rationale behind is obvious: an activated retina needs more blood perfusion. Immersing one hand in cold water causes vessel constriction in various body parts, including the eye. Cooling the eye directly would rather increase the choroidal blood flow, as its function among others is to maintain the temperature balance of the eye. However, some of these provocation influence more than one factor: for example, an isometric exercise increases the blood pressure, but also decreases the IOP and changes the vascular resistance in the eye. The latter is due to the activation of the sympathetic nervous system and is particularly pronounced in the choroid.

All these tests are potentially helpful in identifying patients with vascular dysregulation.

S 12 Ocular Pharmacotherapy (Eye Medications)

When you hold a small bottle (sometimes called an eyedropper bottle) containing eye medication in you hand, you could easily overlook the immense research that has gone into the development of that medicine you are about to apply.

The Search for a Medication. When trying to find new medications, the first step scientists undertake is to search for a substance (molecule) that has a specific, clearly defined effect. This molecule can be found anywhere: as a regular component of the human body, in plants, fungi or bacteria; it may be extracted from inorganic matter or even chemically synthesized. Imagine the following experiment: A smooth muscle cell is isolated and kept alive in a nutrient medium. Adrenaline is then added. Adrenaline is a hormone that is produced in the adrenal glands and circulates in our bodies throughout the bloodstream in a highly diluted form. In our experiment, when adrenaline is added, the muscle cell immediately contracts: this is a defined biological effect. If an entire blood vessel is isolated and once again adrenaline is added to the medium, then all the smooth muscle cells of the vessel will contract and cause vasoconstriction. This is a defined pharmacological effect. In summary, one has a pharmacological substance that exerts a specifically defined effect.

From Active Ingredient to Drug. A substance that has a defined pharmacological effect is not automatically a good drug. A substance that could potentially be used as a medication must exhibit its effect not only *in vitro*, meaning in the lab [Lat. *vitro*: glass], but also inside the human body, or *in vivo* [Lat. *vivum*: living being]. Additionally, the desired effect should be much stronger than any potential side effects, and finally, it should not be toxic in the concentrations required for a therapeutic effect. Other criteria could include the substance being easy to administer and, depending on the indication, have either a short or a protracted effect. If all these requirements are considered, it is no wonder that, from among the large selection of potential medications available, the pharmaceutical industry needs years to introduce one single drug onto the market.

From Drug to the Desired Application Form. Whenever a medication is prescribed, the goal is to deposit it safely at the problem site without unduly burdening the rest of the body. The entire process, ranging from bringing a pharmacologically active substance into the body, distributing it throughout the body, and finally eliminating it from the body, is called pharmacokinetics [Gr. *pharmakon*: drug/Gr. *kinein*: to move].

Depending upon the chemical profile, different drugs have varying affinities to certain body parts. For example, with a drug that is lipophobic [Gr. *lipos*: fat; Gr. *phobos*: fear] or not soluble in fat, only a very small portion reaches the brain because of the blood-brain barrier. The cerebral vessels allow only certain (mostly fat-soluble, lipophilic [Gr. *lipos*: fat; Gr. *philo*: liking] molecules to penetrate through their walls and gain access to the brain. This mechanism can be quite beneficial to the organism, but it can also be a hindrance in medical therapy. The blood-brain barrier poses an obstacle when certain drugs have to be distributed into the brain (such as an antibiotic in cases of encephalitis), especially if they are not available in a lipophilic form.

When a drug is taken in pill form, only a very small portion (about 1%) reaches the eye via the bloodstream. Just as with the brain, water-soluble, hydrophilic [Gr. *hydros*: water; Gr. *philo*: liking] molecules barely reach the intact retina or the optic nerve but are easily delivered to the choroid (cf. S 1). Analogous to the "blood-brain barrier," there is also a "blood-retina barrier." The lens is literally out of reach for most drugs. There is always the option of injecting a drug directly into the eye, resulting in a 100% intraocular distribution. Because this type of administration is very uncomfortable for the patient, it is only used in emergency situations. A drug can also be injected under the conjunctiva (subconjunctival injection) or into the fatty tissue surrounding the eyeball. With this form of application, approximately 10% of the medication is delivered into the eye; the rest is eliminated by the bloodstream. This method is a bit more acceptable to the patient but, nevertheless, it is not suitable for long-term therapy. Whenever possible, the pharmaceutical industry tries to develop ocular medications that can be instilled into the eye as drops.

From Drug to Eyedrops. Certain conditions must be met before a drug can be manufactured and administered to the patient as eyedrops. The most important question deals with the fate of a topically (i.e. locally on the surface) applied drug. Does it penetrate into the eye at all, or is it only washed out through the lacrimal duct where it drains into the pharynx, or does it reach the conjunctival vessels and from here, enter the body's circulation? Eyedrops primarily gain access to the eye via the cornea (cf. S 1). The various layers of the cornea alternate between hydrophobic [Gr. *hydros*: water/Gr. *phobos*: fear] and hydrophilic. This means that in order for a drug to penetrate through the different corneal layers, it must have both water-soluble and fat-soluble characteristics, i.e. be both hydrophilic as well as hydrophobic. Many drugs that could effectively lower the IOP do not meet these requirements. The eye only absorbs between 1% and 5%, even of a "perfect" eyedrop. The majority of that portion not absorbed is drained by the lacrimal duct into the nose and pharynx, from where it enters into the stomach. Another part enters the conjunctival vessels and is transported directly into the bloodstream. Inside the eye, the primary target areas are located in the anterior segment, such as the anterior chamber, iris and ciliary body. It is difficult to exert a therapeutic influence on structures in the eye's posterior portion.

Further Requirements for Eyedrops. A drug available as drops not only has to penetrate the eye, but it must also satisfy other requirements. For example, it should not burn or sting when applied. Certain substances cannot be used for eyedrops because they are only available in solutions that are too acidic or too alkaline.

Additionally, the solution must be colorless, as colors would interfere with vision. A high viscosity is unacceptable because of a glue-like effect on the eyelids. The necessity to satisfy these stringent requirements explains why, from among the huge number of potential drugs, only a few are on the market as eyedrops.

Contraindications for Eyedrops. All types of eyedrops can cause adverse reactions and allergies. In these cases, one must discontinue the therapy. Minor problems, such as a slight and temporary burning sensation, are harmless and will usually disappear within a short time. Since a considerable part of the drug enters the bloodstream, the same contraindications apply as in systemic therapy with the same substance. For example, a patient suffering from asthma should use topically administered beta-blockers only in exceptional circumstances, as drugs of this class can precipitate an asthma attack. Because of possible systemic side effects associated with the use of eyedrops, the patient's general practitioner must know about the specific ophthalmic therapy prescribed. Depending upon the substance, specific contraindications or drug interactions may be present.

Instilling the Eyedrops Correctly. Learning how to properly administer eyedrops is easy, and in most cases, the patient can do it alone. Before the drops are administered for the very first time, the patient should take the eyedropper in one hand and squeeze a drop onto his other hand. This indicates how tightly the bulb must be squeezed before the fluid leaves the dropper, a factor that may vary from bottle to bottle. To instill the drops: The lower eyelid is pulled down while the eye looks up at the ceiling. Next, the bulb is squeezed and at least one drop should fall onto the exposed conjunctiva on the inner side of the lower eyelid (Fig. S 12.1).

The lid is then slowly released and the eye should be closed for about one minute. With each blink of the eye, there is an exchange of the tear film that rapidly drains the drug into the lacrimal duct and into the nasopharynx. The patient should try to refrain from closing the eyelids too tightly as this presses tears (and medica-

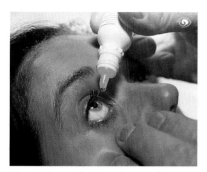

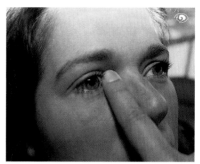

Fig. S 12.1: Administering eyedrops.

Fig. S 12.2: By exerting manual pressure on the lacrimal ducts, the systemic side effects of eye medication can be reduced.

tion) out of the eye. When potential systemic side effects of the drug should be avoided, systemic absorption can be reduced by blocking the lacrimal duct for a short time with the finger. This slows down the rate at which the medication enters the circulatory system (Fig. S 12.2).

If the patient is unsure whether the drug really got into the eye, another drop can be administered without having to worry about the consequences. There will not be an "overdose" because the medication dissolves in the tears, and tears are only present in a very small volume. If the patient instills "too much" of the medication, the tears automatically overflow and the excess runs down the cheek. After instilling the drops, there might be a slight irritation – this is quite normal and should not cause concern. However, a stronger sensation is not only very unpleasant, it also leads to an increased production of tear film, which will drain the drug much faster than usual. It is not harmful if a drop accidentally splashes right onto the cornea, but it is irritating.

Cold drops are less comfortable than tepid drops. The bottle can be warmed by carrying it around in a pocket for about 5 minutes or placed under warm blankets. This slight warming of the eyedrops before administration is especially helpful for babies and children.

The doctor prescribes how often the eyedrops should be administered each day. The pharmaceutical industry strives to develop eyedrops whose effects last for many hours. Nevertheless, there are situations in which very frequent administration, such as every hour, is crucial. This is necessary, for example, in acute intraocular inflammations when an anti-inflammatory drug has to be instilled every hour. Most glaucoma medications have to be given once or twice daily; some older glaucoma preparations have to be applied up to four times a day.

If the ophthalmologist prescribes more than one medication, these should not be instilled at the same time, but the second drug should be applied after an interval of five or, even better, ten minutes. Otherwise there is the risk that the first drug is washed out by the second.

Storing the Eyedrops. The pharmaceutical industry offers drugs that have been especially manufactured so that: a) they form a stable solution (without any tendency to form sediments on the bottom of the bottle); b) the medically active molecule does not break down (for example, by light exposure); and c) they are free from all microorganisms, such as bacteria. Drugs are manufactured in a sterile environment; however, once the bottle is opened, bacteria can easily enter. To prevent these germs from multiplying, preservatives have been added to the eyedrops. These substances not only inhibit the growth of microorganisms and thus ensure the safe use of the drops for a certain period of time, but also cause shortterm changes in the corneal epithelium which lead to better drug penetration. Because there is never absolute growth inhibition, a bottle of eyedrops should not be used for more than one month after it is initially opened. Unfortunately, some patients develop allergies to the preservatives and many different drugs contain the same type of preservative. For these allergic patients, preservative-free drugs have been developed that are available either in single-dose containers (which are relatively expensive) or in a bottle having an elaborate valve mechanism that prevents external air from entering into the bottle, thus keeping out germs.

The package insert indicates whether eyedrops should be refrigerated. If the patient has any questions about the storage of

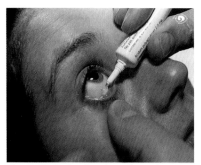

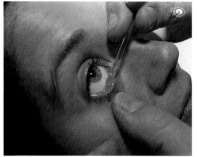

Fig. S 12.3: Application of an ointment.

Fig. S 12. 4: Application of an ophthalmic ointment with a glass spatula.

eyedrops or is unsure about the handling, he should ask his pharmacist, the medication expert.

Ointments and Gels. There are gel-like drugs that have a high viscosity and, upon application into the eye, become more fluid and function just like drops. Under certain circumstances, a gel might be more comfortable to use and could also have a longer-lasting effect. In theory, administering an ointment would be the perfect solution for topical ocular therapy: the ointment is comfortable for the patient to use; the drug stays longer on the eye's surface and can thus exert the desired therapeutic effect for a prolonged period. Nevertheless, the real disadvantages are that there is a reduction of visual acuity because of the "ointment film" and ointments can cause the eyelids and eyelashes to stick together. For these reasons, ointments are generally applied just before going to sleep or to patients whose eyes are bandaged. Ointments play only a minor role in glaucoma therapy.

An ointment is applied in just the same manner as drops: The patient looks up, pulls down on the lower lid with a finger, and squeezes a strip of ointment (approximately 5 mm long) into the exposed conjunctiva (Fig. S 12.3). A blunt spatula made of glass or plastic may also be used to administer the ointment within the lower lid (Fig. S 12.4).

Superficially Acting Eye Medication. There are also substances that do not need to penetrate the eye but rather which are administered, for example, in inflammations of the outer surface of the eye (conjunctivitis) and its appendages. Another example for this group of drugs would be an ointment used against chronic blepharitis (inflammation of the eyelid and its glands); these creams are gently rubbed into the skin of the lid margin. There are also "artificial tears" that are instilled by those suffering from dry eye syndrome. It is important that these drugs have a good local tolerability and exert their effect for an extended time.

S 13 How do Lasers Function?

A laser produces a special type of light that is frequently used in technology and medicine. Before the nature of laser light is considered, some basic fundamentals about light will be presented.

Light. Light is an electromagnetic oscillation (or vibration). All of space is filled with magnetic and electric fields.

An oscillating electric field creates a magnetic field that oscillates perpendicularly at the same frequency and at the same wavelength, and vice versa.

These oscillations are a form of energy, an energy that travels in the form of an electromagnetic wave at the speed of light. The energy contained in an electromagnetic wave travels until it is absorbed when the wave encounters some absorbing medium. As an example of an energy source, consider the sun: The sun radiates (emits) many different electromagnetic waves, some of which reach the earth where they provide light and warmth. The energy of the sun is transported to the earth via the electromagnetic waves and is partially absobed by the earth and its surrounding objects. Part is also reflected to continue along its path until it is eventually absorbed.

The radiated energy not only has a wave-like character, it also has a corpuscular form. This means that this energy can be considered both as waves and also as very tiny particles (called photons) that move with incredible speed [Gr. *phos*: light]. A photon possesses a defined energy, i.e. each transports a defined quantum of

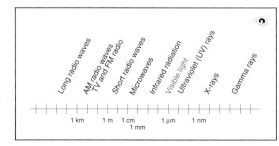

Fig. S 13.1: Visible light is a small segment of the broad spectrum of electromagnetic waves.

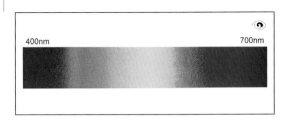

Fig. S 13.2: The various wavelengths are subjectively perceived as colors.

400nm   700nm

energy. If one considers the energy quanta radiated by the sun, then one finds a wide spectrum of photon energies ranging from high to low, as depicted in Figure S 13.1.

High energy radiation is found in the form of gamma rays, low energy as microwaves. Human eyes, however, are sensitive to only a small portion of this spectrum, and this is what is called light (Fig. S 13.2). The human eye is able to differentiate various wavelengths within this small portion, and these are perceived as assorted colors. Blue light, for example, has a higher energy level than red light. Correspondingly, blue light has a higher oscillatory frequency and thus a shorter wavelength than red light.

Take the light radiated (emitted) by a light bulb: it contains all the colors as well as much infrared light, i.e. light that has a wavelength too long to be perceived by human eyes, but which can be felt as heat. Light quanta that are emitted by a light bulb represent a diverse mix: they are released at random times and with varying wavelengths in all directions (Fig. S 13.3). From this mixture (which is perceived as white light), various colors can be selected. For example, using a color filter permits only light of a certain wavelength, i.e. a certain color, to be transmitted (Fig. S 13.4).

Should one place a pinhole in the path of this single-colored (monochromatic) light, then only some of the light can pass through, namely, those photons that oscillate together in a related, specific phase (Fig. S 13.5).

The light which has been refined in this highly selective fashion has roughly the same properties as laser light. However, light produced this way is fairly inefficient since at the end, only a tiny portion of the original light radiated by the light bulb remains. But with lasers, this process is much more efficient.

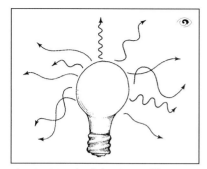

Fig. S 13.3: The light given off by a light bulb has differing wavelengths that go off in various directions.

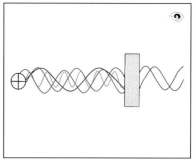

Fig. S 13.4: Using a color filter on a regular light bulb, monochromatic light can be produced.

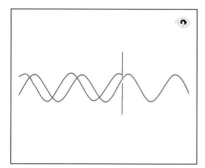

Fig. S 13.5: … if a small aperture diaphragm (e.g. pinhole) is used, light similar to that produced by a laser is produced.

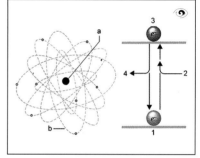

Fig. S 13.6: Left: a) atomic nucleus, b) electrons. Right: An electron (1) is excited – by absorbing incoming energy (2) – to a higher energy level (3). When light is emitted (4), it falls back to its original, lower level.

How Light is Created. An atom can be "excited" by energy, i.e. when it is excited, one or more of its electrons are no longer at the lowest energy level, but are now found in a higher level. In a light bulb, energy from the electrical current is passed on to the atoms of the filament. At a later – but random – time (usually split seconds later), the electrons in the filament atoms again fall down to a lower energy level (Fig. S 13.6). The energy difference is emitted as electromagnetic radiation, i.e. in the form of light and heat. The precise time and direction that a photon is radiated are subject to the laws of randomness.

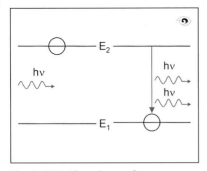

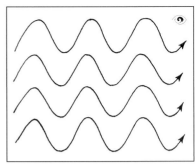

Fig. S 13.7: The release of energy can be stimulated by a photon that has the same energy.

Fig. S 13.8: Laser light is monochromatic, coherent and in phase.

How Laser Light is Created. If an "excited" atom is struck by a photon which carries precisely the amount of energy that the atom is set to emit, this energy is not released at just any time, but precisely at that moment when the atom is struck by the photon (Fig. 13.7). In this case, the energy release is no longer random but rather stimulated. Hence the term "laser": light amplification by stimulated emission of radiation, which implies that the light output will be amplified by the stimulated release of further light quanta. Since this result, as just described, only occurs when the stored energy is identical with the incoming energy, the amplified radiation has the same wavelength. There is thus a reproduction of light with a completely identical wavelength, and this is described as being monochromatic [Gr. *monos*: alone, single/Gr. *chroma*: color]. Light from a laser is thus always and completely monochromatic.

The photons released by the atoms do not go off in just any direction or phase, but take on the wave characteristics of the stimulating photon. To summarize the most important qualities of laser light, it is: a) monochromatic, b) coherent [Lat. *cohere*: coherent, connected] and c) in phase. The last characteristic indicates that there are not phase shifts, i.e. the wave fronts do not shift with respect to each other (Fig. S 13.8).

Lasers. For generating laser light, certain media are required. Argon gas, for example, can be made to produce laser light. The medium employed gives the laser its name: there are thus argon lasers, krypton lasers, etc. To excite the atoms, energy is needed, and when this energy is brought into the medium, it is termed "pumping." A medium can be pumped in a number of different ways, frequently using flashes of light (Fig. S 13.9). To generate laser light, the medium is placed between special mirrors, and the light being amplified bounces back and forth between them. The stimulation is amplified in a sort of chain reaction. A portion of the laser light exits through one of the mirrors, which is partially transparent, and this light can then be used for the desired purpose (Fig. S 13.10).

Laser light is and remains light. It does not consist of a mixture of many different kinds of photons, but rather it is an ordered quantity of photons that have the same energy and which can be considered "clones" of each other.

The Advantages of Laser Light. Since laser light is very uniform, it is much easier to utilize. Advantages of lasers include the possibility of knowing precisely how and where the light will be absorbed, its ability to be better focused, etc. Simply stated, a laser is merely light that is convenient to use as a tool (Fig. S 13.11).

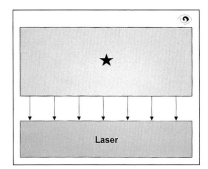

Fig. S 13.9: The laser medium (red) is "pumped" with energy from a source (*). Many sources can provide the energy, e.g. a xenon lamp.

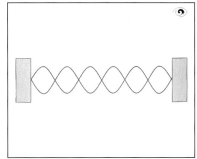

Fig. S 13.10: Laser light travels back and forth between two mirrors; if one is somewhat transparent, laser light is delivered (not shown).

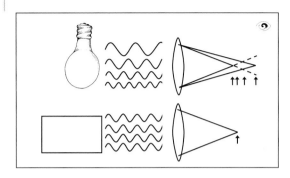

Fig. S 13.11: Light from a bulb (above) cannot be focused as well as laser light (below).

Biological Effects of Laser Light. Just as with other light, laser light can pass through (penetrate) transparent media, e.g. the cornea or the lens, and become absorbed by pigments, for example, the pigment epithelium of the retina. When the light is absorbed, its energy is transferred to the medium, i.e. warming takes place. With laser light, one can thus heat up the pigment layer of the retina so intensely that the retina lying immediately above it is "cooked," so to speak. This means that the protein molecules are dramatically altered, and this is termed denaturing. When this effect occurs in biological tissue, for example, in the retina, then it is termed coagulation [Lat. *coagulare*: to make clots]. Nature "heals" this damage with scar tissue. It is thus used to create scarring in a poorly perfused part of the retina (e.g. in diabetic retinopathy, cf. S 7). A slight, local coagulation can also cause the retina to adhere to the pigment layer just below it. This effect is used to "seal" retinal holes when seeking to prevent retinal detachment (Fig. S 13.12).

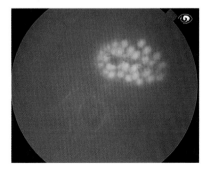

Fig. S 13.12: Laser impacts shot around a retinal hole.

The "Laser Scalpel." Laser light is not only used for coagulating purposes. When laser energy is strongly focused spatially and temporally, the light becomes absorbed by a medium that is normally transparent. Since much energy is concentrated at a very small spot very quickly, there is no time for the medium to transport the energy away in the form of heat. Small explosions are thus generated, causing a "photodisruption" [Gr. *photon*: light/Lat. *disruptere*: tear apart]. These micro-ruptures [Gr. *micros*: small] can be used to disrupt undesired vitreous body strands, or to "laser" a small hole in the iris (iridotomy, cf. Chapter 7.3.1).

It should be mentioned here that the field of medical laser applications is most indebted to the great researcher and pioneer, Prof. Franz Fankhauser, from Bern, Switzerland.

Transparent media, such as the cornea, are not equally transparent for all wavelengths [Lat. *transperere*: let pass]. Were one to use ultraviolet (UV) light with its very short wavelength, the greatest part of this light's energy would be transferred to the corneal surface. This effect occurs when snow skiing on a sunny day without the protection of proper sunglasses: intense eye irritation develops. The ultraviolet light damages the corneal surface and after a while, the eyes feel sore, red and irritated. A similar but even more intense effect can be used to change the thickness of the cornea: When high energy ultraviolet light is concentrated on the cornea, this energy is so intensely absorbed at the surface that it causes corneal material to vaporize. Through this intentional ablation, the thickness of the cornea can be decreased. If this thinning takes place more in the center than in the periphery, the focusing power of the cornea decreases. This results in either a partial or complete correction of myopia (cf. S 4). These UV rays are generated by excimer lasers. The name derives from the way the laser light is created, i.e. with an "excited dimer" [Gr. *di*: two/Gr. *meros*: part].

Such an optical correction is technically most fascinating and can be very precisely performed because it is guided by a computer. Nevertheless, one should remember the following: in myopia, the eye is usually too long. By thinning the cornea, the eye still remains too long; the focusing error is just less manifest. The healthy cornea is already very thin, normally around ½ mm. The thinning of the cornea is technically feasible and, in the short-term, well tolerated. Nevertheless, there is still not enough known about the long-term consequences of this operation. Therefore, caution is still most indicated in this relatively new procedure (cf. S 4).

Laser light is thus a special light that is a great tool in ophthalmology and in many other medical fields, as well. Unfortunately, it must be said that laser light is basically used to destroy tissue. However, such intended destruction is useful in many diseases. In this sense, laser treatment also has a solid, if limited, place in glaucoma therapy.

Appendices

The appendices contain reference information. Appendix 1 is a glossary defining many of the specialized terms used throughout this book. Appendix 2 is a list of glaucoma medications based on their mechanism of action. Here one can look up a particular drug, find out the active ingredient and in which forms it can be administered (e.g. drops, ointments, tablets). Appendix 3 lists other sources of information about specific topics. Appendix 4 provides a website which also includes addresses for those with vision impairment. Appendix 5 describes the actual status of eye care in many developing countries. Appendix 6 gratefully acknowledges those people (and institutions) who have contributed to the making of this book, all unflagging in their enthusiastic support.

A 1 Glossary

Note: italicized words represent entries in the Glossary to which the reader is referred

Accommodation	In this context, the ability of the eye to change its focal length by altering the shape of the *lens*, thereby enabling either near or far objects to be sharply focused on the retina
Aceclidine	A topical synthetic *cholinergic agonist* used to reduce *intraocular* pressure in *glaucoma*
Acetazolamide	A *carbonic anhydrase* inhibitor
Acetylcholine	A *cholinergic agonist* acting at the nerve ends (synapses) of the *parasympathetic nervous system*
Acetylsalicylic acid	Pain reliever, inhibits inflammation and *coagulation* (also known by the common name of aspirin, often abbreviated as ASA)
Acupuncture	Chinese method of treatment in which very thin needles are inserted into the body at specific locations (acupuncture points) in order to achieve a therapeutic effect by establishing a harmonic balance in the body
Adaptation	In this context, adjustment of the eye to varying light conditions (bright or dark adaptation) by changing the *pupil* size and switching from *cone* to *rod* vision; the *iris* thus acts as an optical diaphragm
Adenine	Purine base, DNA component; together with deoxyribose or ribose, it forms *nucleosides*
Adrenalin	Hormone produced by the adrenal glands and a neurotransmitter; powerful stimulant of the adrenergic receptors in the *sympathetic nervous system*; increases the pulse rate and cardiac output
Adrenergic	Agent that mimics the effects of *epinephrine*
Adenosine triphosphate	Cf. *ATP*
After-cataract	Clouding of the *lens* capsule after a *cataract* operation, often leading to poorer vision
After-cataract discission	Elimination of the *after-cataract* via disruption of the clouded *lens* capsule using a *laser*
Agonist	A drug that has an affinity for, and stimulates, the physiological activity at cell receptors in a manner similar to a naturally occurring substance

Albinism	Disturbance of melanin formation. Affected individuals are conspicuous due to their white hair and light pink skin. They suffer from an aversion to light, often have poor vision and quivering eyes due to an underdevelopment of the *macula*. Because of a lack of *pigment*, the *iris* appears blue or red
Alkaloid	A substance derived from a plant that has non-acidic (basic) chemical characteristics, e.g. *pilocarpine*, morphine, codeine
Allele	Alternate forms of a genetic characteristic
Alpha receptor	Cf. *receptor*
Amblyopia	Developmentally related vision impairment without visible *pathological* changes
AMD	Age-related Macular Degeneration: *sclerosis* of the *macula* due to hemorrhaging between *Bruch's membrane* and the *pigment* epithelium; occurs after the age of 40 (cf. *macular degeneration*)
Amino acids	Fundamental building blocks from which all proteins are constructed. To date, 25 different amino acids have been found in man
Amotio retinae	Detachment of the *retina*
Anatomy	Study of the body's *morphology* and structure
Anesthetic, Anesthesia	A substance that produces numbness or insensitivity to pain, or such a condition
Angina pectoris	Acute insufficiency of the blood supply to the heart muscle, which leads to sudden, excruciating pain that lasts from seconds to minutes. The pain is usually localized to the chest area, but may radiate to the arms, shoulder and neck regions
Angiography	Method of displaying the blood vessels via x-rays using a contrast medium
Angle-block glaucoma	Form of *glaucoma* in which the outflow path of the *aqueous humor*, the *trabecular meshwork*, is completely or partially blocked by the *periphery* of the *iris*
Aniridia	Absence of the *iris*
Anorexia nervosa	A *pathological* aversion to food
Anterior chamber	Space behind the *cornea* and in front of the *iris* that is filled with *aqueous humor*
Anterior chamber angle	Angle formed by the interior of the *cornea* and

	the front of the *iris* in the *anterior chamber*; site of the *trabecular meshwork*
Anthroposophic medicine	A form of medicine that seeks to create a humanistic extension of conventional medicine; this group understands disease as arising from a complex interaction of physical and psychological processes in humans
Antibiotic	Medication for treating bacterial infections
Anticoagulant	*Coagulation* inhibiting, "blood thinning" medication
Antiphospholipid-syndrome	*Autoimmune disease* in which antibodies are formed against the body's own *phospholipids*, often leading to severe *thromboses* and *ischemic* attacks resulting in organ damage
Aphakia	Absence of the *lens* in the eye
Apoptosis	"Programmed" (in the sense of purposely directed by the body) cell death
Applanation	Cf. *Goldmann applanation tonometry* Applanation tonometry
Application	In this context, administration or use of a medication topically
Apraclonidine	An improvement of the drug, *clonidine*, which is less fat-soluble than the parent compound; used in the treatment of *open-angle glaucoma* and *ocular hypertension*; applied topically
Aqueous humor	Liquid produced by the ciliary body of the *posterior chamber*; fills the *anterior* and *posterior chambers* of the eye
Argon laser iridoplasty	coagulation of the peripheral iris tissue, leading to shrinkage and pulling of the iris out of then-chamber angle.
Argon laser trabeculoplasty	Cf. *trabeculoplasty*
Arteriole	A small *artery*
Arteriosclerosis	*Pathological* thickening and stiffening of the *arterial* wall that can lead to a heart attack, stroke, etc.
Arteritis cranialis	Cf. *Giant cell arteritis*
Arteritis temporalis	Cf. *Giant cell arteritis*
Artery	Blood vessel that transports blood away from the heart
Astigmatism	A lack of sharp focus in different eye meridians, e.g. due to *corneal* astigmatism = corneal deformation

Astrocyte	Nerve cell characterized by fibrous, plasmic or fibroplasmic processes
Atherosclerosis	The most common form of *arteriosclerosis* in which fat deposits form on the innermost layer of the *arteries*. This results in chronic alterations of the vessel walls and finally to a type of chronic inflammation
ATP	Adenosine triphosphate; the primary energy carrier in intermediary metabolism. ATP is synthesized in the *mitochondria* of humans and animals
Atrophy	Loss of tissue that is caused by a reduced blood supply, loss of nerve innervation or a lack of use
Atropine	*Parasympathomimetic* agent. When locally applied to the eye, it causes a prolonged *dilation* of the *pupil*
Autogenic training	Psychological relaxation therapy
Autoimmune diseases	Group of diseases in which the body perceives its own structures as being "foreign" and attacks them
Autonomic nervous system	Also called the vegetative nervous system. The nervous system not under conscious control, responsible for maintaining basic and vital body functions, such as heartbeat, digestion, etc. Subgroups of this system include the *sympathetic, parasympathetic* and the intramural nervous systems
Autoregulation	The ability of a tissue to maintain its perfusion independent of the blood pressure (and of the eye pressure)
Avascular	Not having any blood vessels
Axenfeld-Rieger syndrome	Also called posterior embryotoxon. A developmental abnormality characterized by a prominent white *Schwalbe's ring* and *iris* strands that partially obscure the *chamber angle*, often leading to juvenile *glaucoma*
Axon	Nerve fiber extending from the nerve cell body to the distal nerve ending (*dendrite*)
Axoplasm	The plasma of a nerve fiber
Bebie curve	Cumulative *visual field* defect curve
Beta-blocker	Substance that blocks the beta-*receptors*
Beta-receptor	Cf. *receptor*

Betaxolol	Cardio-selective *beta-blocker* used to treat *ocular hypertension* and *open-angle glaucoma*
Bicarbonate	Salt containing the HCO_3^- ion
Bicycle ergometry	This instrument measures and records the output and corresponding changes in the circulatory capacity with a device that produces a variable load and is attached to a bicycle (may also be combined with an electrocardiogram, and
simulation	then it is referred to as an exercise EKG)
Binocular vision	Vision using both eyes, three dimensional vision; syn. *stereoscopic vision*
Bland	Normal, mild
Blue-field entoptic	Procedure for measuring the blood circulation in the *retina*, based on the *entoptic phenomenon*
Branch vein thrombosis	*Thrombosis* – or occlusion – of a branch *vein*
Bright adaptation	Cf. *adaptation*
Brimonidine	*Adrenergic* agent having a high degree of alpha-2 selectivity
Brinzolamide	*Carbonic anhydrase inhibitor*
Bronchospasm	Contraction of the bronchial smooth muscles, e.g. asthmatic attack. Can be triggered or exacerbated by *beta-blockers* in *predisposed* individuals.
Bruch's membrane	Also known as the basal lamina of the *choroid*: transparent inner layer of the *choroid* in contact with the *pigment* layer of the *retina*;
Bulbus oculi	Eyeball
Buphthalmia, buphthalmus	*Congenital* or *infantile glaucoma*
Calcium antagonist	Medication that prevents calcium from entering the cells and thereby inhibits contractions of the vascular muscles; the blood vessels thus dilate after administration of calcium antagonists
Capillary	Smallest blood vessel forming the connection between *arterioles* and *venules*
Capillary microscopy	Microscopic examination of the blood flow through *capillaries*, e.g. in the nailfold or in the *conjunctiva* of the eye
Carbachol	*Cholinergic* agent
Carbonate dehydratase	Syn: *carbonic anhydrase*
Carbonic anhydrase	*Enzyme* that catalyzes the reaction of carbon dioxide and water into *bicarbonate* and vice versa
Carteolol	*Beta-blocker* with intrinsic activity, i.e. this sub-

	stance not only blocks the *sympathetic nervous system*, but also slightly stimulates it
Caspase	*Enzyme* with which a cell can digest itself
Cataract	Partial or complete clouding of the *lens*
Causal, causal connection	The origin of something, that which produces an effect
CDI	Color Doppler Imaging; cf. *color duplex sonography*
Central serous chorioretinopathy	Serous detachment of the *retinal pigment epithelium* of unknown origin (presumably caused by a disturbances of the *choroidal* blood circulation), which leads to visual disturbances in the form of central *scotomata* or blurred vision. Young men are primarily affected; the rate of spontaneous recovery is high
Central vein thrombosis	Occlusion of the central *retinal vein*
Cholinergic	Agent that mimics the effects of *acetylcholine*
Choroid	Dark, vascular membrane lying between the *sclera* and the *retina*
Chromosomes	Strand-like carriers of genetic hereditary factors located in the cell nucleus and primarily composed of DNA
Church window phenomenon	Phenomenon observed with *pigment dispersion syndrome* and *pigmentary glaucoma*: Due to its rubbing against the *zonular fibers*, the *iris* loses *pigment* from its posterior surface giving rise to lighter, non-pigmented areas that *radiate*, spoke-like, from the *pupil*. When light shines into the eye, it is reflected by the eye *fundus*, but it can now leave the eye not only through the *pupil* but also through these *iris* defects, resulting in a resemblance to a church window
Ciliary body glaucoma	Connects the *choroid* with the circumference of the *iris*. It has protrusions or folds on its internal surface, called ciliary processes, which secrete the *aqueous humor*
Ciliolenticular block	Rare, acute form of *glaucoma* in which the *ciliary body* touches the *lens* and the *aqueous humor* is pressed into the vitreous space. The *iris* and *lens* are then pushed towards the front of the eye and the *anterior chamber angle* is blocked
Clonidine	Alpha-2 selective *adrenergic* agent

Coagulation	Clumping; purposeful destruction of tissue with electrical (surgical diathermy) current
Collagen	Extracellular proteins; major components of connective tissue
Collagenous	Pertaining to collagen
Color duplex sonography	Special ultrasound procedure which depicts, in color codes, the direction of the blood flow in the heart and vessels; the flow velocity can also be determined
Cones	Cf. *photoreceptors*
Congenital glaucoma	A rare form of *glaucoma* characterized by underdevelopment of the *anterior chamber angle* during fetal development
Conjunctiva	Outermost layer covering the *sclera* and the inner surface of the eyelids
Conjunctivitis	Inflammation of the *conjunctiva*
Constriction	Pulling together or narrowing
Contraction, contracting	Shortening or creating tension
Contraindication	The potential development of an undesirable side-effect making a proposed line of treatment inadvisable
CO_2	Chemical formula for carbon dioxide
Cornea	The anterior convex and transparent continuation of the sclera.
Corpuscular, corpuscle	A small mass or body, a particle
Corticoid	Hormone formed in the adrenal cortex. There are several groups of corticoids all of which originally start with cholesterol: mineralocorticoids, *glucocorticoids* and sex hormones. *Glucocorticoids* influence hydrocarbon metabolism, while mineralocorticoids regulate the electrolyte concentration in blood. Syn: corticosteroid
Cox-2 inhibitor	Agent that specifically inhibits the effects of those *prostaglandins* involved in inflammatory processes but not those necessary for formation of the gastric mucosa (exerts a protective effect on the stomach)
Cryocoagulation	Tissue destruction using freezing applications; syn. cryocautery
Cyclodialysis	*Intraocular* pressure-reducing operation where the *ciliary body* is removed, thereby forming a direct connection between the *anterior chamber* and the *choroid*. Since it is difficult to control the extent of the pressure-reducing effect, this

	once widely used technique is now only rarely performed
Cyclophotocoagulation	*Intraocular* pressure-reducing intervention in which the *aqueous humor* producing *ciliary body* is partially destroyed using a *laser*
Cytochrome	Protein of the respiratory chain (cytochrome system) in the *mitochondria*; in this chain of reactions, electrons are transferred resulting in energy production
Cytosine	Purine base, *DNA* component, together with deoxyribose or ribose, it forms *nucleosides*
Cytostatic	An agent that can inhibit cell division, such as of tumor cells (or in this context, to prevent scar tissue formation or bleb closure)
Dark adaptation	Cf. *adaptation*
Deep sclerectomy	type of glaucoma opration where there is no initial penetration into the anterior chamber, and the part of the sclera thickness is removed to enhance the diffusion of humor out of the anterior chamber.
Demyelinating disease	Disease that causes destruction of the *myelin sheath* in the central nervous system (cf. *multiple sclerosis*)
Dendrite	Extension or branch of a nerve cell located at its distal end
Descemet's membrane	Inner layer of the *cornea*, lies directly behind the *endothelium*
Diabetes mellitus	Disease characterized by increased levels of *glucose* (sugar) in the blood and urine due to a relative lack of *insulin*
Diabetic retinopathy	*Retinal* damage caused by *diabetes*
Diastole, diastolic	Relaxation phase during the heart cycle
Diathermy	Warmth in the tissues below the skin produced by a high frequency electrical current
Diclofenamide	*Carbonic anhydrase inhibitor*
Diffusion	Transport process caused by an *osmotic* concentration difference; the substance is transported from a high concentration area to a low concentration area, resulting in an equilibrium in the concentration
Digitalis	Medication originally derived from the foxglove plant and used in the treatment of *heart*

	failure (cardiac insufficiency); enhances the pumping capacity of the heart. Cf. *heart failure*
Digoxin	*Digitalis* preparation
Dilation	Widening (e.g. of the *pupil*)
Diopter	Unit used in ophthalmology for measuring the focusing power of a *lens* or an optical system
Dipivefrin	Ester and *pro-drug* of *epinephrine*; used to lower *intraocular pressure* by diminishing the production of the *aqueous humor* in the *ciliary body* and increasing outflow through the *trabecular meshwork*
Diuretic	Agent that causes an increased production and excretion of urine
DNA	Deoxyribonucleic acid; carrier of hereditary information and genetic material; has a double helical structure
Dorzolamide	*Carbonic anhydrase inhibitor* used in the treatment of *open-angle glaucoma* and *ocular hypertension*
Drusen	Clumps of fatty deposits in the *papilla* or between the *pigment epithelium* and the *choroid*; present in increased quantities in *AMD*
Dysregulation	Faulty regulation
Ectoderm	Outer embryonic tissue which forms external surface structures, parts of the sensory organs and the central nervous system
Edema	Swelling caused by the accumulation of fluid in a tissue
Eicosanoid	Hormone-like, highly effective extra-cellular transmitter substance. In contrast to hormones, the blood does not transport eicosanoids to a distant site of action, but rather they exert their effects in and around the tissues where they are locally formed. There are three subgroups of eicosanoids: *prostaglandins*, leukotrienes and thromboxanes
Electrophysiology	Branch of science dealing with the conduction and utilization of electrical phenomena in the body. Cf. *ERG, VEP*
Electroretinography	Cf. *ERG*
Embolism	Obstruction or occlusion of a blood vessel by an *embolus*

Embolus	A detached *thrombus* or other particle carried by the blood
Emmetropia	Normal vision
Empty sella	The sella turcica is a depression in the base of the skull which normally "seats" the pituitary gland. In the "empty sella" syndrome, x-rays do not show the pituitary gland at this location and the sella ("saddle") appears empty
Emulsion	Mixture of two or more liquids that are not soluble in each other
Endoderm	Innermost embryonic tissue layer that gives rise to the *epithelium* of the respiratory tract, bladder, urethra, liver, pancreas thyroid gland, etc.
Endothelin	Extremely potent vasoconstrictor in the body, produced by endothelial cells of the vessels
Endothelin blocker	Substance that inhibits the effects of *endothelin* by blocking the *endothelin* receptors
Endothelium	Single layer internal lining of the blood vessels and body cavities
Entoptic phenomena	Optical perception arising from the body itself (e.g. floaters)
Enzyme	Substance, similar to a catalyst, that accelerates chemical reactions in the body
Epinephrine	Cf. *adrenaline*; syn. adrenaline
Epithelium	Outermost (covering) cell layer of tissue
ERG	Electroretinography. A technique that displays and records electrical fields produced by the *retina* and *pigment epithelium*
Excavation	Hollowed out area or site
Expression	Cf. *gene expression*
Extracellular	Lying or occurring outside of the cell
Exude	Excrete, secrete
Fenestrated	Windowed, i.e. having a small opening or pores
Fibrin	A protein required for blood *coagulation*
Fistula	Filtering bleb
Flicker light	rapid on-off change of the light.
Fludrocortisone	Mineralocorticoid
Fluorescein	A fluorescing substance. It is used to temporarily stain the cornea (e.g. in *intraocular applanation* pressure measurements); also used in angiography where it is especially useful in displaying *retinal* blood vessels (cf. *fluorescein angiography*)

Fluorescein angiography	Display of the *retinal* blood vessels using *fluorescein* dye
Foramen	Hole, opening, aperture
Frequency doubling technology	takes advantage of flickering light perception to test the visual function.
Fundus	Posterior surface of the eye as seen with an *ophthalmoscope*

Ganglion	An aggregation of nerve cells having a nodular shape and functioning as a junction
Ganglion cell	Nerve cell
Gene	Hereditary tendency, factor of heredity
Gene expression	Transformation of genetic information into a genetic product
Genetic code	Order, sequence of the *DNA* bases
Genetics	Study of heredity
Genome	All the *genes* of an organism
Giant cell arteritis	*Autoimmune* vasculitis (blood vessel inflammation) of the large and medium-sized *arteries*, usually occurring in advanced age. The superficial temporal artery (temple artery) is often affected. Frequently other *arteries*, especially the ophthalmic and posterior ciliary arteries, are also involved. In the eye, this often leads to an *ischemia* of the *papilla*, and rarely to occlusion of the central retinal artery
Glaucoma	Group of eye diseases that often, but not always, appear in association with elevated *intraocular pressure*
Glaucoma attack	Medical emergency; a sudden, massive increase in intraocular pressure that arises due to a blockage in the outflow of the *aqueous humor*. The eye is very red and the disease is usually accompanied by severe pain and generalized symptoms, such as headache, nausea and vomiting
Glaucoma chronicum simplex	Cf. *primary open angle glaucoma*
Glaucomatous damage	Glaucomatous damage is characterized by the loss of *retinal* nerve cells, nerve fibers and *astrocytes* of the *papilla*. Due to the loss of nerve fibers, defects arise in the *visual field* of which the patient, in the initial stages of the disease, is unaware

Gliosis-like alterations	Fine shiny areas present on the *retina*, associated with vascular dysregulation
Glucocorticoid	Cf. *corticoid*
Glucose	Special form of sugar (especially used in this context as blood sugar)
Glycerin	Cf. *osmotic agent*
Glycosylation	The addition of *glucose* to protein molecules
Goldmann applanation tonometry	Measuring intraocular pressure by applying a force strong enough to flatten a defined corneal area using a special prism.
Gonioscopy	Examination of the *anterior chamber angle*
Goniotomy	Surgical opening of the *trabecular meshwork* up to *Schlemm's canal*, performed in *congenital* and *juvenile glaucoma* to lower the *intraocular pressure*. This procedure improves or enables the outflow of the *aqueous humor* (cf. *trabeculotomy*)
Granule	A grain-like particle
Guanine	Purine base, *DNA* component, together with deoxyribose or ribose, it forms *nucleosides*
H+	Hydrogen ion
H_2CO_3	cf. *Bicarbonate*
Halo	A rainbow-colored ring perceived around a light source
Heart failure	When the heart, as a pump, fails to maintain adequate blood circulation; syn. cardiac insufficiency
Hematocrit	That portion of the whole blood composed of blood cells
Hemorrhage	Bleeding
Heterochromy	When the *irises* of one person display a different color
Heterochromic cyclitis	Acute *iridocyclitis* in association with *heterochromy*; syn. Fuch's heterochromic cyclitis
Hg	Chemical symbol for mercury; syn. hydrargyrum
Histology	Science of microscopic anatomy of body tissues
H_2O	Chemical formula for water
Homeopathy	Alternative healing method. Based on the belief that a disease can be healed using a very diluted (potentiated) substance that evokes the same disease symptoms in a healthy person

HRF	Heidelberg Retina Flowmeter. Instrument used in scanning *laser Doppler flowmetry*
HRT	In this context, used for Heidelberg Retina Tomography; instrument used in *laser scanning tomography*. (Outside of this context, HRT is a common abbreviation for hormone replacement therapy)
Hydrophilic	Literally, water loving, i.e. a substance that easily dissolves (is soluble) in water
Hydrophobic	Literally, water afraid, i.e. a substance that does not easily dissolve in water
Hyperglycemia	Abnormally high blood *glucose* levels
Hyperlipidemia	Abnormally high blood lipid (fat) levels
Hypermetropic	Cf. *hyperopic*
Hyperopic	Far-sighted
Hypertension (hypertonia)	Arterial hypertension = elevated blood pressure; (cf. hypertension, ocular)
Hypertension, ocular	Elevated *intraocular pressure* without *glaucomatous damage*. Even though patients having ocular hypertension develop glaucomatous damage more frequently than the average population, this is not an inevitable consequence of high ocular pressure; syn. elevated, high *intraocular pressure*
Hypoglycemia	Abnormally low blood *glucose* levels
Hypophysis	Cf. *pituitary gland*
Hypotension (hypotonia)	*Arterial* hypotension = low blood pressure
Hypotension, ocular	Low *intraocular pressure*
Hypotension, orthostatic	Cf. *orthostatic hypotension*
Hypoxanthine	A product of *ATP* degradation
Indocyanine green	*Fluorescing* dye especially effective in depicting *choroidal* blood vessels
Indomethacin	Pain-relieving medication that inhibits *prostaglandin* synthesis
Infantile glaucoma	*Congenital glaucoma* in the broadest sense; the *chamber angle* is insufficiently developed (but still more developed than in *congenital glaucoma*), and this leads to elevated *intraocular pressure* during the first years of life
Infarct, Infarction	Death of a tissue due to obstruction or closure of a blood vessel
Infrared radiation	Invisible electromagnetic radiation perceived as heat

Inhibit, inhibitor	Interfering with a specific biological activity, or a substance that does this
Innervation, innervated	The supply of nerve fibers to a tissue; connected to the nervous system
Insulin	Hormone secreted by the islet cells of the *pancreas*; aids the uptake of *glucose* into the cells from the blood
Intermittent	Sporadically occurring (and then disappearing between episodes)
Intima	Innermost layer of an *artery*
Intraocular	Located within the eye
Intravenous	Within a *vein* or introduced into a *vein*
Ion channel	Channel through which electrically charged particles can enter or exit
Iridectomy	Operation that removes a piece of the *iris periphery*, thereby creating a new passage between the *posterior* and *anterior chambers*; the *aqueous humor* can then flow more directly into the *trabecular meshwork*
Iridocyclitis	Inflammation of the *iris* and *ciliary body*
Iridotomy	Operation using a *laser* that creates a hole in the *iris periphery* through which the *aqueous humor* can flow from the *posterior* to the *anterior chambers* (cf. *iridectomy*)
Iris	Circular membrane in front of the *lens,* patent in the center by the area called the *pupil.* The iris has a variable pigmentation that leads to different eye colors
Iris bombé	A condition in which the *peripheral iris* circularly adheres to the *lens* surface, e.g. following an infection. This prevents the passage of the *aqueous humor* from the *posterior* to the *anterior chamber*. As a result, *intraocular pressure* rises and then pushes the *peripheral iris* forward, in a bulging fashion, thereby blocking the *anterior chamber angle*; syn: umbrella iris
Iris diagnostics	Alternative medicine method in which physical and psychological illnesses can be diagnosed from observations made on the *iris*. It has not been scientifically substantiated
Ischemia	Inadequate blood perfusion to a tissue
Isopter	In a visual field examination, a line that connects all test locations from the same stimulus

Juvenile	Young, not yet mature or fully developed
Juvenile glaucoma	A form of *glaucoma* arising from insufficient maturation of the *anterior chamber angle*. The drainage function of the *trabecular meshwork* is well enough developed though that elevated *intraocular pressure* occurs only in later childhood years, thus defining the difference between this disease and *congenital* or *infantile glaucoma*
Kneipp cure	A treatment method that consists of (alternating) spray treatments with water, mechanical stimulation (water walking), compresses and baths with therapeutic ingredients
Krukenberg spindle tomography	Spindle or triangular-shaped *pigment* deposit on the inner surface of the *cornea* occurring in the *pigment dispersion syndrome*
Lamina cribrosa	Sieve-like portion of the *sclera* through which the optic nerve fibers enter and leave the eye
Laser	<u>L</u>ight <u>a</u>mplification by <u>s</u>timulated <u>e</u>mission of <u>r</u>adiation; coherent ray of single colored light generated by special techniques; used in medicine for cutting, coagulating and scanning tissue
Laser Doppler flowmetry	Procedure which makes it possible to display the blood flow in the *capillary* region of the *retina* and optic nerves using a *laser*
Laser Doppler velocimetry	Measurement of the blood flow velocity in a blood vessel using a *laser*
Laser scanning	Imaging of a tissue by scanning with a ray of *laser* light
Latanoprost	*Prostaglandin* analog used in the treatment of *open-angle glaucoma* and *ocular hypertension*
Latency time extension	"Delayed" reaction of the visual cortex to a *retinal* stimulation (see also *VEP*)
Lens	Interior lens of the eye; responsible for *accommodation*
Leukocyte	White blood cell
Levobonolol	Beta-blocker
Limbus	Literally, boundary wall; in this context, the transition from the *cornea* to the *sclera*
Lipid	Fatty substance and source of body energy; major constituent of cell structure

Local anesthesia	Induction of numbness or insensitivity to pain at a specific site or area
Lumen	Inner vessel opening or diameter
Lupus erythematosus	Generalized *autoimmune disease* showing a diverse clinical picture: arthritis (joint inflammations), dermatological symptoms, neurological disturbances, kidney problems, blood changes, etc.
Lymphocytes	Subgroup of *leukocytes* responsible for fighting infections
Macula, macula lutea	Literally, yellow spot; in this context, that site in the middle of the *retina* where vision is the sharpest. In the center of the macula is the central fovea, which contains only *cones*
Macular degeneration	Loss or reduction of *macular* function, often age-related
Macular edema	Collection of fluid in the area of the *macula*
Maculopathy	*Pathological*, non-inflammatory change in the *macula*
Magnetic resonance	Imaging procedure in which the orbits of hydrogen atoms are influenced in their orientation by an applied magnetic field and then changed with a short high frequency pulse so that the protons send out electromagnetic waves when they return to their original orientation. Using computerized analysis, these resonance signals are detected and measured in various positions, thereby providing information about the composition of the individual tissues or body layers; syn. nuclear spin tomography
Malignant	Severe form, virulent, frequently fatal
Malignant glaucoma	Cf. *ciliolenticular block glaucoma*
Mannitol	*Osmotic* agent
MAO inhibitor	Monoamine oxidase inhibitor; medication used in the treatment of depression. Monoamine oxidase breaks down catecholamines (e.g. *noradrenaline*, serotonin); MAO inhibitors prevent this reaction
MD	In this context, abbr. for mean defect. Concept encountered in *perimetry*, indicates the mean value of the *visual field* damage averaged over the test locations

Melanin	Brownish-black *pigment* responsible for the color found in skin, hair, *choroid* and *iris*
Melanocyte	*Melanin*-producing cells
Membrane	Thin layer of tissue; border layer
Membrane potential	Electrical voltage potential which arises across a *membrane* (e.g. a cell membrane) that separates two different ionic solutions from each other
Mesoderm	Middle of three primary germ layers of embryonic tissue from which the skeleton, muscles, heart, blood vessels, etc. are formed
Metamorphopsia	Visual disturbance in which images are distorted
Methazolamide	A *carbonic anhydrase inhibitor*
Miosis	*Constriction* of the *pupil*
Miotic	*Pupil*-constricting medication
Mitochondria	Cellular organelles, the "power plants" of the cell in which *glucose* and fat are converted to energy
Mitochondriopathies	Group of diseases that arise from one or several mutations of the mitochondrial *DNA*
Mitomycin C	*Cytostatic* agent
mmHg	Abbr. for millimeters of *mercury* (in a column); unit in which *intraocular* (or blood) *pressure* is measured
Molecule	Chemical compound composed of two or more atoms
Monochromatic	Single-colored
Monocular	One-eyed
Morbus	Disease
Morbus Crohn	Non-specific, probably autoimmune inflammation that can affect all parts of the gastrointestinal tract, but most often involves the lower small and large intestines; syn. Crohn's Disease
Morphology	Study of body form and structure
MRI	<u>M</u>agnetic <u>R</u>esonance <u>I</u>maging. Cf. *magnetic resonance*
Mucopolysaccharide	Amino sugars that are linked together to form large molecules
Multiple sclerosis	Inflammatory, demyelinating disease of unknown origin; patches of *sclerosis* and demyelinization (plaques) arise in the central nervous system which cause numerous and varied deficiencies
Mouches volantes	Floaters; perception of forms resembling "fly-

	ing mosquitoes" caused by age-related structural alterations of the *vitreous body*
Mutation	A variable alteration in the genetic material: Just as a whole *chromosome* can change or be lost, only a single gene or a single purine base can be affected by a mutation. The cause for mutations are manifold and not always recognizable (one then speaks of a spontaneous mutation); mutations can also occur during cell division or, for example, due to radiation damage
Mydriasis	*Dilation* of the *pupils*
Mydriatic	Agent that *dilates* the *pupils*
Myelin	Lipoprotein (cf. *myelin sheath*)
Myelin sheath	Isolating sheath of *myelin* that coats nerve fibers; syn: medullary sheath
Myocardium	Heart muscle
Myopic	Near-sighted
Necrosis	Cell death
Neodynium:YAG laser	The type of *laser* in which light is produced by a Neodymium: Yttrium-Aluminum-Garnet medium
Neovascularization	Growth of new blood vessels
Neovascularization glaucoma	Form of *glaucoma* in which newly-formed blood vessels grow into the *anterior chamber angle*, thereby blocking the *aqueous humor* outflow
Nerve Fiber Analyzer	Nerve Fiber Analyzer GDx®. Instrument used for analyzing the thickness of a nerve fiber layer
Nervus opticus	Optic nerve
Neurofibromatosis	Disease in which benign tumors, usually arising from the *myelin sheath*, lead to compression symptoms and neurological deficiencies. Neurofibromas may be associated with other symptoms (e.g. *pigment* spots, skeletal changes, etc.). If a certain number of signs and symptoms are concurrently present, one speaks of neurofibromatosis generalisata (also known as von Recklinghausen's disease)
Neuron	Nerve cell
Neuroprotection	Safeguarding a nerve cell against the effects of harmful influences
Neuroretinal rim	That region of the *papilla* filled with nerve fibers

Neurovascular coupling	practically instant dilation of the blood vessels in neural tissue, following activation of neighbouring neural cells
Nifedipine	*Calcium antagonist*
Nilvadipine	*Calcium antagonist*
Non-responder	Patient who is not helped by a certain medication
Noradrenaline	Neurotransmitter in the *sympathetic nervous system*
Norepinephrine	Syn. *noradrenaline*
Normal pressure glaucoma	Cf. *open-angle glaucoma*, primary
Nucleoside	Formed when deoxyribose or ribose bonds with a purine base
Occiput, occipital	Back part of the head; lying at the back of the head
Octopus®	Automated *perimetry* instrument
Ocular Blood Flow System (OBF)	Procedure that measures variations in the *intraocular* pressure due to the arterial pulse. *Capillary* perfusion can be calculated from the size of the pressure fluctuations
Ocular hypertension	cf. *hypertension, ocular*
Ocular vasospastic syndrome	Term introduced to describe the eye's involvement in the *vasospastic syndrome*. The main characteristics are (stress-induced) diffuse *visual field* defects with preserved *visual acuity* that respond well to treatment with *calcium antagonists*
Oculus	Eye
Ocusert	*Intraocular pressure*-reducing medication in which the active ingredient, *pilocarpine*, is enclosed within a polymer and gradually released over days (depot effect)
Oncologist	A physician specializing in the treatment of *malignant* tumors
Oncotic pressure	*Osmotic* pressure in tissues, exerts a suction effect; to prevent swelling, proteins in the blood extract fluid from the tissues into the circulatory system
Open-angle glaucoma, primary	Form of glaucoma in which the *anterior chamber angle* appears normal. Access to the *trabecular meshwork* is thus free and the outflow resistance must be due to changes in the *meshwork*

itself. Primary open angle glaucoma is further subdivided in medical textbooks: chronic open angle glaucoma with *elevated intraocular pressure* and in normal pressure (tension) glaucoma. A patient with normal pressure glaucoma exhibits *glaucomatous damage* even though the *intraocular pressure* never exceeds the normal upper level, set at 21 mmHg; there is no sharp border between high and normal pressure glaucoma

Opacity Lens Meter (OLM®)	Instrument used to quantify lens *opacification* (cloudiness)
Ophthalmologist	A physician specializing in the eye, its diseases and treatment
Ophthalmology	The medical specialty dealing with the eye
Ophthalmoscope	Instrument that allows a direct view of the eye.
Opsin	A protein that, together with *retinal*, forms *rhodopsin*
Optical coherence tomography	imaging principle based on the interference of the light backscattered from the tissue of interest.
Optic disc	Cf. *papilla*
Optic nerve head	Cf. *papilla*
Oral	Through the mouth; relating to the mouth
Orbit, orbita	Eye socket
Orthoptics	Study of eye movements and *binocular* vision, and treatment of corresponding defects
Orthostatic	Erect posture or position
Orthostatic hypotension	Excessive drop in blood pressure due to changing from a lying to a standing position
Osmosis	When two solutions are separated by a membrane that blocks the passage of molecules but not solvents, the solvent travels from the lower concentration side to the higher concentration (to dilute it)
Osmotic	Agent that promotes *osmosis*
Oxidation damage	*Pathological* oxidation caused by free *oxygen radicals*
Oxygen radical	Oxygen atom that possesses a free (unpaired) electron and is thus very reactive
Pachymetry	measurement of the corneal thickness.
Pancreas	A gland located between the small intestine and

	the spleen; it produces and secretes *insulin* and other hormones
Papilla	The site where the axons of the *retinal* ganglion cells converge and then leave the eye; syn. *optic nerve head, optic disc*
Papillary excavation	*Physiological* (normal) or *pathological* (loss of tissue) depression in the center of the *papilla.*
Parasympathetic nervous system	Part of the *autonomic nervous system*. Stimulation of the parasympathetic nervous system promotes activity in the gastrointestinal tract. In the eye, it can cause *pupillary constriction*. In general, the parasympathetic and *sympathetic nervous systems* oppose each other. The parasympathetic system is active during rest (rest and digest) (*cf. sympathetic nervous system*)
Paresthesia	Abnormal physical sensation, e.g. prickling, burning, or tingling in the hands
Pathologic	Pertaining to illness and disease
Pathology	The medical science dealing with all aspects of disease: its nature, cause, development and morphology
Perfusion	Circulation of blood through a vessel
Peri-	"Around"
Perimeter	Instrument for measuring a *visual field*
Perimetry	*Visual field* examination
Periphery	At the edge, located away from the center
Permeate, permeation	To penetrate or penetration
PET	<u>P</u>ositron <u>E</u>mission <u>T</u>omography. Imaging procedure in which the patient swallows a substance that emits positrons. The distribution of the medication in the body can then be displayed using computer tomography
Peter's anomaly	Congenital deformity where there is centralized opacification of the *cornea* and other malformations in the eye; often associated with *glaucoma* and diseases of the central nervous and cardiovascular systems; syn. *anterior chamber* cleavage syndrome
PEX	Cf. *pseudoexfoliation syndrome*
PG	Abbr. for *prostaglandin*
Phacoemulsification	*Cataract* liquefaction by ultrasound
Pharmacokinetics	Relating to the absorption, distribution, metabolism and elimination of a drug by the organism

Phospholipid	A phosphorous-containing *lipid*; major *lipid* form found in all cell membranes
Photocoagulation	Tissue destruction by light (usually with a *laser*)
Photodynamic therapy	Treatment for wet *AMD*. A light-sensitive substance (benzoporphyrin) is intravenously injected and preferentially adheres to the walls of newly formed blood vessels. Upon activation by *laser* light, *thromboses* are formed in these vessels, thereby effectively closing them
Photon	Smallest unit of light
Photoreceptors	Light-sensitive sensory cells of the *retina*. One distinguishes between *rods* (responsible for dusk and night vision) and *cones* (responsible for daylight and color vision)
Phototransduction	Procedure in which a pulse of light is converted into a nerve impulse
pH value	Symbol for the negative logarithm of the hydrogen ion ($H+$) concentration. The pH value indicates whether a solution is acidic (pH < 7), basic (pH > 7) or neutral (pH = 7)
Physiological	Normal, healthy, the opposite of *pathological*
Physiology	The science of normal functioning and vital processes in the body
Phytotherapy	Treatment with plants and plant extracts
Pigment	A substance that blocks or absorbs part of the light spectrum; dye
Pigmentary glaucoma	Form of *glaucoma* occurring in association with a *pigment dispersion syndrome*; there are so many deposits of pigment at the *anterior chamber angle* that the outflow of the *aqueous humor* through the *trabecular meshwork* is blocked
Pigment dispersion syndrome	A *pathological* condition wherein *melanin* deposits are lodged on those parts of the eye in contact with the *aqueous humor*, thereby impeding its outflow (cf. *pigmentary glaucoma, church window phenomenon, Krukenberg's spindle*)
Pigment layer	*Pigment*-rich layer between the *retina* and the *choroid*
Pilocarpine	*Cholinergic* agent that is also an *alkaloid*
Pituitary gland	Hormone-producing gland located at the base of the brain in the sella turcica (cf. *empty sella*)
Plaques	Cf. *senile plaques*
Plasma	The liquid, non-cellular portion of blood

Plateau iris	Usually in-born anatomical variation in which the *peripheral iris* is especially close to the *trabecular meshwork*.
POAG	Abbr. for Primary Open-Angle Glaucoma; cf. *open-angle glaucoma, primary*
Polymer	Substance composed of several molecules
Posterior chamber	Space behind the *iris* and in front of the intraocular *lens*
Postoperative	After an operation
Postsynaptic	After the *synaptic* gap; located on the organ reacting to the stimulus
Predisposition	Tendency or characteristic that makes the occurrence of a disease more likely
Preeclampsia	A rare but very dangerous complication of pregnancy resulting in high blood pressure, combined with extensive *edema* and elevated
metastasizing	protein concentration in the urine. *Vasospasms* of the brain vessels appear to form an important component of the disease
Presynaptic	Before the *synaptic* gap; located on the nerve ending
Presbyopia	Far-sightedness associated with middle age
Primary open angle glaucoma	Cf. *open-angle glaucoma*, primary; abbr. *POAG*
Pro-drug	Medication where the active ingredient is coupled to a carrier from which it must be separated at its site of action. This principle can reduce side effects
syndrome	rated at its site of action. This principle can reduce side effects
Proliferative	Rampant growth
Propanolol	*Beta-blocker*
Prophylaxis, prophylactic	Preventive measure, preventing
Prostaglandin	A member of the *eicosanoids*, hormone-like substances that are responsible for numerous cell and tissue functions. For example, they can influence the blood flow to a tissue, increase body temperature, stimulate birth contractions, etc.
Prostate carcinoma,	Tumor of the prostate gland from which malignancies spread to other body organs and parts
Protein	Complex molecules and principle constituent of all cell protoplasm. Consists primarily of a-amino acids in peptide bonds
Provocation tests	deliberately placing a system out of balance, to explore the response.

Pseudoexfoliation	*Glaucoma* that occurs in association with a *pseudoexfoliation syndrome* in which protein deposits in the *anterior chamber angle* are so extensive that the *aqueous humor* cannot flow out through the *trabecular meshwork*
Pseudoexfoliation glaucoma	Deposits of abnormal protein (probably arising from the blood) in all parts of the eye that are bathed by the *aqueous humor* (cf. *pseudoexfoliation glaucoma*)
Pseudophakia	Condition in which the natural intraocular *lens* has been replaced by an artificial *lens*
Psychosomatics	The study of the psychological influences in the context of explaining physical ailments or disturbances, in which these influences are held to be the cause of such illness
Pupil	Round opening in the center of the *iris* through which light rays enter the eye
Pupillary block	In this condition, the normal outflow of the *aqueous humor* from the *posterior chamber* through the *pupil* into the *anterior chamber* is blocked. The pressure that builds up in the *posterior chamber* displaces the *iris periphery* anteriorly (forward), thereby effectively blocking the *anterior chamber angle* and preventing the outflow of the *aqueous humor*. Older, farsighted patients are especially predisposed to pupillary block
Quantitative	Having to do with numbers and amounts
Radial	Radiating
Radiate	Spreading out in all directions from a center, as spokes on a wheel
Radiation	In *ophthalmology*, visible radiation is meant; the posterior portion of the optic pathway
Radical	Cf. *oxygen radical*
Raynaud's Disease	Characterized by *vasoconstrictive* attacks of the finger arteries; first, there is a blanching, then the fingers turn blue and finally red, when blood flow returns. When the illness persists for a prolonged period, blood vessel damage and subsequent tissue death may appear. Women are affected much more frequently than men

Refracting	Measuring or determining the *refraction*, i.e. the ability of the eye to focus
Refraction	Focusing power of the eye or an optical system
Reoperation	A second (or more) operative procedure for the same problem
Resorption	The absorption of a substance into a tissue
Reperfusion	Renewed blood flow after a period of reduced circulation
Reperfusion damage	Damage that arises primarily because of oxidative stress during *reperfusion*
Responder	A person who reacts favorably to a specific medication
Retina	That layer of nerve cells at the back of the eye responsible for vision and which contains *rods* and *cones*
Retinal	Pertaining to the *retina*; also a substance produced by the body from retinol (vitamin A) and which, together with *opsin*, forms *rhodopsin*. There are two configurations for retinal: 11-cis and all-trans
Retinal angiospasm	*Pathological* constriction of a *retinal* blood vessel
Retinitis pigmentosa	Collective term for a series of *retinal* diseases that lead to severe loss of vision and of the *visual field* and to night blindness. In the classical form of retinitis pigmentosa, *pigment* deposits are found in the *retina* which slowly advance from the *periphery* to the center
Retinopathy	Non-inflammatory *retinal* disease
Retro-, Retrobulbar	Behind, behind the eyeball
Retrobulbar anesthesia	*Anesthetic* injected behind the eyeball that prevents transmission of pain impulses from the nerves; the optic nerve is numbed and the eye muscles are immobilized
Retrobulbar neuritis	Inflammation of the optic nerve behind the eyeball; syn: neuritis nervi optici
Reversible	Capable of being changed in the opposite direction; said of diseases or chemical reactions
Receptor	A structure that receives signals at the target organ
Recidivism, recidivating	Relapse of a disease
Rheumatoid arthritis	Chronic inflammatory disease of the joints probably based on autoimmune mechanisms in which an inflammation of a joint capsule leads

	to inflammations of the joints, ligaments and bursae
Rhodopsin	Visual *pigment* comprised of *opsin* and 11-cis *retinal* which is stored as a membrane protein in the *rods* and *cones*. When a light impulse reaches rhodopsin, 11-cis *retinal* changes into all-trans *retinal*, thereby splitting *opsin* from *retinal*. This, in turn, generates an electrical nerve impulse that is transferred to the brain via the optic nerve. Subsequently, all-trans *retinal* is retransformed into 11-cis *retinal*
Ribosome	Cell granule that is the site of protein synthesis (protein production)
RNA	Ribonucleic acid; "Copies" of *DNA* required for protein synthesis
Rod	Cf. *photoreceptors*
Rubeosis iridis	*Pathologic* new blood vessel formation on the *iris* (cf. *neovascularization*)
Rudimentary	Under-developed, stunted
RVA	Device for measuring the diameter of retinal vessels
Saccade	Abrupt, involuntary rapid eye movements
Saccadic suppression	Unnoticed image suppression occurring concurrent to a *saccade* and lasting but a split second
Scanning	Probing point by point
Schlemm's canal	Canal lying behind the *trabecular meshwork* in the *anterior chamber angle*; the *aqueous humor* is produced by the *ciliary body* and leaves the eye through this canal
Schwalbe's ring	Dividing line between the *cornea* and trabecular *endothelium*, composed of collagen
Sclera	Tough, white outer layer of the eyeball
Scleral flap excision	Technique used in a *trabeculectomy* in which a small flap of tissue, similar to an animal door that can flap open, is excised from the sclera
Sclerectomy, deep	A special type of *glaucoma* operation in which an inner part of the *sclera* is removed to create a passage for the *aqueous humor*. In contrast to a *trabeculectomy*, there is no direct opening into the *anterior chamber*.
Sclerosis	Hardening of a tissue
Scotoma, scotomata	Isolated defect(s) in the *visual field*
Secondary glaucoma	*Glaucoma* which is not a primary disease but

	rather which arises secondary to some other disease, injury or operation
Secretion, secreting	Substance released by a gland, releasing
Sediment	Precipitate
Selective laser trabeculo-plasty	selectively targeting the pigmented cell of the trabecular meshwork using special types of laser.
Semi-	Partial
Semi-permeable	Allowing water and some (usually smaller) molecules to pass
Senile plaques	Lumpy, fatty deposits in the *papilla* or between the *pigment epithelium* and *choroid*. Possible precursor of *AMD*
Short wavelength auto-mated perimetry (SWAP)	automated perimetry with blue stimulus on yellow background.
Sign	Objective symptom of disease
SmartLens™	Contact lens for continuous measurement of the *intraocular* pressure
Soma, somatic	Body, relating to the body
SPECT	Abbr. for Single Photon Emission Computer Tomography, an imaging procedure in which the activity of a tissue (e.g. heart, brain) can be examined using gamma rays
Stereoscopic vision	Cf. *binocular vision*
Sterile	Aseptic, free of living microorganisms and spores
Steroid	Cf. *corticoid*
Stimulus	An action or activity that can evoke or elicit a response in a receptor
Strabismus	Deviation of one or both eyes, as in crossed eyes. In contradistinction to the eyes working in unison
Stroma	Tissue structure or framework of an organ
Sub-	Under or below
Subconjunctival anesthesia	*Anesthetic* injected under the *conjunctiva* of the eye; pain impulses are blocked during the operation but the patient can still see and slightly move the eye muscles (cf. *retrobulbar anesthesia*)
Suppression	Inhibition, as of a secretion
Sympathetic nervous system	Part of the *autonomic nervous system*. Stimulation of the sympathetic nervous system leads to an increase in blood pressure, pulse and respiration and to *dilation* of the *pupils*, while simultaneously inhibiting the gastrointestinal activity.

	The actions of the sympathetic and *parasympathetic nervous systems* oppose each other. The sympathetic nervous system is active in times of stress (fight or flight) (cf. *parasympathetic nervous system*)
Sympatholytic	An agent that suppresses or inhibits the activity of the *sympathetic nervous system*
Sympathomimetic	An agent that promotes or enhances the activity of the *sympathetic nervous system*
Symptom	Subjective report of a patient's disease or condition
Synapse	Functional membrane-to-membrane contact between a nerve cell and any other cell
Syndrome	Aggregation or complex of several signs and symptoms
Synechia	Adhesion, especially of the *iris* to the *cornea* or the *lens*
Synthesis	Production, composition
Systemic	Generalized, regarding an organ system
Systole, systolic	The *contraction* phase of the heartbeat
Tachycardia	Rapid heartbeat
Tenon	The connective tissue envelope surrounding the eyeball and eye muscles
Tenon's capsule	Cf. *Tenon*
Tension, - tony	Pressure
Tetracaine	Local *anesthetic* agent applied topically to the eyeball and *conjunctiva*
Thermocoagulation	Destruction of tissue by applying heat
Thermography	Technique with which the infrared radiation (warmth) given off by the body can be measured and displayed
Thrombocyte	Blood platelet
Thrombocyte aggregation inhibitor	Medication that inhibits blood *coagulation* by preventing the blood platelets from clumping together (cf. *anticoagulant*)
Thrombosis	Formation of a (blood vessel blocking) *thrombus*
Thrombus	Blood clot
Thymine	Purine base, *DNA* component, together with deoxyribose or ribose, it forms *nucleosides*
Timolol	*Beta-blocker*
Tinnitus	Ringing in the ears
Tonometry	Measuring *intraocular* pressure

Toxic	Poisonous
Trabecular meshwork	A meshwork of *collagen* fibers located in the *anterior chamber angle* through which the *aqueous humor* flows out
Trabeculectomy	Operation performed to reduce the *intraocular* pressure: the *aqueous humor* is channeled out of the eye through a newly formed *scleral* tunnel. This induces the formation of a bleb.
Trabeculoplasty	*Intraocular* pressure-reducing operation in which a bundle of argon *laser* light is focused circularly into the *trabecular meshwork*. After a certain time, the scars thus created can lead to a decrease in the *intraocular* pressure
Trabeculotomy	*Intraocular* pressure-reducing intervention in *congenital* and *infantile glaucoma*. To enable or improve the outflow of the *aqueous humor*, the inner wall of *Schlemm's canal* and the *trabecular meshwork* are cut with a trabeculotome (cf. also *goniotomy*)
Trans-	Across, through
Transillumination	Light shining through a substance or tissue
Transscleral	Through the *sclera*
Triplet	In this context, a group of 3 bases that code for an amino acid
Ulcer	A lesion on the surface of the skin or mucous membrane caused by a superficial loss of tissue, usually accompanied by an inflammatory reaction
Ulceration	Formation of an ulcer
Ulcerative colitis	Inflammatory disease of the large intestines; possibly due to an autoimmune process or psychological factors
Unoprostone	*Prostaglandin* derivative used as a medication for reducing *intraocular* pressure
Uvea	Vascular tunic and middle layer of the eye, comprised of the *choroid, ciliary body* and *iris*
Vas	Vessel
Vasoactive	Acting on or at a vessel. A vasoactive substance is one that can influence the vessel diameter
Vasoconstrictor, vasoconstriction	Agent and act of narrowing a blood vessel's diameter
Vasospasm	Cramp-like *constriction* of a vessel

Vasospastic syndrome	Syndrome in which the patient reacts to stimuli, such as stress or cold, with vascular *constriction* more intensely than would a normal person
Vein	Blood vessel that transports blood back to the heart
Venous stasis syndrome	Obstruction of the *retinal* vein outflow by blood congestion. In severe cases, associated with retinal *ischemia* and *hemorrhage*; also known as a venous thrombosis
Venule	A small *vein*
VEP	<u>V</u>isual <u>E</u>voked <u>P</u>otential. Electrodes placed at the back of the head measure the electrical field changes that occur in the *visual cortex*; this provides a picture of the brain potentials that are elicited by *retinal* illumination
Video capillary microscopy	Procedure with which the blood flow through the smallest blood vessels (*capillaries*) can be depicted using a microscope and recorded for more precise analysis with a camera. For practical reasons, the examination is usually performed on the *capillaries* in the nailfold of the fingers
Viscocanalostomy	*Intraocular* pressure-reducing operation in which *Schlemm's canal* is flushed with a viscous substance that stretches it
Viscous	Slow-flowing, sticky
Visual	Having to do with seeing
Visual acuity	Sharpness or distinctness of vision, visual resolution
Visual cortex	Located at the back of the head, that part of the brain in which visual information is processed
Visual evoked potential	Cf. VEP
Visual field	That space or area seen by a fixed (non-moving) eye.
Visual training	Combination of eye training and relaxation training of the whole body. A beneficial influence on the progression of eye disease has yet to be proven
Vitreous, vitreous body	Transparent gel-like medium which fills the interior of the eyeball between the *lens* and the *retina*
Vortex, vortex vein	*Scleral veins* having a shape of a vortex or whorl
Zonular fibers	Fibers that attach the *intraocular lens* to the *ciliary body* and hold the *lens* in place

A 2 Catalog of Medications

Catalogue of medications listed in this book. However, not all are available worldwide.

Medications that reduce intraocular pressure

	Active ingredient	Eye Drops	Ointment	Tablets
Beta Blockers				
Arteoptic 0.5%, 1%, 2%	Carteolol	X		
Arteoptic SDU 1%	Carteolol	X		
Arutimol 0.25%, 0.5%	Timolol	X		
Arutimol SDU 0.25%, 0.5%	Timolol	X		
Betamann 0.1%, 0.3%, 0.6%	Metipranolol	X		
Beta-Ophthiole 0.1%, 0.3%, 0.6%	Metipranolol	X		
Betimol 0.25%, 0.5	Timolol	X		
Betoptima	Betaxolol	X		
Betoptic	Betaxolol	X		
Betoptic S	Betaxolol	X		
Betoptic S SDU	Betaxolol	X		
Chibro-Timoptol 0.1%, 0.25%, 0.5%	Timolol	X		
Dispatim 0.25%, 0.5%	Timolol	X		
Dispatim 0.25%, 0.5% SDU	Timolol	X		
Duratimol 0.1%, 0.25%, 0.5%	Timolol	X		
Glauconex 0.25%, 0.5%	Befunolol	X		
Glauco-Stulln	Pindolol	X		
Nyolol Gel 0.1%	Timolol	X		
Ocupress 1%	Carteolol	X		
Oftan Timolol 0.25%, 0.5%	Timolol	X		
Pindoptan 0.5%, 1%	Pindolol	X		
Teoptic 1%, 2%	Carteolol	X		
Timo-Comod 0.1%, 0.25%, 0.5% SDU	Timolol	X		
TimoEDO 0.25%, 0.5% SDU	Timolol	X		
Timoftal 0.25%, 0.5%	Timolol	X		
Timohexal 0.1%, 0.25%, 0.5%	Timolol	X		
Timolol-POS 0.1%, 0.25%, 0.5%	Timolol	X		
Timolol-ratiopharm 0.25%, 0.5%	Timolol	X		
Timomann 0.1%, 0.25%, 0.5%	Timolol	X		
Tim-Ophthal 0.1%, 0.25%, 0.5%	Timolol	X		

	Active ingredient	Eye Drops	Ointment	Tablets
Tim-Ophthal 0.1%, 0.25%, 0.5% SDU	Timolol	X		
Timoptic-XE 0.25%, 0.5%	Timolol		X	
Timoptic 0.1%, 0.25%, 0.5%	Timolol	X		
Timoptol 0.1%, 0.23%, 0.5%	Timolol	X		
Timoptol-XE 0.25%. 0.5%	Timolol	X		
Timosine	Timolol	X		
Timo-Stulln 0.25%, 0.5% SDU	Timolol	X		
Timisol 0.1%, 0.25%, 0.5%	Timolol	X		
Timisol SDU 0.25%, 0.5%	Timolol	X		
Turoptin 0.1%, 0.3%, 0.6%	Metipranolol	X		
Vistagan 0.1%, 0.25%, 0.5%	Levobunolol	X		

Beta Blockers + Pilocarpine

	Active ingredient	Eye Drops	Ointment	Tablets
Arteopilo 2%	Carteolol/ Pilocarpine	X		
Betacarpin	Metipranolol/ Pilocarpine	X		
Fotil	Timolol/ Pilocarpine	X		
Fotil-forte	Timolol/ Pilocarpine	X		
Normoglaucon	Metipranolol/ Pilocarpine	X		
Ripix	Metipranolol/ Pilocarpine	X		
Timpilo 2%, 4%	Timolol/ Pilocarpine	X		

Beta Blockers + Carbonic Anhydrase Inhibitors

	Active ingredient	Eye Drops	Ointment	Tablets
Cosopt	Timolol/ Dorzolamide	X		

Carbonic Anhydrase Inhibitors

	Active ingredient	Eye Drops	Ointment	Tablets
Acetazolamid "Agepha"	Acetazolamide			X
Azopt	Brinzolamide	X		
Diamox 250 mg, 500mg	Acetazolamide			X
Diclofenamid 50 mg	Diclofenamide			X

	Active ingredient	Eye Drops	Ointment	Tablets
Diuramid	Acetazolamide			X
Glaupax 250 mg	Acetazolamide			X
Trusopt	Dorzolamide	X		

Miotic Agents

	Active ingredient	Eye Drops	Ointment	Tablets
Borocarpin 0.5%, 1%, 2%	Pilocarpine	X		
Carbamann 1%, 2%, 3%	Carbachol	X		
Glaucadrine	Aceclidine/			
	Adrenaline	X		
Glaucostat	Aceclidine	X		
Isopto Carpine				
0.5%, 1%, 2%, 3%, 4%, 6%, 8%	Pilocarpine	X		
Isopto Carbachol				
0.75%, 1.5%, 2.25%, 3%	Carbachol	X		
Isopto-Pilocarpin				
0.5%, 1%, 2%, 3%, 4%	Pilocarpin	X		
Jestril viskos	Carbachol	X		
Miocarpine 1%, 2%, 4%, 6%	Pilocarpine	X		
Phospholinjodid 0.06%, 0.125%	Ecothiopathodid	X		
Pilocarpin ankerpharm 1%, 2%	Pilocarpine		X	
Pilocarpin "Agepha" 1%, 2%	Pilocarpine	X		
Pilocarpin "Blache" 2%, 3%	Pilocarpine		X	
Pilocarpin "Puroptal" 1%, 2%	Pilocarpine	X		
Pilocarpol 1%, 2%	Pilocarpine	X		
Piloftal 2%	Pilocarpine	X		
Pilogel	Pilocarpine		X	
Pilopos 0.5%, 1%, 2%, 3%	Pilocarpine	X		
Pilopos 2%	Pilocarpine		X	
Pilostigmin Puroptal	Pilocarpine/			
	Synstigmine	X		
Pilo-Stulln 0.25% SDU	Pilocarpine	X		
Pilo-Stulln 1%	Pilocarpine	X		
Spersacarbachol 1.5%, 3%	Carbachol	X		
Spersacarpine				
0.25%, 0.5%, 1%, 2%, 3%	Pilocarpine	X		
Spersacarpine 2%	Pilocarpine		X	
Vistacarpin N Liquifilm	Pilocarpine	X		

	Active ingredient	Eye Drops	Ointment	Tablets

Adrenaline and Congeners

	Active ingredient	Eye Drops	Ointment	Tablets
Diopine 0.1%	Dipivefrine	X		
Epifrin 0.1%	Dipivefrine	X		
Glaucon 1%, 2%	Epinephrine	X		
Glaucothil 0.1%	Epinephrine	X		
Links-Glaukosan	Epinephrine	X		
Suprexo	Epinephrine/ Guanethidine	X		
Thiloadren N	Dipivefrine/ Pilocarpine	X		
Thilodigon 0.5%	Dipivefrine/ Guanethidine	X		

Alpha-2 Agonists

	Active ingredient	Eye Drops	Ointment	Tablets
Alphagan 0.2%	Brimonidine	X		
ruclonin 1/8%, 1/16%	Clonidine	X		
Clonid-Ophthal 1/8%, 1/16%	Clonidine	X		
Clonid-Ophthal 1/8% SDU	Clonidine	X		
Dispaclonidin 1/8%	Clonidine	X		
Iopidine 0.5%	Apraclonidine	X		
Isoglaucon ¼%, 1/8%, 1/16%	Clonidine	X		

Alpha-2 Agonists and Beta Blocker

	Active ingredient	Eye Drops	Ointment	Tablets
Combigan	Brimodine/Timolol	X		

Eicosanoids

	Active ingredient	Eye Drops	Ointment	Tablets
Xalatan	Latanoprost	X		
Travatan	Travatoprost	X		
Lumigan	Bimatoprost	X		

Eicosanoids and Beta Blockers

	Active ingredient	Eye Drops	Ointment	Tablets
Xalacom	Latanoprost/Timolol	X		

Docosanoids

	Active ingredient	Eye Drops	Ointment	Tablets
Rescula 0.15%	Unoprostone isopropyl	X		

	Active ingregient	Drops for oral use	Tablets	Injection
Medications to improve ocular circulation in patients with vascular dysregulation				
Magnesium	e.g. Magnesium-L-aspartat-hydro-chlorid-trihydrat		X	
Low dose calcium-channel blockers				
Nifedipin	e.g. Nifedipine	X		
To increase blood pressure				
Salt tablets	NaCl		X	
Mineralocorticoids	Fludrocortisone		X	
To protect mitochondrias				
Ginkgo	Ginkgo 120 mg		X	

A 3 Additional Reading Material

The amount of information on glaucoma that has been published within the past years is so vast that it would be impossible to mention (or read) everything available. There are tens of thousands of original research papers that discuss the various aspects of glaucoma. What the authors seek to provide is a list of those resources that might prove helpful to the reader.

Textbooks

General Books on Ophthalmology –

books that would be useful to the reader not familiar with ophthalmology:

Spalton DJ, Hitchings RA, Hunter PA: In: Atlas of clinical ophthalmology. New York (etc.): Gower Medical Publishing; 1984.

Kanski JJ: Clinical ophthalmology: A systematic approach. 3rd ed. Oxford; Boston: Butterworth-Heinemann; 1994.

Duane TD, Tasman W (ed): In: Duane's Clinical Ophthalmology: Philadelphia (etc.): Lippincott; 1995.

Albert DM, Jakobiec FA (eds.): In: Atlas of Clinical Ophthalmology. Philadelphia: WB Saunders; 1996.

Mandava S: Color Atlas of Ophthalmology. New York: Thieme; 1999.

Yanoff M, Duker JS, AugsbergerJJ, *et.al.* (eds.): Ophthalmology. Philadelphia, London: Mosby; 1999.

Albert DM, Jakobiec FA (eds.): Principles and Practice of Ophthalmology. Philadelphia: WB Saunders; 2000.

Parrish K II (ed.): Atlas of Ophthalmology. (The University of Miami, Bascom Palmer Eye Institute atlas of color ophthalmology). Philadelphia, PA: Current Medicine; 2000.

Interesting Issues in Ophthalmology –

are discussed in the following books:

Kanski JJ: The Eye in Systemic Disease. London; Boston: Butterworth-Heinemann; 1990.

Fraunfelder FT: Current Ocular Therapy. Philadelphia: WB Saunders; 1990.

Spencer WH (ed.): Ophthalmic Pathology: An Atlas and Textbook. 4th ed. Philadelphia: WB Saunders; 1996.

Fechner PU, Teichmann KD: Ocular Therapeutics: Pharmacology and Clinical Application. Thorofare NJ: Slack; 1997.

Rhee DJ, Deramo VA: Wills Eye Manual: Office and Emergency Room Diagnosis and Treatment of Eye Disease. Philadelphia: Lippincott, Williams & Wilkins; 1999.

Rhee DJ, Deramo VA: The Wills Eye Drug Guide: Diagnostic and Therapeutic Medications. Philadelphia: Lippincott, Williams & Wilkins; 2001).

Fankhauser F, Kwasniewska S. Lasers in ophthalmology. The Hague: Kugler Publications; 2003.

Textbooks on Glaucoma –

a small selection is mentioned, without attempting to be comprehensive:

Béchetoille A: In: Les Glaucomes. Vol. 2 Paris: Angers: SI Japperenard; 2000.

Ritch R, Shields MB, Krupin T (eds.). In: The Glaucomas. St. Louis [etc.]: Mosby; 1996.

Béchetoille A (ed.). Glaucomes à Pression Normale [Normal Pressure Glaucomas]. Symposium international glaucomes à pression normale, 23–24 juin 1989. Angers: SI Japperenard; 1990.

Sampaolesi R: Glaucoma. 2ª ed. Buenos Aires [et al.]: Editorial Medica Panamericana; 1991.

Shields MB: In: Textbook of Glaucoma. Baltimore: Williams & Wilkins; 1997.

Van Buskirk EM, Shields MB (eds.): 100 Years of Progress in Glaucoma. Philadelphia: Lippincott-Raven; 1997.

Bavishi AK, Nagpal PN: Glaucoma, Changing Concepts in Management. – Ahmedabad: Bhargavi printers, Ranip; 1998.

European Glaucoma Society: Terminology and Guidelines of Glaucoma. Savona, Italy: Editrice DOGMA®; 1998.

Fehér J (ed.): Glaucoma. Budapest: Akadmiai Kiado; 1998.

Stamper RL, Lieberman MF, Drake MV (eds.). In: Becker-Shaffer's Diagnosis and Therapy of the Glaucomas. St. Louis [etc.]: Mosby; 1999.

Zimmermann TJ, Kooner KS (eds.): Clinical Pathways in Glaucoma. New York: Thieme; 2001.

Specific Aspects of Glaucoma –

are covered in the following books:

Jerndal T, Hansson HA, Bill A: In: Goniodysgenesis: A new Perspective on Glaucoma. Copenhagen: Scriptor; 1978.

Sherwood MB, Spaeth GL (eds.). In: Complications of Glaucoma Therapy. Thorofare NJ: Slack; 1990.

Drance SM, Van Buskirk EM, Neufeld AH (eds.). In: Pharmacology of Glaucoma. Baltimore [etc.]: Williams & Wilkins; 1992.

Minckler DS, Van Buskirk ME, Wright, KW: In: Color Atlas of Ophthalmic Surgery. Glaucoma. Philadelphia: Lippincott; 1992.

Thomas JV (ed.), Belcher CD III, Simmons RJ (assoc. eds.): In: Glaucoma Surgery. St. Louis [etc.]: Mosby; 1992.

Varma R, Spaeth GL, Parker KW: In: The Optic Nerve in Glaucoma. Philadelphia: Lippincott; 1993.

Alward WL. In: Color Atlas of Gonioscopy. San Francisco: Foundation of the American Academy of Ophthalmology; 2000.

Drance SM (ed). In: Optic Nerve in Glaucoma. Amsterdam [etc.]: Kugler; 1995.

Drance SM (ed.). In: Vascular Risk Factors and Neuroprotection in Glaucoma: Update 1996. Amsterdam [etc.]: Kugler; 1997.

Bisantis C, Carella G: Vascular System of the Optic Nerve and Perioptic Area. Viterbo: Stampa United Printing; 1998.

Weinreb RN, Mills RP (eds.): Glaucoma Surgery: Principles and Techniques. 2nd ed. San Francisco, CA: American Academy of Ophthalmology; 1998.

Gramer E, Grehn F (eds.). In: Pathogenesis and Risk Factors of Glaucoma. Berlin [etc.]: Springer; 1999.

Books from the Basel Research Group –

written, as is this book, by staff of the University Eye Clinic in Basel:

Kaiser HJ, Flammer J, Hendrickson P. (eds.): Ocular Blood Flow: New Insights into the Pathogenesis of Ocular Diseases. Basel: Karger; 1996.

Haefliger IO, Flammer J (eds.): Nitric Oxide and Endothelin in the Pathogenesis of Glaucoma. Philadelphia. Lippincott-Raven; 1998.

Kaiser HJ, Flammer J: Visual Field Atlas. University Eye Clinic, 1992. Basel: Buser Druck; 1999.

Orgül S, Flammer J (eds.): Pharmacotherapy in Glaucoma. Bern: Huber; 2000.

Shaarawy T, Flammer J. Glaucoma therapy–current issues and controversies. London: Martin Dunitz - Taylor & Francis Group; 2004.

Vision –

the following provide more insight on this topic:

Zeki S: A Vision of the Brain. Oxford [etc.]: Blackwell Scientific Publications; 1993.

Rodieck RW: The First Steps in Seeing. Sunderland, Mass.: Sinauer; 1998.

Automatic Perimetry –

a subject described in more detail in these books:

Drance SM, Anderson DR (eds.): Automatic Perimetry in Glaucoma. Orlando: Grune & Stratton; 1985.

Whalen WR and Spaeth GL (eds.): Computerized Visual Fields: What they are and how to use them. Thorofare: Slack; 1985.

Lachenmayr B, Vivell PMO: Perimetrie. Stuttgart [etc.]: Thieme; 1992.

Anderson DR, Patella VM: Automated Static Perimetry. Mosby; 1998.

Octopus: Visual Field Digest. 4th ed. Schlieren [etc.]: Interzeag; 1998.

Weijland A, Fankhauser F, Bebie H, Flammer J: Automated Perimetry – Visual Field Digest. 5th ed.: Haag Streit International; 2004.

Unique Works from Books and Journals –

Frequency of Glaucoma –

information can be found in:

Shiose Y, Kitazawa Y, Tsukahara S, *et al.* Epidemiology of glaucoma in Japan — a nationwide glaucoma survey. *Jpn J Ophthalmol* 1991;35(2): 133–155.

Mitchell P, Smith W, Attebo K, Healy PR. Prevalence of open-angle glaucoma in Australia: The Blue Mountains Eye Study. *Ophthalmology* 1996;103:1661–1669.

Quigley HA. Number of people with glaucoma worldwide. *Br J Ophthalmol* 1996;80:389–393.

Hattenhauer MG, Johnson DH, Ing HH, *et al.* The probability of blindness from open-angle glaucoma. *Ophthalmology* 1998;105:2099–2104.

Buhrmann RR, Quigley HA, Barron Y, *et al.* Prevalence of glaucoma in a rural East African population. *Invest Ophthalmol Vis Sci* 2000;41:40–48.

King AJ, Reddy A, Thompson JR, Rosenthal AR. The rates of blindness and of partial sight registration in glaucoma patients. *Eye* 2000;14(Pt 4):613–9.

Quigley HA, Buhrmann RR, West SK, *et al.* Long term results of glaucoma surgery among participants in an east African population survey. *Br J Ophthalmol* 2000;84(8):860–4.

Schoff EO, Hattenhauer MG, Ing HH, *et al.*: Estimated incidence of open-angle glaucoma in Olmsted County, Minnesota. *Ophthalmology* 2001; 108(5):882-886.

Voogd SD, Ikram MK, Wolfs RC, Jansonius NM, Hofman A, de Jong PT. Incidence of Open-Angle Glaucoma in a General Elderly Population The Rotterdam Study. Ophthalmology. 2005 Jul 21; [Epub ahead of print]

Anton A, Andrada MT, Mujica V, Calle MA, Portela J, Mayo A. Prevalence of primary open-angle glaucoma in a Spanish population: the Segovia study. J Glaucoma. 2004 Oct;13(5):371–6.

Iwase A, Suzuki Y, Araie M, Yamamoto T, Abe H, Shirato S, Kuwayama Y, Mishima HK, Shimizu H, Tomita G, Inoue Y, Kitazawa Y; Tajimi Study Group, Japan Glaucoma Society. The prevalence of primary open-angle glaucoma in Japanese: the Tajimi Study. Ophthalmology. 2004 Sep; 111(9):1641–8.

Varma R, Ying-Lai M, Francis BA, Nguyen BB, Deneen J, Wilson MR, Azen SP; Los Angeles Latino Eye Study Group. Prevalence of open-angle glaucoma and ocular hypertension in Latinos: the Los Angeles Latino Eye Study. Ophthalmology. 2004 Aug;111(8):1439–48.

Morphological Aspects of Glaucoma –
more on this topic in:

Naumann GOH: Glaukome und Hypertoniesyndrome. In: Naumann, GOH.: Pathologie des Auges II. – 2. Aufl. – Berlin [etc.]: Springer, 1997. – (Spezielle pathologische Anatomie; Bd. 12).

Lütjen-Drecoll E: Functional morphology of the trabecular meshwork in primate eyes. *Prog Retin Eye Res* 1999;18(1): 91–119.

Jonas JB, Budde WM: Diagnosis and pathogenesis of glaucomatous optic neuropathy: morphological aspects. In: *Prog Retin Eye Res* 2000;19(1): 1–40.

Yucel YH, Zhang Q, Gupta N, Kaufman PL, Weinreb RN. Loss of neurons in magnocellular and parvocellular layers of the lateral geniculate nucleus in glaucoma. *Arch Ophthalmol* 2000;118(3):378–84.

Gherghel D, Orgül S, Prünte C, Gugleta K, Lübeck P, Gekkieva M, Flammer J: Interocular differences in optic disc topographic parameters in normal subjects. *Curr Eye Res* 2000;20:276–282.

Artes PH, Chauhan BC. Longitudinal changes in the visual field and optic disc in glaucoma. Prog Retin Eye Res. 2005 May;24(3):333–54.

Risks for Glaucoma –
including the glaucoma risk in general is described in:

Drance SM, Buskirk Van EM, Neufeld AH (eds.): In: Pharmacology of Glaucoma. Flammer J, Gasser P, Prünte Ch, Yao K: The probable involvement of factors other than intraocular pressure in the pathogenesis of glaucoma; p. 273–283. Baltimore: William & Wilkins;1992.

Sponsel WE, Ritch R, Stamper R, Higginbotham EJ, Anderson DR, Wilson MR, Zimmerman TJ: Prevent Blindness America visual field screening study. The Prevent Blindness America Glaucoma Advisory Committee [see comments]. *Am J Ophthalmol* 1995;120(6):699–708.

Stewart WC: The effect of lifestyle on the relative risk to develop open-angle glaucoma. *Curr Opin Ophthalmol* 1995;6(2): 3–9.

Hiller R, Podgor MJ, Sperduto RD, Wilson PW, Chew EY, D'Agostino RB: High intraocular pressure and survival: the Framingham Studies. *Am J Ophthalmol* 1999;128(4):440–445.

Wax MB: Is there a role for the immune system in glaucomatous optic neuropathy? *Curr Opin Ophthalmol* 2000;11(2):145–50.

Mojon DS, Hess CW, Goldblum D, Bohnke M, Koerner F, Mathis J: Primary open-angle glaucoma is associated with sleep apnea syndrome. *Ophthalmologica* 2000;214(2):115–118.

Friedman DS, Wilson MR, Liebmann JM, Fechtner RD, Weinreb RN. An evidence-based assessment of risk factors for the progression of ocular hypertension and glaucoma. Am J Ophthalmol. 2004 Sep;138(3 Suppl):S19–31.

Gherghel D, Hosking SL, Orgul S. Autonomic nervous system, circadian rhythms, and primary open-angle glaucoma. Surv Ophthalmol. 2004 Sep-Oct;49(5):491–508.

Origin of Increased Pressure –

some special aspects are covered in:

Krieglstein GK (ed.): In: Glaucoma update III. Sampaolesi R: Congenital glaucoma. Long-term results of surgery. Berlin [etc.]: Springer; 1987.

Kondo T, Miura M: Mathematical analysis of the pupillary block. *Glaucoma* 1989; 11:176–180.

Orgül S, Hendrickson P, Flammer J: Anterior chamber depth and pigment dispersion syndrome. *Am J Ophthalmol* 1994;117(5):575–577.

Zaltas MM, Schuhman JS: Malignant glaucoma: theory and therapy, from past to present. *Semin Ophthalmol* 1994;9(4):243–247.

Bachmann JA: Juvenile onset primary open-angle glaucoma: three case studies and review. *J Am Optom Assoc* 1998;69(12):785–795.

Naumann GO, Schlötzer-Schrehardt U, Küchle M: Pseudoexfoliation syndrome for the comprehensive ophthalmologist. Intraocular and systemic manifestations. *Ophthalmology* 1998;105(6):951–968.

Ritch R: Pigment dispersion syndrome. *Am J Ophthalmol* 1998;126(3): 442–445.

Eye Pressure and Visual Field Damage –
there are only a few works covering this relationship; some of these are:

Niesel P, Flammer J: Correlations between intraocular pressure, visual field and acuity, based on 11 years observations of treated chronic glaucomas. *Int Ophthalmol* 1980;3:31–35.

Weber I, Koll W, Krieglstein GK: Intraocular pressure and visual field decay in chronic glaucoma. *Ger J Ophthalmol* 1993;2:165–169.

Teus MA, Castejon MA, Calvo MA, Perez-Salaices P, Marcos A: Intraocular pressure as a risk factor for visual field loss in pseudoexfoliative and in primary open-angle glaucoma. *Ophthalmology* 1998;105(12):2225–9; discussion 2229–30.

Danias J, Podos SM: Comparison of glaucomatous progression between untreated patients with normal-tension glaucoma and patients with therapeutically reduced intraocular pressures: the effectiveness of intraocular pressure reduction in the treatment of normal-tension glaucoma (multiple letters). *Am J Ophthalmol* 1999;127:623–625.

Mitchell P, Wang JJ, Hourihan F: The relationship between glaucoma and pseudoexfoliation: the Blue Mountains Eye Study. *Arch Ophthalmol* 1999;117(10):1319–24.

The AGIS Investigators: The advanced glaucoma intervention study (AGIS): 7. The relationship between control of intraocular pressure and visual field deterioration. *Am J Ophthalmol* 2000;130(4):429–440.

Kass MA, Heuer DK, Higginbotham EJ *et al.*: The ocular hypertension treatment study. *Arch Ophthalmol* 2002;120:701–713.

Ocular perfusion –
Methods for measurement are described in:

Riva CE, Petrig B: Blue field entoptic phenomenon and blood velocity in the retinal capillaries. *J Opt Soc Am* 1980;70:1234–8.

Prünte C, Niesel P: Quantification of choroidal blood-flow parameters using indocyanine green video-fluorescence angiography and statistical picture analysis. *Graefes Arch Clin Exp Ophthalmol* 1988;226:55–8.

Sponsel WE, DePaul KL, Kaufman PL: Correlation of visual function and retinal leukocyte velocity in glaucoma. *Am J Ophthalmol* 1990;109:49–54.

Wolf S, Arend O, Sponsel WE, Schulte K, Cantor LB, Reim M: Retinal hemodynamics using scanning laser ophthalmoscopy and hemorheology in chronic open-angle glaucoma. *Ophthalmology* 1993;100:1561–6.

Munch K, Vilser W, Senff I: [Adaptive algorithm for automatic measurement of retinal vascular diameter]. *Biomed Tech (Berl)* 1995;40:322–5.

Prünte C, Flammer J, Markstein R, Rudin M: Quantification of optic nerve blood flow changes using magnetic resonance imaging. *Invest Ophthalmol Vis Sci* 1995;36:247–51.

Michelson G, Schmauss B, Langhans MJ, Harazny J, Groh MJ: Principle, validity, and reliability of scanning laser Doppler flowmetry. *J Glaucoma* 1996;5:99–105.

Kaiser HJ, Schoetzau A, Stümpfig D, Flammer J: Blood-flow velocities of the extraocular vessels in patients with high-tension and normal-tension primary open-angle glaucoma. *Am J Ophthalmol* 1997;123:320–7.

Petrig BL, Lorenz B, Cranstoun SD, Riva CE: [Measuring leukocyte velocity in macular capillaries using a miniaturized blue field simulator: effect of aperture of the pupil]. *Klin Monatsbl Augenheilkd* 1997;210:305–7.

Fontana L, Poinoosawmy D, Bunce CV, O'Brien C, Hitchings RA: Pulsatile ocular blood flow investigation in asymmetric normal tension glaucoma and normal subjects [see comments]. *Br J Ophthalmol* 1998;82(7):731–6.

Michelson G, Welzenbach J, Pal I, Harazny J: Automatic full field analysis of perfusion images gained by scanning laser Doppler flowmetry. *Br J Ophthalmol* 1998;82:1294–300.

Anderson DR: Introductory comments on blood flow autoregulation in the optic nerve head and vascular risk factors in glaucoma. *Surv Ophthalmol* 1999;43 Suppl 1:S5–9.

Arend O, Harris A, Martin BJ, Remky A: Scanning laser ophthalmoscopy-based evaluation of epipapillary velocities: method and physiologic variability. *Surv Ophthalmol* 1999;44 Suppl 1:S3–9.

Gasser P, Orgül S, Dubler B, Bucheli B, Flammer J: Relation between blood flow velocities in the ophthalmic artery and in nailfold capillaries. *Br J Ophthalmol* 1999;83:505.

Gugleta K, Orgül S, Flammer J: Is corneal temperature correlated with blood-flow veocity in the ophthalmic artery? *Curr Eye Res* 1999;19:496–501.

Hiroshiba N, Ogura Y, Sasai K, *et al.*: Radiation-induced leukocyte entrapment in the rat retinal microcirculation. *Invest Ophthalmol Vis Sci* 1999;40:1217–22.

Koçak I, Orgül S, Flammer J: Variability in the Measurement of Corneal Temperature Using a Noncontact In-frared Thermometer. *Ophthalmologica* 1999;213:345–349.

Petrig BL, Riva CE, Hayreh SS: Laser Doppler flowmetry and optic nerve head blood flow. *Am J Ophthalmol* 1999;127:413–25.

Senn B, Orgül S, Keller U, Dickermann D, Dubler B, Vavrecka J, Gasser P, KaiserHJ, Flammer J: Retro-bulbar and Peripheral Capillary Blood Flow in Hypercholesterolemic Subjects. *Am J Ophthalmol* 1999;128:310–316.

Hayashi N, Tomita G, Kitazawa Y: Optic disc blood flow measured by scanning laser-Doppler flowmetry using a new analysis program. *Jpn J Ophthalmol* 2000;44(5):573–574.

Straubhaar M, Orgül S, Gugleta K, Schötzau A, Erb C, Flammer J: Choroidal laser Doppler flowmetry in healthy subjects. *Arch Ophthalmol* 2000;118:211–5.

Osusky R, Rohr P, Schötzau A, Flammer J: Nocturnal Dip in the Optic Nerve Head Perfusion. *Jpn J Ophthalmol* 2000;44:128–131.

Gekkieva M, Orgül S, Gherghel D, Gugleta K, Prünte C, Flammer J: The Influence of Sex Difference in Measurements with the Langham Ocular Blood Flow System. *Jpn J Ophthalmol* 2001;45:528–532.

Gugleta K, Orgül S, Flammer I, Gherghel D, Flammer J: Reliability of confocal choroidal laser Doppler flowmetry. *Invest Ophthalmol Vis Sci* 2002;43:723–8.

Preitner A, Orgul S, Prunte C, Flammer J. Measurement procedures in confocal choroidal laser Doppler flowmetry. Curr Eye Res. 2004 Apr;28(4):233–40.

Riva CE, Logean E, Falsini B. Visually evoked hemodynamical response and assessment of neurovascular coupling in the optic nerve and retina. Prog Retin Eye Res. 2005 Mar;24(2):183–215.

Cioffi GA, Alm A. Measurement of ocular blood flow. J Glaucoma. 2001 Oct;10(5 Suppl 1):S62–4.

Vascular Factors –
and their significance for glaucomatous damage are described in:

Drance SM, Sweeney VP, Morgan RW, Feldman F: Studies of factors involved in the production of low-tension glaucoma. *Arch Ophthalmol* 1973;89:457–465.

Flammer J, Guthauser F, Mahler F: Do ocular vasospasms help cause low-tension glaucoma? In: *Doc Ophthalmol Proc Ser* 1987;49: 397–399.

Gasser P, Flammer J: Influence of vasospasm on visual function. *Doc Ophthalmol* 1987;66:3–18.

Mahler F, Saner H, Wurbel H, Flammer J: Local cooling test for clinical capillaroscopy in Raynaud's phenomenon, unstable angina, and vasospastic visual disorders. *VASA* 1989;18:201–204.

Béchetoille, A: In: Glaucome à pression normale = Normal pressure glaucoma. Flammer J: Vasospasm as a potential factor in the pathogenesis of normal tension glaucoma; p. 187–194. Angers: Sl Japperenard; 1990.

Gasser P, Flammer J: Blood-cell velocity in the nailfold capillaries of patients with normal-tension or high-tension glaucoma. *Am J Ophthalmol* 1991;111:585–588.

Flammer J: Psychophysical mechanisms and treatment of vasospastic disorders in normal-tension glaucoma. In: Bull belge Ophthalmol, *Bull Soc Belge Ophthalmol* 1992;244:129–34.

Drance, SM, Buskirk Van EM, Neufeld AH (eds.): In: Pharmacology of Glaucoma. Flammer J, Gasser P, Prünte Ch, Yao K: The probable involvement of factors other than intraocular pressure in the pathogenesis of glaucoma; p. 273–283. Baltimore: William & Wilkins; 1992.

Graf Th, Flammer J, Prünte Ch, Hendrickson P: Gliosis-Like retinal alterations in glaucoma patients. *J Glaucoma* 1993;2:257–259.

Kaiser HJ, Flammer J, Burckhardt D: Silent myocardial ischemia in glaucoma patients. *Ophthalmologica* 1993;207(1):6–7.

Flammer J: The vascular concept of glaucoma. *Surv Ophthalmol* 1994;38 Supple:S3–6.

Schwartz, B: Circulatory defects of the optic disk and retina in ocular hypertension and high pressure open-angle glaucoma. *Surv Ophthalmol* 1994; 38[Suppl.]:S23–S34.

Kaiser HJ, Flammer J, Wenk M, Lüscher T: Endothelin-1 plasma levels in normal-tension glaucoma: abnormal response to postural changes. *Graefes Arch Clin Exp Ophthalmol* 1995;233(8):484–488.

Orgül S, Flammer J: Perilimbal aneurysms of conjunctival vessels in glaucoma patients. *German J Ophthalmol* 1995;4:94–96.

Anderson DR, Davis EB: Glaucoma, capillaries and pericytes. 1. Blood flow regulation. *Ophthalmologica* 1996;210:257–262.

Kaiser H J, Flammer J, Hendrickson Ph (eds.): In: Ocular blood flow. Flammer J: To what extend are vascular factors involved in the pathogenesis of glaucoma? p. 12–39. Basel: Karger; 1996.

Flammer J, Messerli J, Haefliger I: Sehstörungen durch vaskuläre Dysregulationen. In: Therap Umschau 1996;53:37–42.

Gass A, Flammer J, Linder L, Romeiro SC, Gasser P, Haefeli WE: Inverse correlation between endothelin-1-induced peripheral microvascular vasoconstriction and blood pressure in glaucoma patients. *Graefes Arch Clin Exp Ophthalmol* 1997;235(10):634–638.

Kaiser HJ, Schötzau A, Flammer J: Blood flow velocity in the extraocular vessels in chronic smokers. *Br J Ophthalmol* 1997;81(2):133–135.

Kaiser HJ, Schoetzau A, Stümpfig D, Flammer J: Blood-flow velocities of the extraocular vessels in patients with high-tension and normal-tension primary open-angle glaucoma. *Am J Ophthalmol* 1997;123(3):320–327.

Sponsel WE, Kaufman PL, Blum FG Jr: Association of retinal capillary perfusion with visual status during chronic glaucoma therapy. *Ophthalmology* 1997;104(6):1026–32.

Flammer J, Orgül S: Optic nerve blood-flow abnormalities in glaucoma. *Progr Retin Eye Res* 1998;17:267–289.

Trible JR, Anderson DR: Factors associated with retrobulbar hemodynamic measurements at variable intraocular pressure. *J Glaucoma* 1998;7(1):33–8.

Flammer J, Haefliger IO, Orgül S, Resink T: Vascular dysregulation: a principal risk factor for glaucomatous damage? *J Glaucoma* 1999;8:212–219.

Girardin F, Orgül S, Erb C, Flammer J: Relationship between corneal temperature and finger temperature. *Arch Ophthalmol* 1999;117(2):166–169.

Bohdanecka Z, Orgül S, Meyer AB, Prünte Ch, Flammer J: Relationship between blood flow velocities in retrobulbar vessels and laser Doppler flowmetry at the optic disk in glaucoma patients. *Ophthalmologica* 1999;213(3):145–149.

Haefliger IO, Dettmann E, Liu R, Meyer P, Prünte Ch, Messerli J, Flammer J: Potential role of nitric oxide and endothelin in the pathogenesis of glaucoma. *Surv Ophthalmol* 1999;43[Suppl 1]:S51–58.

Senn B, Orgül S, Keller U, *et al.*: Retrobulbar and peripheral capillary blood flow in hypercholesterolemic subjects. *Am J Ophthalmol* 1999;128(3):310–316.

Schumann J, Orgül S, Gugleta K, Dubler B, Flammer J. Interocular difference in progression of glaucoma correlates with intraocular differences in retrobulbar circulation. *Am J Ophthalmol* 2000;129(6):728–733.

Sonnsjö B, Dokmo Y, Krakau T: Disc haemorrhages, precursors of open angle glaucoma. *Prog Retin Eye Res* 2002;21:35–56.

Flammer J, Orgül S, Costa VP, Orzalesi N, Krieglstein GK, Metzner Serra L,

Renard JP, Stefansson E: The impact of ocular blood flow in glaucoma. *Prog Retin Eye Res* 2002;21:359–393.

Golubnitschaja O, Wunderlich K, Decker C, Mönkemann H, Schild HH, Flammer J: Molecular imaging of perfusion disturbances in glaucoma. *Amino Acids* (in print).

Grieshaber MC, Flammer J. Blood flow in glaucoma. Curr Opin Ophthalmol. 2005 Apr;16(2):79–83.

Satilmis M, Orgul S, Doubler B, Flammer J. Rate of progression of glaucoma correlates with retrobulbar circulation and intraocular pressure. Am J Ophthalmol. 2003 May;135(5):664–9.

Emre M, Orgul S, Haufschild T, Shaw SG, Flammer J. Increased plasma endothelin-1 levels in patients with progressive open angle glaucoma. Br J Ophthalmol. 2005 Jan;89(1):60–3.

Gottanka J, Kuhlmann A, Scholz M, Johnson DH, Lutjen-Drecoll E. Pathophysiologic changes in the optic nerves of eyes with primary open angle and pseudoexfoliation glaucoma. Invest Ophthalmol Vis Sci. 2005 Nov;46(11):4170–81.

Vascular Dysregulations –
the general medical importance of this problem is described in:

O'Brien C: Vasospasm and glaucoma [editorial; comment]. *Br J Ophthalmol* 1998;82(8):855–6.

Gasser P, Orgül S, Dubler B, Bucheli B, Flammer J: Relation between blood flow velocities in the ophthalmic artery and in nailfold capillaries. *Br J Ophthalmol* 1999;83(4):505.

Gherghel D, Orgül S, Dubler B, Lubeck P, Gugleta K, Flammer J: Is vascular regulation in the central retinal artery altered in persons with vasospasm? *Arch Ophthalmol* 1999;117(10):1359–1362.

Romerio SC, Linder L, Flammer J, Haefeli WE: Correlation between apolipoprotein B and endothelin-1-induced vasoconstriction in humans. *Peptides* 2000;21(6): 871–4.

Flammer J, Pache M, Resink T: Vasospasm, its Role in the Pathogenesis of Diseases with Particular Reference to the Eye. *Prog Retin Eye Res* 2001;20:319–349.

Flammer J, Kaiser HJ, Haufschild T: Susac syndrome: a vasospastic disorder? *Eur J Ophthalmol* 2001;11,2:175–179.

Pache M, Kräuchi K, Cajochen C, Wirz-Justice A, Dubler B, Flammer J, Kaiser HJ: Cold feet and prolonged sleep-onset latency in vasospastic syndrome. *The Lancet* 2001;385:125–126.

Flammer J: Glaucomatous optic neuropathy: a reperfusion injury. *Klin Monatsbl Augenheilkd* 2001:218(5):290–1.

Hasler PW, Orgül S, Gugleta K, Vogten H, Zhao X, Gherghel D, Flammer J: Vascular dysregulation in the choroid of subjects with acral vasospasm. *Arch Ophthalmol* 2002;120:302–7.

Flammer J, Orgül S, Costa VP, Orzalesi N, Krieglstein GK, Metzner Serra L, Renard JP, Stefansson E: The impact of ocular blood flow in glaucoma. *Prog Retin Eye Res* (in print).

Buckley C, Hadoke PWF, Henry E, O'Brien C: Systemic vascular endothelial cell dysfunction in normal pressure glaucoma. *Br J Ophthalmol* 2002;86:227–232.

Wunderlich K, Zimmerman C, Gutmann H, Teuchner B, Flammer J, Drewe J. Vasospastic persons exhibit differential expression of ABC-transport proteins. Mol Vis. 2003 Dec 31;9:756–61.

Gugleta K, Orgul S, Hasler PW, Picornell T, Gherghel D, Flammer J. Choroidal vascular reaction to hand-grip stress in subjects with vasospasm and its relevance in glaucoma. Invest Ophthalmol Vis Sci. 2003 Apr;44(4):1573–80.

Emre M, Orgul S, Gugleta K, Flammer J. Ocular blood flow alteration in glaucoma is related to systemic vascular dysregulation. Br J Ophthalmol. 2004 May;88(5):662–6.

Teuchner B, Orgul S, Ulmer H, Haufschild T, Flammer J. Reduced thirst in patients with a vasospastic syndrome. Acta Ophthalmol Scand. 2004 Dec;82(6):738–40.

Gugleta K, Orgul S, Hasler PW, Flammer J. Circulatory response to blood gas perturbations in vasospastic subjects. Invest Ophthalmol Vis Sci, in press

Normal Tension Glaucoma –

a special type of primary open angle glaucoma that is especially seen in association with vascular risk factors and discussed in:

Orgül S, Flammer J: Interocular visual-field and intraocular-pressure asymmetries in normal-tension-glaucoma. *Eur J Ophthalmol* 1994;4(4):199–201.

Cartwright MJ, Grajewski AL, Friedberg ML, Anderson DR, Richards DW: Immune-related disease and normal-tension glaucoma. A case-control study [see comments]. *Arch Ophthalmol* 1992;110(4):500–2.

Orgül S, Gaspar AZ, Hendrickson P, Flammer J. Comparison of the severity of normal-tension glaucoma in men and women. *Ophthalmologica* 1994;208(3):142–144.

Orgül S, Gass A, Flammer J: Optic disc cupping in arteritic anterior ischemic optic neuropathy. *Ophthalmologica* 1994;208(6):336–338.

Yamazaki Y, Drance SM: The relationship between progression of visual field defects and retrobulbar circulation in patients with glaucoma. *Am J Ophthalmol* 1997;124(3):287–295.

Orgül S, Prünte C, Flammer J: Endothelium-derived vasoactive substances relevant to normal-tension glaucoma. *Curr Opin Ophthalmol* 1998;9(2): 88–94.

Kamal D, Hitchings R: Normal tension glaucoma – a practical approach. *Br J Ophthalmol* 1998;82(7):835–840.

Van Buskirk EM: The tale of normal-tension glaucoma. *J Glaucoma* 1998;7(6):363–365.

Gugleta K, Orgül S, Flammer J: Asymmetry in intraocular pressure and retinal nerve fiber layer thickness in normal-tension glaucoma. *Ophthalmologica* 1999;213(4):219–223.

Drance, SM: The collaborative normal-tension glaucoma study and some of its lessons. *Can J Ophthalmol* 1999;34(1):1–6.

Henry E, Newby DE, Webb DJ, O'Brien C: Peripheral endothelial dysfunction in normal pressure glaucoma. *Invest Ophthalmol Vis Sci* 1999; 40(8):1710–4.

Erb C, Batra A, Lietz A, Bayer AU, Flammer J, Thiel HJ: Psychological characteristics of patients with normal-tension glaucoma. *Graefe's Arch Clin Exp Ophthalmol* 1999;237:753–757.

Ishida K, Yamamoto T, Sugiyama K, Kitazawa Y: Disk hemorrhage is a significantly negative prognostic factor in normal-tension glaucoma [see comments]. *Am J Ophthalmol* 2000;129(6):707–14.

Kashiwagi K, Tsumura T, Ishii H, Ijiri H, Tamura K, Tsukahara S: Circadian rhythm of autonomic nervous function in patients with normal-tension glaucoma compared with normal subjects using ambulatory electrocardiography. *J Glaucoma* 2000;9(3):239–46.

Sugiyama T, Schwartz B, Takamoto T, Azuma I: Evaluation of the circulation in the retina, peripapillary choroid and optic disk in normal-tension glaucoma. *Ophthalmic Res* 2000;32(2-3):79–86.

Opial D, Boehnke M, Tadesse S, Lietz-Partzsch A, Flammer J, Munier F, Mermoud A, Hirano M, Flückiger F, Mojon DS: Leber's hereditary optic neuropathy mitochondrial DNA mutations in normal-tension glaucoma. *Graefe's Arch Clin Exp Ophthalmol* 2001;239:437–440.

Anderson DR; Normal Tension Glaucoma Study. Collaborative normal tension glaucoma study. Curr Opin Ophthalmol. 2003 Apr;14(2):86–90.

Pournaras CJ, Riva CE, Bresson-Dumont H, De Gottrau P, Bechetoille A. Regulation of optic nerve head blood flow in normal tension glaucoma patients. Eur J Ophthalmol. 2004 May-Jun;14(3):226–35.

Significance of the Blood Pressure –
the importance of low blood pressure has been emphasized for decades:

Kaiser HJ, Flammer J: Systemic hypotension: a risk factor for glaucomatous damage? *Ophthalmologica* 1991;203(3):105–108.

Kaiser HJ, Flammer J, Graf T, Stümpfig D: Systemic blood pressure in glaucoma patients. *Graefes Arch Clin Exp Ophthalmol* 1993;231:677–680.

Tielsch JM, Katz J, Sommer A, Quigley HA, Javitt JC: Hypertension, perfusion pressure and primary open-angle glaucoma. A population-based assessment. *Arch Ophthalmol* 1995;113(2):216–221.

Gugleta K, Orgül S, Stümpfig D, Dubler B, Flammer J: Fludrocortisone in the treatment of systemic hypotension in primary open-angle glaucoma patients. *Int Ophthalmol* 2000;23(1):25–30.

Osusky R, Rohr P, Schotzau A, Flammer J: Nocturnal dip in the optic nerve head perfusion. *Jpn J Ophthalmol* 2000; 44:128–131.

Gherghel D, Orgül S, Gugleta K, Gekkieva M, Flammer J: Relationship Between Ocular Perfusion Pressure and Retrobulbar Blood Flow in Patients With Glaucoma With Progressive Damage. *Am J of Ophthalmol* 2000;130(5):597–605.

Gherghel D, Orgül S, Gugleta K, Flammer J: Retrobulbar blood flow in glaucoma patients with nocturnal over-dipping in systemic blood pressure. *Am J Ophthalmol* 2001;5:641–7.

Fuchsjager-Mayrl G, Wally B, Georgopoulos M, Rainer G, Kircher K, Buehl W, Amoako-Mensah T, Eichler HG, Vass C, Schmetterer L. Ocular blood flow and systemic blood pressure in patients with primary open-angle glaucoma and ocular hypertension. Invest Ophthalmol Vis Sci. 2004 Mar;45(3):834–9.

Psychological Issues and Eye Diseases –
emotional stress can evoke ocular symptoms in predisposed individuals:

Bunce C, Hitchings R: Glaucoma and quality-of-life [letter; comment]. *Ophthalmology* 1999;106(3):440.

Erb C, Batra A, Lietz A, Bayer AU, Flammer J, Thiel HJ. Psychological characteristics of patients with normal-tension glaucoma. *Graefes Arch Clin Exp Ophthalmol* 1999;237:753–757.

Perimetry –
this tool is one of the primary bases for diagnosis and following the course of glaucoma. The development of perimetry is closely linked to the history of glaucoma:

Goldmann H: Grundlagen exakter Perimetrie. *Ophthalmologica* 1945;109 [Separatum](2–3):5.

Fankhauser F, Koch P, Roulier A: On automation of perimetry. In: *Albrecht Von Graefes Arch Klin Exp Ophthalmol* 1972;184:126–150.

Flammer J, Drance SM, Augustiny L, Funkhauser A: Quantification of glaucomatous visual field defects with automated perimetry. *Invest Ophthalmol Vis Sci* 1985;26(2):176–181.

Flammer J: The concept of visual field indices. *Graefes Arch Clin Exp Ophthalmol* 1986;224(5):389–392.

Flammer J, Jenni A, Bebié H, Keller B: The octopus glaucoma G1 program. *Glaucoma* 1987;9:67–72

Bebie H, Flammer J, Bebie T: The cumulative defect curve: separation of local and diffuse components of visual field damage. *Graefes Arch Clin Exp Ophthalmol* 1989;227(1):9–12.

O'Brien C, Poinoosawmy D, Wu J, Hitchings R: Evaluation of the Humphrey FASTPAC threshold program in glaucoma [see comments]. *Br J Ophthalmol* 1994;78(7):516–9.

Viswanathan AC, Hitchings RA, Fitzke FW: How often do patients need visual field tests? *Graefes Arch Clin Exp Ophthalmol* 1997;235(9):563–8.

Chauhan BC. Detection of glaucoma: the role of new functional and structural tests. Curr Opin Ophthalmol. 2004 Apr;15(2):93–5.

Girkin CA. Relationship between structure of optic nerve/nerve fiber layer and functional measurements in glaucoma. Curr Opin Ophthalmol. 2004 Apr;15(2):96–101.

Genetics of Glaucoma
Even though still in an early stage of development, this area will become increasingly important in years to come:

Anderson KL, Lewis RA, Bejjani BA, *et al.*: A gene for primary congenital glaucoma is not linked to the locus on chromosome 1q for autosomal dominant juvenile-onset open angle glaucoma. *J Glaucoma* 1996;5(6):416–21.

Sarfarazi M: Recent advances in molecular genetics of glaucomas. *Hum Mol Genet* 1997;6(10):1667–1677.

Wolfs RCW, Klaver CCW, Ramrattan RS *et al.*: Genetic risk of primary open-angle glaucoma. *Arch Ophthalmol* 1998;116:1640–1645.

Craig JE, Mackey DA: Glaucoma genetics: where are we? Where will we go? *Curr Opin Ophthalmol* 1999;10(2):126–134.

Angius A, Spinelli P, Ghilotti G, *et al.*: Myocilin Gln368stop mutation and advanced age as risk factors for late-onset primary open-angle glaucoma. *Arch Ophthalmol* 2000;118(5):674–9.

Huang W, Jaroszewski J, Ortego J, Escribano J, Coca-Prados M: Expression of the TIGR gene in the iris, ciliary body, and trabecular meshwork of the human eye. *Ophthalmic Genet* 2000;21(3):155–69.

Kubota R, Mashima Y, Ohtake Y, *et al.*: Novel mutations in the myocilin gene in Japanese glaucoma patients. *Hum Mutat* 2000;16(3):270.

Shimizu S, Lichter PR, Johnson AT, *et al.*: Age-dependent prevalence of mutations at the GLC1A locus in primary open-angle glaucoma. *Am J Ophthalmol* 2000;130(2):165–77.

Golubnitschaja-Labudova O, Liu R, Decker C, Zhu P, Haefliger IO, Flammer J: Altered gene expression in lymphocytes of patients with normal-tension glaucoma. *Curr Eye Res* 2000;21:867–76.

Moenkemann H, Flammer J, Wunderlich K, Breipohl W, Schild HH, Golubnitschaja O. Increased DNA breaks and up-regulation of both G(1) and G(2) checkpoint genes p21(WAF1/CIP1) and 14-3-3 sigma in circulating leukocytes of glaucoma patients and vasospastic individuals. Amino Acids. 2005 Mar;28(2):199–205.

Yeghiazaryan K, Flammer J, Wunderlich K, Schild HH, Orgul S, Golubnitschaja O. An enhanced expression of ABC 1 transporter in circulating leukocytes as a potential molecular marker for the diagnostics of glaucoma. Amino Acids. 2005 Mar;28(2):207–11.

Golubnitschaja O, Yeghiazaryan K, Liu R, Monkemann H, Leppert D, Schild H, Haefliger IO, Flammer J. Increased expression of matrix metalloproteinases in mononuclear blood cells of normal-tension glaucoma patients. J Glaucoma. 2004 Feb;13(1):66–72.

Golubnitschaja O, Wunderlich K, Decker C, Monkemann H, Schild HH, Flammer J. Molecular imaging of perfusion disturbances in glaucoma. Amino Acids. 2002;23(1-3):293–9.

Martin KR, Quigley HA. Gene therapy for optic nerve disease. Eye. 2004 Nov;18(11):1049–55.

Frezzotti R, Renieri A, Frezzotti P. Adult-onset primary glaucoma and molecular genetics: a review. Eur J Ophthalmol. 2004 May-Jun;14(3):220–5.

Therapy for Reducing Intraocular Pressure –

The basis of glaucoma treatment. Whether medication-based, laser-based or surgery-based, the literature is abundant. Here is a selection of publications that deal with treatment options; those that are medication-based are classified according to their substance group.

Medication-based therapy:

Beta-blockers

Kaufmann HE: Timolol. A beta adrenergic blocking agent for the treatment of glaucoma. *Arch Ophthalmol* 1977;95:601.

Flammer J, Robert Y, Gloor B: The influence of pindolol and timolol treatment on the visual fields of glaucoma patients. *J Ocul Pharmacol* 1986;2(4): 305–311.

Messmer C, Flammer J, Stümpfig D: Influence of betaxolol and timolol on the visual fields of patients with glaucoma. *Am J Ophthalmol* 1991;112(6): 678–681.

Zimmerman TJ: Topical ophthalmic beta blockers: a comparative review. *J Ocul Pharmacol* 1993;9(4):373–384.

Kaspar J, Champion C, Flammer J, Haefliger IO: Vasorelaxing Properties of Carteolol in isolated porcine ciliary arteries. *Klin Monatsbl Augenheilkd* 2000;216:318–320.

Lübeck P, Orgül S, Gugleta K, Gherghel D, Gekkieva M, Flammer J: Effect of Timolol on anterior optic nerve blood flow in patients with primary open-angle glaucoma as assessed by the Heidelberg retina flowmeter. *J of Glaucoma* 2000;10:13–17.

Brogiolo G, Flammer J, Haefliger IO: The beta-blocker carteolol inhibits contractions induced by KCl in pig ciliary arteries: an effect modulated by extracellular Ca++. *Klin Monatsbl Augenheilkd* 2002;219:268–72.

Morf T, Beny JL, Flammer J, Haefliger IO: Effect of palmitoleic acid on bradykinin-induced endothelium-de-pendent relaxation in isolated pig ciliary artery. *Klin Monatsbl Augenheilkd* 2002;219:284–288.

van der Valk R, Webers CA, Schouten JS, Zeegers MP, Hendrikse F, Prins MH. Intraocular pressure-lowering effects of all commonly used glaucoma drugs: a meta-analysis of randomized clinical trials. Ophthalmology. 2005 Jul;112(7):1177–85.

Carbonic Anhydrase Inhibitors

Becker B: Decrease in intraocular pressure in men by a carbonic anhydrase inhibitor, diamox. *Am J Ophthalmol* 1954;37:13.

Flammer J, Drance SM: The effect of acetazolamide on the differential threshold. *Arch Ophthalmol* 1983;101:1378–1380.

Pfeiffer, N: Dorzolamide: development and clinical application of a topical carbonic anhydrase inhibitor. *Surv Ophthalmol* 1997;42(2):137–151.

Pillunat LE, Bohm AG, Koller AU, Schmidt KG, Klemm M, Richard G: Effect of topical dorzolamide on optic nerve head blood flow. *Graefes Arch Clin Exp Ophthalmol* 1999;237(6):495–500.

Sugrue MF: Pharmacological and ocular hypotensive properties of topical carbonic anhydrase inhibitors. *Prog Retin Eye Res* 2000;19(1):87–112.

Cvetkovic RS, Perry CM. Brinzolamide : a review of its use in the management of primary open-angle glaucoma and ocular hypertension. Drugs Aging. 2003;20(12):919–47.

Alpha-2-Agonists

Stewart WC: Perspectives in the medical treatment of glaucoma. *Curr Opin Ophthalmol* 1999;10(2):99–108.

DeSantis L: Preclinical overview of brinzolamide. *Surv Ophthalmol* 2000; 44[Suppl 2]:S119–129.

Liu R, Flammer J, Haefliger IO: Brimonidine and inhibition of nitrite production in isolated porcine ciliary processes. *Klin Monatsbl Augenheilkd* 2001;218:348–350.

Liu R, Wu R, Flammer J, Haefliger IO: Inhibition by Brimonidine of Forskolin-Induced Nitrite Production in Isolated Pig Ciliary Processes. *Invest Ophthalmol Vis Sci* (in print).

Wheeler L, WoldeMussie E, Lai R. Role of alpha-2 agonists in neuroprotection. Surv Ophthalmol. 2003 Apr;48 Suppl 1:S47–51.

Prostaglandin Analogs

Alm A: Prostaglandin derivates as ocular hypotensive agents. *Prog Retin Eye Res* 1998;17(3):291–312.

Eisenberg DL, Camras CB: A preliminary risk-benefit assessment of latanoprost and unoprostone in open-angle glaucoma and ocular hypertension. *Drug Saf* 1999;20(6):505–514.

Linden C, Alm A: Prostaglandin analogues in the treatment of glaucoma. *Drugs Aging* 1999;14(5):387–398.

Brogiolo G, Flammer J, Haefliger IO: Latanoprost is a vasoconstrictor in isolated porcine ciliary arteries. *Klin Monatsbl Augenheilkd* 2001;218: 373–375.

El Sherbini ME, Gekkieva M, Flammer J, Haefliger IO. Effect of Xalatan® and Cosopt® on the vascular tone of quiescent isolated pig ciliary arteries. *Klin Monatsbl Augenheilkd* 2002;219:273–276.

Simmons ST, Dirks MS, Noecker RJ. Bimatoprost versus latanoprost in lowering intraocular pressure in glaucoma and ocular hypertension: results from parallel-group comparison trials. Adv Ther. 2004 Jul-Aug;21(4):247–62.

Perry CM, McGavin JK, Culy CR, Ibbotson T. Latanoprost : an update of its use in glaucoma and ocular hypertension. Drugs Aging. 2003;20(8):597–630.

Al-Jazzaf AM, DeSantis L, Netland PA. Travoprost: a potent ocular hypotensive agent. Drugs Today (Barc). 2003 Jan;39(1):61–74.

Docosanoids

Beano F, Orgül S, Stümpfig D, Gugleta K, Flammer J: An evaluation of the effect of unoprostone isopropyl 0.15% on ocular hemodynamics in normal-tension glaucoma patients. *Graefe's Arch Clin Exp Ophthalmol* 2001;239: 81–86.

Laser Therapy:

Wise JB: Glaucoma treatment by trabecular tightening with the argon laser. *Ophthalmology* 1979;81:69–78.

Trokel, SL (ed.): In: Yag laser ophthalmic microsurgery. Fankhauser F: The Q-switched laser: principles and clinical results. p. 101–146. Conn: Appleton-Century-Crofts; 1983.

Fankhauser F, Durr U, Giger H, Pol P, Kwasniewska S: Lasers, optical systems and safety in ophthalmology: a review. *Graefes Arch Clin Exp Ophthalmol* 1996;234(8):473–487.

Ang LP, Aung T, Chew PT: Acute primary angle closure in an Asian population: long-term outcome of the fellow eye after prophylactic laser peripheral iridotomy. *Ophthalmology* 2000;107(11):2092–6.

Jacobi PC, Dietlein TS, Colling T, Krieglstein GK: Photoablative laser-grid trabeculectomy in glaucoma filtering surgery: histology and outflow facility measurements in porcine cadaver eyes. *Ophthalmic Surg Lasers* 2000;31(1):49–54.

Nolan WP, Foster PJ, Devereux JG, Uranchimeg D, Johnson GJ, Baasanhu J: YAG laser iridotomy treatment for primary angle closure in east Asian eyes. *Br J Ophthalmol* 2000;84(11):1255–9.

Holz HA, Lim MC. Glaucoma lasers: a review of the newer techniques. Curr Opin Ophthalmol. 2005 Apr;16(2):89–93.

Lai JS, Tham CC, Chua JK, Poon AS, Chan JC, Lam SW, Lam DS. To compare argon laser peripheral iridoplasty (ALPI) against systemic medications in treatment of acute primary angle-closure: mid-term results. Eye. 2005 Jul 8; [Epub ahead of print]

Harasymowycz PJ, Papamatheakis DG, Latina M, De Leon M, Lesk MR, Damji KF. Selective laser trabeculoplasty (SLT) complicated by intraocular pressure elevation in eyes with heavily pigmented trabecular meshworks. Am J Ophthalmol. 2005 Jun;139(6):1110–3

Noureddin BN, Zein W, Haddad C, Ma'luf R, Bashshur Z. Diode laser transcleral cyclophotocoagulation for refractory glaucoma: a 1 year follow-up of patients treated using an aggressive protocol. Eye. 2005 Apr 29; [Epub ahead of print]

Surgical Therapy:

Krupin T, Kaufman P, Mandell A, Ritch R, Asseff C, Podos SM, Becker B: Filtering valve implant surgery for eyes with neovascular glaucoma. *Am J Ophthalmol* 1980;89(3):338–43.

Kirchhof B: Retinectomy lowers intraocular pressure in otherwise intractable glaucoma: preliminary results. *Ophthalmic Surg* 1994;25(4):262–7.

Perkins TW, Gangnon R, Ladd W, Kaufman PL, Libby CM: Molteno implant with mitomycin C: intermediate-term results. *J Glaucoma* 1998;7(2): 86–92.

Diestelhorst M, Khalili MA, Krieglstein GK: Trabeculectomy: a retrospective follow-up of 700 eyes. *Int Ophthalmol* 1998–99;22(4):211–20.

Azuara-Blanco A, Wilson PR, Spaeth GL, Schmidt CM, Augsburger JJ: Filtration procedures supplemented with mitomycin C in the management of childhood glaucoma. *Br J Ophthalmol* 1999;83(2):151–156.

Karlen ME, Sanchez E, Schnyder CC, Sickenberg M, Mermoud A: Deep sclerectomy with collagen implant: medium term results. *Br J Ophthalmol* 1999;83(1):6–11.

Lai JS, Poon AS, Chua JK, Tham CC, Leung AT, Lam DS: Efficacy and safety of the Ahmed glaucoma valve implant in Chinese eyes with complicated glaucoma. *Br J Ophthalmol* 2000;84(7):718–21.

Membrey WL, Poinoosawmy DP, Bunce C, Hitchings RA: Glaucoma surgery with or without adjunctive antiproliferatives in normal tension glaucoma: 1 intraocular pressure control and complications. *Br J Ophthalmol* 2000;84(6):586–90.

Orgül S, Flammer J. (eds): In: Pharmacotherapy in Glaucoma. Gherghel D, Orgül S, Prünte C, Flammer J: Trabeculectomy with a scleral tunnel technique combined with Mitomycin C; p. 243–250. Bern: Huber; 2000.

Spaeth GL, Marques Pereira ML: How does resetting intraocular pressure help optic nerve function? *Eye* 2000;14(Pt 3b):476–87.

Vysniauskiene I, Shaarawy T, Flammer J, Haefliger IO. Intraocular pressure changes in the contralateral eye after trabeculectomy with mitomycin C. Br J Ophthalmol. 2005 Jul;89(7):809–11.

Shaarawy T, Wu R, Mermoud A, Flammer J, Haefliger IO. Influence of non-penetrating glaucoma surgery on aqueous outflow facility in isolated porcine eyes. Br J Ophthalmol. 2004 Jul;88(7):950–2

Shaarawy T, Flammer J, Haefliger IO. Reducing intraocular pressure: is surgery better than drugs? Eye. 2004 Dec;18(12):1215–24.

Jones E, Clarke J, Khaw PT. Recent advances in trabeculectomy technique. Curr Opin Ophthalmol. 2005 Apr;16(2):107–13.

Flach AJ. Does medical treatment influence the success of trabeculectomy? Trans Am Ophthalmol Soc. 2004;102:219–23

Influencing Eye Perfusion with Drugs –

Guthauser U, Flammer J, Mahler F: The relationship between digital and ocular vasospasm. *Graefes Arch Clin Exp Ophthalmol* 1988;226(3):224–226.

Kitazawa Y, Shirai H, Go FJ: The effect of Ca2(+)-antagonist on visual field in low-tension glaucoma. *Graefes Arch Clin Exp Ophthalmol* 1989;227(5): 408–412.

Gasser P, Flammer J: Short- and long-term effect of nifedipine on the visual field in patients with presumed vasospasm. *J Int Med Res* 1990;18:334–339.

Gaspar AZ, Flammer J, Hendrickson Ph: Influence of nifedipine on the visual fields of patients with optic-nerve-head disease. *Eur J Ophthalmol* 1994;4(1):24–28.

Gaspar AZ, Gasser P, Flammer J: The influence of magnesium on visual field and peripheral vasospasm in glaucoma. *Ophthalmologica* 1995; 209(1):11–13.

Meyer P, Lang MG, Flammer J, Lüscher TF: Effects of calcium channel blockers on the response to endothelin-1, bradykinin and sodium nitroprusside in porcine ciliary arteries. *Exp Eye Res* 1995;60:505–510.

Sawada A, Kitazawa Y, Yamamoto Okabe I, Ichien K: Prevention of visual field defect progression with brovincamine in eyes with normal-tension glaucoma. *Ophthalmology* 1996;103(2):283–288.

Drance, StM (ed.): In: Vascular Risk Factor and Neuroprotection in Glaucoma. Dettmann ES, Flammer J, Haefliger IO: Magnesium and vascular tone modulation; p.79–86. Kugler Publications; 1997.

Yamamoto T, Niwa Y, Kawakami H, Kitazawa Y: The effect of nilvadipine, a calcium-channel blocker, on the hemodynamics of retrobulbar vessels in normal-tension glaucoma. *J Glaucoma* 1998;7(5):301–305.

Niwa Y, Yamamoto T, Harris A, Kagemann L, Kawakami H, Kitazawa Y: Relationship between the effect of carbon dioxide inhalation or nilvadipine on orbital blood flow in normal-tension glaucoma. *J Glaucoma* 2000; 9(3):262–7.

Gugleta K, Orgül S, Stümpfig D, Dubler B, Flammer J: Fludrocortisone in the treatment of systemic hypotension in primary open-angle glaucoma patients. *Int Ophthalmol* 2000;23:25–30.

Spicher T, Orgül S, Gugleta K, Teuchner B, Flammer J: The Effect of Losartan Potassium on Choroidal He-modynamics in Healthy Subjects. *J of Glaucoma* 2002;11:177–182.

Costa VP, Harris A, Stefansson E, Flammer J, Krieglstein GK, Orzalesi N, Heijl A, Renard JP, Serra LM. The effects of antiglaucoma and systemic medications on ocular blood flow. Prog Retin Eye Res. 2003 Nov;22(6):769–805.

Neuroprotection –

An interesting, but still relatively new, approach to preventing glaucomatous damage:

Levin LA: Direct and indirect approaches to neuroprotective therapy of glaucomatous optic neuropathy. *Surv Ophthalmol* 1999;43[Suppl 1]: S98–101.

Osborne NN, Chidlow, Nash MS, Wood JP: The potential of neuroprotection in glaucoma treatment. *Curr Opin Ophthalmol* 1999; 10(2):82–92.

Osborne NN, Ugarte M, Chao M, Chidlow G, Bae JH, Wood JP, Nash MS: Neuroprotection in relation to retinal ischemia and relevance to glaucoma. *Surv Ophthalmol* 1999;43 Suppl 1:S102–28.

Weinreb RN, Levin LA: Is neuroprotection a viable therapy for glaucoma? *Arch Ophthalmol* 1999;117(11):1540–1544.

Haefliger IO, Fleischhauer JC, Flammer J: In glaucoma, should enthusiasm about neuroprotection be tempered by the experience obtained in other neurodegenerative disorders? *Eye* 2000;14(Pt 3b):464–72.

Schwartz M, Yoles E: Neuroprotection: a new treatment modality for glaucoma? *Curr Opin Ophthalmol* 2000;11(2):107–11.

Toriu N, Akaike A, Yasuyoshi H, Zhang S, Kashii S, Honda Y, Schimazawa, M, Hara H: Lomerizine, a Ca^{2+} channel blocker, reduces glutamate-induced neurotoxicity and ischemia/reperfusion damage in rat retina. *Exp Eye Res* 2000;70(4):475–84.

Flammer J: Glaucomatous optic neuropathy: a reperfusion injury. *Klin Monatsbl Augenheilkd* 2001;218(5):290–1.

Osborne NN, Chidlow G, Layton CJ, Wood JP, Casson RJ, Melena J. Optic nerve and neuroprotection strategies. Eye. 2004 Nov;18(11):1075–84

Schwartz M. Vaccination for glaucoma: dream or reality? Brain Res Bull. 2004 Feb 15;62(6):481–4. Review.

Neufeld AH. Pharmacologic neuroprotection with an inhibitor of nitric oxide synthase for the treatment of glaucoma. Brain Res Bull. 2004 Feb 15;62(6):455–9.

Complimentary Medicine –

Among other sources, information on this topic can be found in:

Kaluza G, Strempel I: Autogenes Training in der Augenheilkunde dargestellt am Beispiel des Glaukoms. Heidelberg: Kaden; 1994.

Chung HS, Harris A, Kristinsson JK, Ciulla TA, Kagemann C, Ritsch R: Ginkgo biloba extract increases ocular blood flow velocity. *J Ocul Pharmacol Ther* 1999;15(3):233–240.

Ritch R: Potential role for Ginkgo biloba extract in the treatment of glaucoma. *Med Hypothesis* 2000;54(2):221–35.

Rhee DJ, Katz LJ, Spaeth GL, Myers JS. Complementary and alternative medicine for glaucoma. Surv Ophthalmol. 2001 Jul-Aug;46(1):43–55.

Basic Research –

The progress of tomorrow is based on the discoveries of today. To prevent or treat glaucoma, one must better understand regulation of the aqueous humor production and its outflow system, as well as ocular perfusion. Works from the Basel Research Group include:

Yao K, Tschudi M, Flammer J, Lüscher TF: Endothelium-dependent regulation of vascular tone of the porcine ophthalmic artery. *Invest Ophthalmol Vis Sci* 1991;32(6):1791–1798.

Haefliger IO, Flammer J, Lüscher TF: Nitric oxide and endothelin-1 are important regulators of human ophthalmic artery. *Invest Ophthalmol Vis Sci* 1992;33(7):2340–2343.

Haefliger IO, Flammer J, Lüscher TF: Heterogeneity of endothelium-dependent regulation in ophthalmic and ciliary arteries. *Invest Ophthalmol Vis Sci* 1993;34(5):1722–1730.

Meyer P, Flammer J, Lüscher TF: Local anesthetic drugs reduce endothelium-dependent relaxations of porcine ciliary arteries. *Invest Ophthalmol Vis Sci* 1993;34(9):2730–2736.

Meyer P, Flammer J, Lüscher TF: Endothelium-dependent regulation of the ophthalmic microcirculation in the perfused porcine eye: role of nitric oxide and endothelins. *Invest Ophthalmol Vis Sci* 1993;34(13):3614–3621.

Meyer P, Lang MG, Flammer J, Lüscher TF: Effects of calcium channel blockers on the response to endothelin-1, bradykinin and sodium nitroprusside in porcine ciliary arteries. *Exp Eye Res* 1995;60(5):505–510.

Meyer P, Flammer J, Lüscher TF: Local action of the renin angiotensin system in the porcine ophthalmic circulation: effects of ACE-inhibitors and angiotensin receptor antagonists. *Invest Ophthalmol Vis Sci* 1995;36(3): 555–562.

Haufschild T, Nava E, Meyer P, Flammer J, Lüscher TF, Haefliger IO: Spontaneous calcium-independent nitric oxide synthase activity in porcine ciliary processes. *Biochem Biophys Res Commun* 1996;222(3):786–789.

Meyer P, Flammer J, Lüscher TF: Effect of dipyridamole on vascular response of porcine ciliary arteries. *Curr Eye Res* 1996;15(4):387–393.

Lang MG, Zhu P, Meyer P, Noll G, Haefliger IO, Flammer J, Lüscher TF: Amlodipine and benazeprilat differently affect the responses to endothelin-1 and bradykinin in porcine ciliary arteries: effects of a low and high dose combination. *Curr Eye Res* 1997;16(3):208–213.

Zhu P, Beny JL, Flammer J, Lüscher TF, Haefliger IO: Relaxation by bradykinin in porcine ciliary artery. Role of nitric oxide and K(+)-channels. *Invest Ophthalmol Vis Sci* 1997;38(9):1761–1767.

Dettmann ES, Lüscher TF, Flammer J, Haefliger IO: Modulation of endothelin-1-induced contractions by magnesium/calcium in porcine ciliary arteries. *Graefes Arch Clin Exp Ophthalmol* 1998;236(1):47–51.

Liu R, Flammer J, Lüscher TF, Haefliger IO: beta-Adrenergic agonist-induced nitrite production in isolated pig ciliary processes. *Graefes Arch Clin Exp Ophthalmol* 1998;236(8):613–616.

Haefliger IO, Dettmann E, Liu R, Meyer P, Prünte C, Messerli J, Flammer J: Potential role of nitric oxide and endothelin in the pathogenesis of glaucoma. *Surv Ophthalmol* 1999;43[Suppl 1]:S51–58.

Liu R, Flammer J, Haefliger IO: Isoproterenol, forskolin, and cAMP-induced nitric oxide production in pig ciliary processes. *Invest Ophthalmol Vis Sci* 1999;40(8):1833–1837.

Meyer P, Champion C, Schlotzer-Schrehardt U, Flammer J, Haefliger IO: Localization of nitric oxide synthase isoforms in porcine ocular tissues. *Curr Eye Res* 1999;18(5):375–380.

Romano C, Li Z, Arendt A, Hargrave PA, Wax MB: Epitope mapping of anti-rhodopsin antibodies from patients with normal pressure glaucoma. *Invest Ophthalmol Vis Sci* 1999;40(6):1275–80.

Zhu P, Dettmann ES, Resink TJ, Lüscher TF, Flammer J, Haefliger IO: Effect of Ox-LDL on endothelium-dependent response in pig ciliary artery: prevention by an ET(A) antagonist. *Invest Ophthalmol Vis Sci* 1999;40(5):1015–1020.

Fleischhauer JC, Beny JL, Flammer J, Haefliger IO: NO/cGMP pathway activation and membrane potential depolarization in pig ciliary epithelium. *Invest Ophthalmol Vis Sci* 2000;41(7):1759–63.

Hernandez MR, Pena JD, Selvidge JA, Salvador-Silva M, Yang P: Hydrostatic pressure stimulates synthesis of elastin in cultured optic nerve head astrocytes. *Glia* 2000;32(2):122–36.

Haufschild T, Tschudi MR, Flammer J, Lüscher TF, Haefliger IO: Nitric oxide production by isolated human and porcine ciliary processes. *Graefe's Arch Clin Exp Ophthalmol* 2000;238(5):448–453.

Morgan JE: Optic nerve head structure in glaucoma: astrocytes as mediators of axonal damage. *Eye* 2000;14(Pt 3b):437–44.

Zhang X, Erb C, Flammer J, Nau WM: Absolute rate constants for the quenching of reactive excited states by melanin and related 5,6-dihydroxyndole metabolites: implications for their antioxidant activity. *Photochem Photobiol* 2000;71(5):524–33.

Hintermann E, Erb C, Talke-Messerer C, Liu R, Tanner H, Flammer J, Eberle AN: Expression of the mela-nin-concentrating hormone receptor in porcine and human ciliary epithelial cells. *Invest Ophthalmol Vis Sci* 2001;42:206–9.

Haefliger IO, Flammer J, Bény JL, Lüscher T: Endothelium-dependent vasoactive modulation in the ophthalmic circulation. *Prog Retin Eye Res* 2001;20:209–225.

Morf T, Zhu P, Flammer J, Haefliger IO: Vasorelaxing effect of the potassium (K+)-channel opener pinacidil in isolated porcine ciliary arteries. *Klin Monatsbl Augenheilkd* 2001;218:338–340.

Fleischhauer J, Bény JL, Flammer J, Haefliger IO: Cyclic AMP and anionic currents in porcine ciliary epithelium. *Klin Monatsbl Augenheilkd* 2001; 218:370–372.

Pellanda N, Flammer J, Haefliger IO: L-NAME and U 46619-induced contractions in isolated porcine ciliary arteries versus vortex veins. *Klin Monatsbl Augenheilkd* 2001;218:366–369.

Liu R, Hintermann E, Erb C, Tanner H, Flammer J, Eberle AN, Haefliger IO: Modulation of Na/K-ATPase activity by isoproterenol and propranolol in human non-pigmented ciliary epithelia cells. *Klin Monatsbl Augenheilkd* 2001;218:363–365.

Fleischhauer JC, Liu R, Elena PP, Flammer J, Haefliger IO: Topical ocular instillation of nitric oxide synthase inhibitors and intraocular pressure in rabbits. *Klin Monatsbl Augenheilkd* 2001;218:351–353.

Nau-Staudt K, Nau WM, Haefliger IO, Flammer J: Lipid peroxidation in porcine irisies: Dependence on pig-mentation. *Curr Eye Res* 2001;22, 3: 229–234.

Morf T, Beny JL, Flammer J, Haefliger IO: Effect of palmitoleic acid on bradykinin-induced endothelium-de-pendent relaxation in isolated pig ciliary artery. *Klin Monatsbl Augenheilkd* 2002;219:284–288.

Liu R, Flammer J, Haefliger IO: Forskolin upregulation of NOS I protein expression in porcine ciliary processes: a new aspect of aqueous humor regulation. *Klin Monatsbl Augenheilkd* 2002;219:281–283.

Savaskan E, Loffler KU, Meier F, Muller-Spahn F, Flammer J, Meyer P. Immunohistochemical localization of angiotensin-converting enzyme, angiotensin II and AT1 receptor in human ocular tissues. Ophthalmic Res. 2004 Nov-Dec;36(6):312–20.

Wu R, Yao K, Flammer J, Haefliger IO. Role of anions in nitric oxide-induced short-circuit current increase in isolated porcine ciliary processes. Invest Ophthalmol Vis Sci. 2004 Sep;45(9):3213–22.

Erb C, Nau-Staudt K, Flammer J, Nau W. Ascorbic acid as a free radical scavenger in porcine and bovine aqueous humour. Ophthalmic Res. 2004 Jan-Feb;36(1):38–42.

Wu R, Flammer J, Yao K, Haefliger IO. Reduction of nitrite production by endothelin-1 in isolated porcine ciliary processes. Exp Eye Res. 2003 Aug;77(2):189–93.

For additional information, please visit:

http://www.ncbi.nlm.nih.gov/entrez/query.fcgi?DB=pubmed

A 4 Online Sites for the Visually Impaired

There are many resources available on the internet that provide eye health information. This list provides a few of the informative sources available online.

Below you will find a selection and short description of links to general information sites, organizations, and associations that provide information about glaucoma and related diseases of the eye:

- **http://www.glaucoma-association.com** International charity based in England, which since its formation in 1974 has supported the need of people suffering with Glaucoma through the provision of literature and a patient's telephone help line.
- **http://www.glaucomaresearch.ch** Homepage of the Dept. of Ophthalmology of the University Hospital Basel.
- **www.glaucomafoundation.org** The Glaucoma Foundation is committed to educating the public by pinpointing helpful new treatments and cures.
- **http://www.hicom.net/~oedipus/blind.html.** 'The Blindness Related Resources' is an online technology resource centre for blind and visually impaired. Includes a Glaucoma Home Page.
- **http://myeyenet.com/links/visuallyimpaired.html** The Eye Net is a comprehensive source of useful information and products or equipment of use for the visually impaired.
- **www.glaukompatienten.ch** A homepage for patients in German and French language
- **http://monsite.wanadoo.fr/france_glaucome** Association for patients in France.
- **http://www.nei.nih.gov/health/maculardegen/ armd_facts.asp** For patients with age-related macular degeneration.

If you like to contact us, please use the following email: info@glaucoma-meeting.ch

A 5   Ophthalmology in Developing Countries

Throughout the world, there are more than 40 million people who are blind; glaucoma is one of the major causes. This figure, from the World Health Organization (WHO), cites 80% of those afflicted with blindness as living in developing countries. Additionally, the WHO estimates that there are 180 million people who are visually handicapped. Relating this to a temporal dimension, it means that every five seconds, someone loses the ability to see; every minute, a child goes blind. Without effective preventive measures, the number of blind will double, reaching 70 to 80 million, by the year 2020. The direct economic cost of blindness worldwide is estimated at US $25 billion, annually.

Among the blind of the world, 1.5 million are children younger than six years of age. The primary cause of blindness is cataracts, alone responsible for 50% of all cases. Major additional causes include trachoma, glaucoma, diabetes, river blindness (ocular onchocerciasis), leprosy and infectious diseases. About 75% of all cases could have been prevented or could still be cured with surgery or medication. Glaucoma is included among these cases. Glaucoma is widespread throughout the world and, because of inadequate treatment and health care, still leads to blindness in developing countries. Patients often seek medical attention only when it is too late, after irreversible damage has already occurred. To improve this tragic situation, the WHO, federal governments and relief organizations have

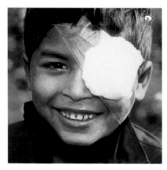
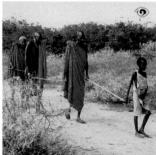
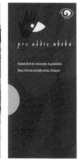

joined to institute an international program, Vision 2020, The Right to Sight. The program's goal is to fight the major causes of blindness by training professional caregivers, especially ophthalmologists, and by making instruments and financial resources available.

Should you wish to actively contribute to fighting blindness, your financial support to one of the following organizations would be most welcome and appreciated:

Christian Blind Mission International, Australia
P.O. Box 5   Phone: +61 3 9817 45 66
1245 Burke Road   Fax: +61 3 9817 61 93
Kew, Victoria 3101   e-mail: cbmiaus@cbmi.org.au
Australia   website: www.cbmi.org.au

Christian Blind Mission International, Canada
P.O. Box 800   Phone: +1 905 640 64 64
3844 Stouffville Road   Fax: +1 905 640 43 32
Stouffville, Ontario L4A 7Z9   e-mail: cbmican@compuserve.com
Canada   website: www.cbmi-can.org

Christian Blind Mission International, New Zealand
27 Gillies Avenue   Phone: +64 9 522 0902
P.O. Box 99820   Fax: +64 9 552 0923
Newmarket   e-mail: cbminz@compuserve.com
Auckland 1031
New Zealand

Christian Blind Mission International, UK
Winship Road   Phone: +44 1223 426 161
Milton   Fax: +44 1223 425 455
Cambridge CB4 6BQ   e-mail: cbm@cbmuk.org.uk
United Kingdom   website: cbmuk.org.uk

Sight Savers
Commonwealth House
Haywards Heath
West Sussex RH 16 3 AZ
United Kindom

Christian Blind Mission International, USA
P.O. Box 19000   Phone: +1 864 239 0065
450 East Park Avenue   Fax: +1 864 239 0069
Greenville, SC 29601   e-mail: cbmiusa@cbmi-usa.org
USA   website: www.cbmi-usa.org

International Eye Foundation (IEF)
7801 Norfolk Ave
Bethesda, Maryland 20814
USA

Pro Addis Abeba, c/o University Eye Clinic Basel
Attn: Prof. Josef Flammer   Phone: +41/61/ 265 86 51
Mittlere Strasse 91   Fax: +41/61/265 86 52
P. O. Box   e-mail: proaddisabeba@bluewin.ch
4012 Basel
Switzerland

All of these organizations will gladly provide you with information describing their activities.

Won't you please help provide all people, no matter where they live, with the same prevention and treatment options that are simply taken for granted by so many?

A 6 Acknowledgments

- The **Schwickert-Stiftung** has generously provided financial support that has made this book possible.
- **Professor Volker Klauss,** M.D., University Eye Clinic Munich, wrote the text regarding ophthalmology in developing countries.
- Our warm thanks also go to the following colleagues who graciously provided photographs and slides for this book:
  - **Asst. Prof. Oliver Arend, M.D.,** University Eye Clinic, Aachen, Germany: Fig. S 11.17
  - **INFEL Publishers Zürich,** Copyright INFEL Zürich, Switzerland: Fig. 2.15
  - **Prof. Jost Jonas, M.D.,** University Eye Clinic, Erlangen, Germany: Fig. 4.14/ 4.15
  - **Asst. Prof. Hanspeter Killer, M.D.,** Eye Clinic Cantonal Hospital Aarau, Switzerland: Figs. S 8.4/S 8.5
  - **Prof. Michael Küchle, M.D.,** University Eye Clinic, Erlangen, Germany: Fig. 3.30
  - **Prof. Jan Müller, M.D.,** Nuclear Medicine Cantonal Hospital Basel, Switzerland: Fig. S 11.5
  - **Prof. Lutz Pillunat, M.D.,** University Eye Clinic Hamburg, Germany: Fig. 3.33
  - **Dr. Luca Remonda,** Radiology Inselspital Bern, Switzerland: Figs. S 11.1 to S 11.4/ S 11.6/S 11.7
  - **Prof. Thérèse Resink, M.D.,** Research Department. Cantonal Hospital Basel, Switzerland: Figs. S 6.2/S 6.4
  - **Asst. Prof. Ulrich Roelcke, M.D.,** Neurology Clinic, Cantonal Hospital Aarau, Switzerland: Fig. S 8.1
  - **Dr. Heinz Peter Schmid,** Ophthalmologist, Biel, Switzerland: Figs. 6.23/6.24
  - **Dr. Walthard Vilser,** IMEDOS, Weimar, Germany: Figs. S 11.36/S 11.37
  - **Prof. Eugen van der Zypen, M.D.,** Anatomical Institute Bern, Switzerland: Figs. 3.12/S 1.9/S 1.15/S 1.20/S 1.22/S 1.35/S 1.46/S 1.49/S 2.2 to S 2.12/S 2.16 to S 2.21/S 9.2/S 9.3
  - **Christoffel Mission for the Blind:** Figs. A 5.1/A 5.2

From the University Eye Clinic Basel, Switzerland:
  - **Asst. Prof. Ernst Büchi, M.D.:** Fig. 5.6
  - **Dr. Konstantin Gugleta:** Figs. S 11.22/S 11.33b/S 11.34/S 11.35
  - **Prof. Hedwig J. Kaiser, M.D.:** Fig. S 1.1
  - **Dr. Peter Meyer:** Figs. 2.4 to 2.6/2.23/3.43/7.12/S 1.17/S 1.36/S 1.37/S 1.38/ S 1.42 to S 1.44/S 1.48/S 1.51/S 2.13 to S 2.15/S 6.1/S 6.3/S 6.5/S 6.8/S 6.9/ S 9.4/S 9.9
  - **Dr. Ines Nuttli:** Fig. S 11.23/S 11.24
  - **Asst. Prof. Christian Prünte, M.D.:** Figs. 4.9/S 5.4 to S 5.8/S 5.12 to S 5.19
  - **Dr. Bettina Schroeder:** Figs. S 9.5/S 9.7/S 9.8/S 11.13/S 11.15
  - **Dr. Tatiana Spicher:** Fig. 6.36
  - **Dr. Barbara Teuchner:** Figs. 6.31/S 11.19 to S 11.21

- Collaboration on the manuscript:
  - **Eve-Marie Becker**
  - **Corinne Egloff**
  - **Sibylle Flammer**
  - **Ines Flammer**
  - **Andreas Flammer**
  - **Dr. Germaine Kreuzer**

Please let us know
what you think of this book!

Dear Reader:

The book you are holding is a collaborative effort – it has been read and reread many times by many people. Nevertheless, it is still the first English edition, and we are aware that there are probably still areas that need attention and even perhaps a mistake or two has slipped by our notice. Because we are planning further translations, we would be most grateful for feedback from you, the reader.

What did you like about the book? Which parts do you feel warrant more detail? Which areas did you find tedious or did you feel too much detail was provided? Did you discover a mistake? Did we use terms that were too difficult or not explained? And have you had personal experiences that contradict that which is written or described in this book?

We would appreciate all forms of comments and suggestions. You may contact us:

- By post-mail to: Secretary to Prof. Josef Flammer, University Eye Clinic, Mittlere Strasse 91, Postfach, CH-4031 Basel, Switzerland
- By fax: ++41/61/265-8652
- Or by e-mail: Josef.Flammer@uhbs.ch

Please provide us with your name and address so we can contact you should we need more information about your comments.

Many thanks,

The Authors

Index